Editorial Board

Professional Aspects of Nurse Anesthesia Practice

Professional Aspects of Nurse Anesthesia Practice

by

American Association of Nurse Anesthetists

Edited by

Scot D. Foster, CRNA, PhD
Associate Clinical Professor and Director of Education
University of California Los Angeles/Olive View Medical Center
Program of Nurse Anesthesia
Los Angeles, California

Lorraine M. Jordan, CRNA, MS
Director of Education and Research
American Association of Nurse Anesthetists
Park Ridge, Illinois

F. A. Davis Company Philadelphia

F. A. Davis Company
1915 Arch Street
Philadelphia, PA 19103

Printed in the United States of America

Last digit indicates print number: 10 9 8 7 6 5 4 3 2

Acquisitions Editor: Alan Sorkowitz
Production Editor: Arofan Gregory
Cover Design By: Donald B. Freggens, Jr.

As new scientific information becomes available through basic and clinical research, recommended treatments and drug therapies undergo changes. The author(s) and publisher have done everything possible to make this book accurate, up to date, and in accord with accepted standards at the time of publication. The authors, editors, and publisher are not responsible for errors or omissions or for consequences from application of the book, and make no warranty, expressed or implied, in regard to the contents of the book. Any practice described in this book should be applied by the reader in accordance with professional standards of care used in regard to the unique circumstances that may apply in each situation. The reader is advised always to check product information (package inserts) for changes and new information regarding dose and contraindications before administering any drug. Caution is especially urged when using new or infrequently ordered drugs.

Library of Congress Cataloging-in-Publication Data

Professional aspects of nurse anesthesia practice / by American Association of Nurse Anesthetists ; edited by Scot D. Foster, Lorraine M. Jordan.
p. cm.
Includes bibliographical references and index.
ISBN 0-8036-0134-4
1. Nurse anesthetists—United States. 2. Nurse anesthetists—Practice—United States.
I. Foster, Scot Douglas. II. Jordan, Lorraine M. III. American Association of Nurse Anesthetists.
[DNLM: 1. Nurse Anesthetists. 2. Professional Practice—standards—United States.
3. Quality Assurance, Health Care—United States. WY 151 P964 1994]
RD82.P76 1994
617.9′6—dc20
DNLM/DLC
for Library of Congress 93-31370
CIP

Dedication

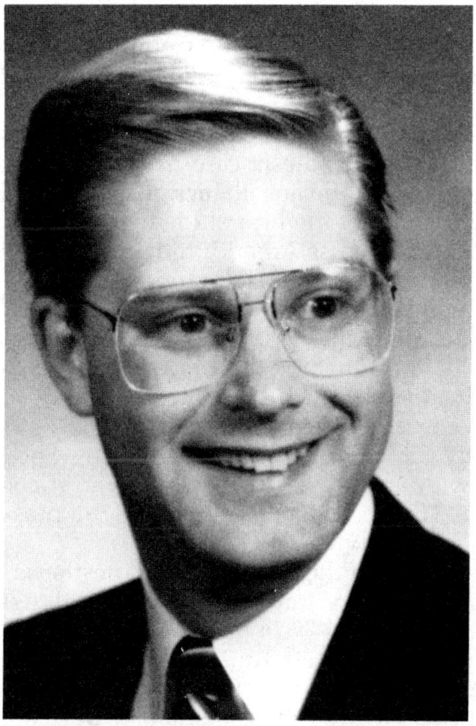

David B. Stasiak, CRNA, MEd, MSN
1956–1992

"Whatever you can do or dream you can—begin it.
Boldness has genius, power, and magic in it."
Goethe

This book is dedicated to the memory of David B. Stasiak, CRNA, MEd, MSN, outstanding nurse anesthetist, exemplary educator, respected administrator, recognized association leader, loving family member, and devoted friend. David touched many lives during his own short lifetime and was one of those individuals who truly made a difference.

David believed in giving something back to the profession that had nurtured him. He was completing his second-year term on the Board of Directors of the American Association of Nurse Anesthetists at the time of his death. He had chaired the AANA Public Relations Committee and was influential in guiding the Association's patient information campaign. In his native Michigan, David was an active association leader, having served as president of the Michigan Association of Nurse Anesthetists.

To quote David: "Conceptually, our profession must focus on the social, political-legal, economic, technologic, educational, and philosophical forces impacting contemporary healthcare today."

David's career spanned both the clinical practice and teaching arenas. He engaged in private anesthesia practice in Detroit area hospitals and served as an adjunct faculty member for the University of Detroit/McAuley School of Nursing. He held the posts of Administrative Director of Nurse Anesthesia for St. Joseph Mercy Hospital—Pontiac and Director of the Graduate Program in Nurse Anesthesiology at University of Detroit Mercy College. He also served as Anesthesia Services Director at Bi-County Community Hospital and early in his career had been clinical education coordinator of the Henry Ford Hospital/University of Detroit Program of Nurse Anesthesia.

He was a role model to his colleagues and a mentor to his students. He believed that to meet the anesthesia care needs of the country—and CRNAs administer more than half of the anesthetics given in the United States yearly—the profession had to "attract the best students." And, to use his words, "our students are our future." Across America today, there are more than 200 nurse anesthetists in practice who were David's students.

The pursuit of education was paramount to David. At the time of his death he was pursuing a doctorate in Nursing from Wayne State University College of Nursing. He was a 1977 graduate of the Grace Hospital School of Nursing and a 1979 graduate (with distinction) in anesthesia from Wayne State University, where he earned two master's degrees.

David was active in the Transcultural Nursing Society, a discipline that combines nursing with anthropology, participating in conferences both in the Netherlands and the United States. He served as the president of the Michigan Transcultural Nursing Society.

He was also a member of the International Anesthesia Research Society, the American Nurses Association, and the International Association for Human Caring. He was listed in *Who's Who in American Nursing* and was a member of the nursing honor society, Sigma Theta Tau.

David lectured extensively and published clinical papers in the *AANA Journal,* among others. He was instrumental in developing national practice guidelines aimed at protecting both nurse anesthetists and their patients.

David's own words aptly describe his beloved chosen profession:

"I believe knowledge and caring are the essence of our nurse anesthesia practice. Vigilance, respect, compassion, integrity, and excellence . . . guide the quality care we deliver to our patients.

Our profession has a proud and distinguished heritage. Let's continue to build on our knowledge and the care constructs established over 100 years ago that will guide our profession into the next millennium."

It is most appropriate that the AANA Board of Directors has dedicated this first AANA professional aspects book to David. It is hoped that this book will stand as a lasting memorial to one who gave so much to Nurse Anesthesia.

Preface

The American Association of Nurse Anesthetists and the editors of and contributors to *Professional Aspects of Nurse Anesthesia Practice* are proud to introduce the first edition of this text: a book that we hope will improve the appreciation of and participation by student nurse anesthetists and CRNAs alike in the professional issues of nurse anesthesia. First, a round of kudos for those involved in its publication: the twenty-five noted experts who have taken the time to make their important contributions; the 1990 AANA Education Committee, who planned the text and ably served as the editorial board; and the AANA Department of Education and Research staff, who supplied much of the clerical effort.

The impetus behind publication of this book came from several sources. Primary among them was the fact that a compendium of professional issues about nurse anesthesia was not available to those students contemplating or currently studying the discipline. The *National Commission of Nurse Anesthesia Education* strongly encouraged publication of a text that could be used in school curricula throughout the nation. Also, the *AANA Strategic Plan for the 1990's,* developed by the American Association of Nurse Anesthetists, called for wider dissemination of material and participation of members in issues related to the profession; activities which this text comprehensively describes. Consequently, the writing of this book was undertaken by the Education Committee of the American Association of Nurse Anesthetists.

We hope this book will serve as a credible and comprehensive description of the discipline of nurse anesthesia for those registered nurses considering entry into the profession as well as for students currently enrolled in educational programs. The content will also serve the practicing CRNA who is seeking a better understanding of the profession, needs practical direction in changing personal practice settings, is assuming new practice roles, or desires to become more professionally involved.

The content of the text has been provided primarily by CRNAs from all practice settings, who have demonstrated substantial expertise in specific areas of professional endeavor. Each chapter has undergone peer review and meticulous editing for format, writing style, and content. The book is divided into seven major headings, covering such topics as defining CRNA practice, rights and responsibilities of professional practice, the health care delivery system, professional practice patterns, assessing and selecting employment options, legal aspects of anesthesia practice, assessing quality in practice, and the continuing challenges of professional practice.

Chapter highlights include qualifications and capabilities of the CRNA, professional roles, committing to professional involvement, the AANA as a professional organization, the regulation of practice (governmental and nongovernmental), standards of care, reimbursement, asserting influence in health care policy, assessing and selecting practice settings, negotiating contracts, establishing functional practice roles, the anatomy of malpractice litigation, the documentation of patient care, measuring of clinical competence, continuous quality improvement, ethical decision making, and chemical dependency.

We hope that this book is a resounding success for several reasons. First, members of this profession have long been aware that we will grow and prosper only when all CRNAs fully understand the roles, rights, and responsibilities of global participation in a wide range of professional activites. In today's climate of rapid change in health care, it is not sufficient for CRNAs to view their professional roles solely within the confines of clinical practice. The progress this profession has made over the last century has been based both on demonstrated excellence in clinical practice **and** participation in the "political-social arena" of health care delivery. Appreciation of this concept is especially critical for the succeeding generation of CRNAs.

Second, we hope the text will stand as further evidence that CRNAs are assuming expanded responsibilities for contributing to the professional literature relative to advanced nursing practice and perhaps the policies that will affect its future direction. Not only are CRNAs becoming recognized as authorities in many areas of clinical practice, but also as professionals able to provide accurate and insightful chronologies of their history, developmental patterns, sociological perspectives, and specific clinical contributions to the health care delivery system at large. Perhaps the greatest contribution of the text will be to solidify the commitment of present students and future practitioners to professional service and the recognition that this unique and formidable challenge requires special diligence and commitment.

Scot D. Foster, CRNA, PhD
Senior Editor

Contributors

John G. Aker, CRNA, MS
Department of Anesthesiology
Research Medical Center
Kansas City, Missouri

Gene A. Blumenreich, JD
General Counsel for American Association of Nurse Anesthetists
Boston, Massachusetts

Nancy Bruton-Maree, CRNA, MS
Program Director
Raleigh School of Nurse Anesthesia
University of North Carolina at Greensboro
Raleigh, North Carolina

Linda L. Callahan, CRNA, MA
Assistant Director of Education
Kaiser Permanente School of Nurse Anesthesia
Los Angeles, California

Scot D. Foster, CRNA, PhD
Associate Clinical Professor and Director of Education
University of California Los Angeles/Olive View Medical Center
Program of Nurse Anesthesia
Los Angeles, California

John F. Garde, CRNA, MS
Executive Director
American Association of Nurse Anesthetists
Park Ridge, Illinois

Ira P. Gunn, MLN, CRNA, FAAN
Nurse Anesthesia Consultant and Clinical Adjunct Professor
School of Nursing and Allied Health
University of Texas at El Paso
El Paso, Texas

Mark C. Hamelink, CRNA, MSN
Lakeshore Anesthesia, PC
South Haven, Michigan

Lorraine M. Jordan, CRNA, MS
Director of Education and Research
American Association of Nurse Anesthetists
Park Ridge, Illinois

Gary P. Kraus, MBA, JD
Assistant Attorney General
State of Missouri
Jefferson City, Missouri

Jonathan T. Lord, MD
Executive Vice President for Clinical Services
Sunhealth
Charlotte, North Carolina

Cathy A. Mastropietro, CRNA, MSN
Project Director
National Commission of Nurse Anesthesia Education
American Association of Nurse Anesthetists
Park Ridge, Illinois

Tom L. McKibban, CRNA, MS
Butler County Anesthesia Associates
El Dorado, Kansas

Ron McManus, BS, MTh, DMin, PhD
Associate Provost
Professor of Religion and Psychology
Texas Wesleyan University
Fort Worth, Texas

Kathleen A. Michels, RN, JD
Director of Federal Government Affairs
American Association of Nurse Anesthetists
Washington, District of Columbia

Diana S. Quinlan, CRNA, MA
Manager, Department of Pediatric Anesthesiology
Nemours Children's Clinic
Jacksonville, Florida

Rita M. Rupp, RN, MA
Executive Staff to the Executive Director
American Association of Nurse Anesthetists
Park Ridge, Illinois

Daniel C. Simonson, BSN, CRNA
Managing Partner and Anesthetist
The Spokane Eye Surgery Center
Spokane, Washington

Janet M. Simpson, CRNA, JD
Holbrook, Heaven, and Jay, P.A.
Kansas City, Kansas

Peter Staver, CRNA, JD
Staver and Souve
Taylor, Michigan

Mitchell H. Tobin, JD
Director of State Government Affairs
American Association of Nurse Anesthetists
Park Ridge, Illinois

Lynne M. Van Wormer, CRNA, BS
Assistant Chief Nurse Anesthetist
Department of Anesthesiology
Albany Medical College
Albany, New York

Kimberly Walker, CRNA, MS
Hermitage, Tennessee

Wynne R. Waugaman, CRNA, PhD
Associate Professor of Clinical Anesthesiology
University of California Los Angeles School of Medicine
Los Angeles, California

Karen Zaglaniczny, CRNA, PhD
Assistant Professor
College of Pharmacy and Allied Health
Wayne State University
Educational Coordinator
Department of Anesthesia Services
Detroit Receiving Hospital
Detriot, Michigan

Contents

ONE

Defining Practice of the Certified Registered Nurse Anesthetist

1

Qualifications and Capabilities of the Certified Registered Nurse Anesthetist

Lorraine M. Jordan

OUTLINE

OBJECTIVES

On completing this chapter, the reader will be able to:

1. List the qualifications a nurse must have to become a CRNA.
2. Identify the range of clinical capabilities CRNAs use in their practice.
3. List criteria for certification as a CRNA.
4. List criteria that a CRNA must fulfill to become recertified.
5. Describe key components that relate to the scope of practice for nurse anesthetists.

Certified Registered Nurse Anesthetists (CRNAs) are a highly successful group of advanced practice nurses who have provided anesthesia services in the United States for more than 100 years. In fact, the development of the nurse anesthesia specialty precedes that of physician anesthesiology in this country. Today, more than 25,000 CRNAs administer nearly 65 percent of the anesthetics given each year in the United States and are the sole anesthesia providers in 85 percent of rural hospitals.[1] CRNAs administer all types of anesthesia, from minor surgical interventions to major surgery, and practice in every setting in which anesthesia is delivered, including traditional hospital surgical suites and obstetric delivery rooms, physician offices, ambulatory surgical centers, health maintenance organizations (HMOs), preferred provider organizations (PPOs), the Military and Public Health Services, and Veterans Administration medical facilities. Currently, the demand for CRNAs far exceeds the available supply. According to the CRNA Manpower Study from the National Center for Nursing Research, U.S. Office of Health and Human Services, projected CRNA human resources need by the year 2010 will exceed 35,000, an increase of 40 percent over the 25,000 needed in 1990.[2]

PROFESSIONAL DEFINITIONS

A CRNA is a registered nurse who is educationally prepared and competent to engage in the practice of nurse anesthesiology. All CRNAs are responsible and accountable for individual professional practice and are capable of exercising independent judgment within their scope of competence and licensure. They accept the responsibility for rendering professional services and the evaluation of the effects of those services on the patient. The practice of CRNAs is a recognized specialty within the profession of nursing and is *not* a medically delegated act. CRNAs are recognized in all 50 states by designated state licensing or regulatory bodies, primarily boards of nursing.

To be a CRNA one must:

1 Graduate from an approved school of nursing and hold current state licensure as a registered nurse.

2 Graduate from a nurse anesthesia educational program accredited by the American Association of Nurse Anesthetists (AANA) Council on Accreditation of Nurse Anesthesia Educational Programs or its predecessor.

3 Successfully complete the certification examination administered by the AANA Council on Certification of Nurse Anesthetists or its predecessor.

4 Comply with criteria for biennial recertification, as defined by the AANA Council on Recertification of Nurse Anesthetists. These criteria include evidence of (a) current licensure as a registered nurse, (b) active practice as a CRNA, (c) appropriate continuing education, and (d) verification of the absence of mental, physical, and other problems that could interfere with the practice of anesthesia.

SCOPE OF PRACTICE

Anesthesia, or *anesthesiology*, is the art and science of rendering a patient insensible to pain by the administration of anesthetic agents and related drugs and therapeutic procedures. Anesthesia and anesthesia-related care represents those services that anesthesia professionals provide on request, assignment, or referral by the patient, physician, or other health care professionals authorized by law, most often to facilitate diagnosis, therapeutic, or surgical procedures. In other instances, the referral or request for consultation or assistance may be for management of pain associated with obstetric labor and delivery, management of acute or chronic ventilatory problems, or management of acute or chronic pain through the performance of selected diagnostic or therapeutic blocks.

CRNAs practice according to their expertise, state statutes or regulations, and local institutional policy. The scope of practice of CRNAs encompasses the professional functions, privileges, and responsibilities associated with nurse anesthesia practice, specifically in reference to those areas listed earlier. These are performed in collaboration with qualified and legally authorized professional health care providers.

Nurse anesthetists administer anesthesia and anesthesia-related care in four general categories: (1) preanesthetic preparation and evaluation; (2) anesthesia induction, maintenance and emergence; (3) postanesthesia care; and (4) perianesthetic and clinical support functions. Nurse anesthetist scope of practice includes, but is not limited to, the following:

- Performing and documenting a preanesthetic assessment and evaluation of the patient, including requesting consultations and diagnostic studies; selecting, obtaining, ordering, or administering preanesthetic medications and fluids; and obtaining informed consent for anesthesia
- Developing and implementing an anesthetic plan
- Selecting and initiating the planned anesthetic technique, which may include general, regional, and local anesthesia and intravenous sedation
- Selecting, obtaining, or administering the anesthetics, adjuvant drugs, and fluids necessary to manage the anesthetic, to maintain the patient's physiologic homeostasis, and to correct abnormal responses to the anesthesia or surgery
- Selecting, applying, or inserting appropriate noninvasive and invasive monitoring modalities for collecting and interpreting patient physiologic data
- Managing a patient's airway and pulmonary status using endotracheal intubation, mechanical ventilation, pharmacologic support, respiratory therapy, or extubation
- Managing emergence and recovery from anesthesia by selecting, obtaining, ordering, or administering medications, fluids, or ventilatory support in order to maintain homeostasis, to provide relief from pain and anesthesia side effects, or to prevent or manage complications
- Releasing or discharging patients from a postanesthesia care unit or ambulatory surgical setting and providing postanesthesia follow-up evaluation and care related to anesthesia side effects or complications
- Ordering, initiating, or modifying pain relief therapy through the use of drugs, regional anesthetic techniques, or other accepted pain relief modalities, including labor epidural analgesia
- Responding to emergency situations by providing airway management, administering emergency fluids or drugs, or using basic or advanced cardiac life support techniques
- Additional nurse anesthesia responsibilities within the expertise of the individual nurse anesthetist

A BRIEF HISTORICAL PERSPECTIVE

Surgical anesthesia was first brought to the United States in the mid-19th century. Although nurse anesthetists were the first professional group in this country to provide anesthesia, their work was not publicly recognized until the 1953 publication of *The History of Anesthesia, with Emphasis on the Nurse Specialist* by Virginia S. Thatcher.[3] The definitive history of nurse anesthetists was published in 1989, entitled *Watchful Care: A History of America's Nurse Anesthetists*.[4] The reader is encouraged to refer to this text as a comprehensive supplement to the brief history of the profession of nurse anesthesia presented in this section.

The profession of nurse anesthesia developed in response to the growing need surgeons had for anesthesia services. Due to high mortality rates related to anesthesia, reported in the latter third of the 19th century, many surgeons turned to nurses as the providers best suited and available to "specialize" in the field. In the absence of a nurse anesthetist, the provider selected was often a young physician in training who would much rather have been involved in the surgical proceedings and consequently demonstrated little interest in the anesthetic care of patients. In addition, the anesthetist was usually responsible directly to the surgeon, which proved to be an unpopular and poorly compensated role for a physician colleague.

In the years preceding the 20th century, it

was the religious orders of sisters in the profession of anesthesia that truly documented the role of nurse anesthesia providers. In 1877, Sister Mary Bernard of St. Vincent's Hospital in Erie, Pennsylvania became the first identifiable nurse anesthetist. In the late 1800s two sisters of the Third Order of the Hospital Sisters of St. Francis from Germany established a community in Illinois and provided anesthesia in this country. Sister Aldonza Elrich and Sister Vanossa Woenke were trained as nurse anesthetists by surgeons.

One woman in particular, Alice Magaw, drew considerable attention for her work as an anesthetist. Magaw was a nurse anesthetist at St. Mary's Hospital in 1889, in Rochester, Minnesota, and worked with a brilliant surgeon, Dr. William Worrell Mayo. Magaw's impeccable care and superb skills in anesthesia made her well known. Her skill at administering ether as a chloroform anesthesia was remarkable. Magaw's leadership in the field of anesthesia at the Mayo Clinic and her belief that the experience of the anesthetist in identifying and reacting quickly to the condition of the patient is of the greatest importance earned her the title of the "mother of anesthesia."

In 1899, Magaw published a paper in the *Northwestern Lancet* describing her success in providing safe anesthesia for more than 3000 patients. Her success continued over the years. By 1906, Ms. Magaw had administered anesthesia to more than 14,000 patients with no patient mortality. She administered ether via the "open method" in the successful anesthesia care she provided.

Throughout the course of the next 50 years, the profession of nurse anesthetists grew rapidly, and members of this profession provided the most able teachers and clinicians available in anesthesia, both in major medical centers as well as rural health care facilities. CRNAs also become an important component of the health service system of the United States, providing meritorious service in the two world wars.

THE ROLE OF EDUCATION

In 1912, the first organized course in anesthesia for graduate nurses was developed by Mother Magdalene Wiedlocker. Nurse anesthetists' education began largely as preceptorships under the auspices of individuals such as Sister Mary Ethelreda O'Dwyer, Virginia S. Thatcher, Alice Magaw, and Agatha Hodgins. As early as 1933, at the first meeting of the National Association of Nurse Anesthetists (NANA, precursor to AANA) the issue of education was addressed. Gertrude Fife, then president of the NANA, addressed the need for developing standards for educational programs in nurse anesthesia. Additionally, at this meeting a committee was formed to investigate the development of an accredited list of schools. Fife stated that she believed it was the role of the association to supply surgeons and hospitals with names of accredited schools and qualified anesthesia providers.

In 1936, the first recommended curriculum was drafted by the Education Committee of the AANA, chaired by Helen Lamb, who was later to be recognized as one of the most influential early leaders in education. The work of this committee led to recommendations to develop a standardized curriculum and define standards of education. They proposed that the education of nurse anesthetists should include theoretic and practical experience in a program of no less than 6 months, including 95 hours of classroom instruction, 18 hours of recorded operating room classroom instruction, and 325 cases of anesthesia administration. The number of cases were to be broken into the following categories: 250 general anesthesia, 25 obstetric, 25 dental, and 25 either spinal, local, and so on.

As the number of programs of nurse anesthesia began to grow, a body of interested CRNA educators formed within the AANA, called the Assembly of School Faculty. The Assembly of School Faculty recognized the need for programs to be housed and recognized within the academic community, not only to ensure the credibility of programs but also to improve their quality. At the first meeting in 1946, work began on developing a standard curriculum as well as mechanisms to promote to the public the commitment of the profession to educational excellence and accountability. As a result of this work, the first program of nurse anesthesia was accredited in 1952 at Ravenswood Hospital of Anesthesia in Chicago. The visit was successful, and the program was recognized as an accredited program by the AANA.

Nurse anesthesia education has evolved over the years into a very sophisticated educational system, incorporating over 90 programs nationwide, 80 percent of which are housed or affiliated within colleges or universities and offer a master's degree. Twenty percent of programs offer a certificate of completion. Educational standards require that all accredited programs of nurse anesthesia provide a master's degree by 1998. Programs are housed administratively in many academic units within institutions of higher education, the most prevalent of which are schools of allied health, and schools of medicine, nursing, or education. Today there are nearly 2000 nurse anesthesia students enrolled in accredited programs using more than 400 graduate faculty including CRNAs, doctorally prepared basic scientists, anesthesiologists, and other health care providers.

The minimum program length is 24 months. Each program is required to provide an extensive, educationally sound curriculum that combines both academic theory and clinical practice. Students are given the opportunity to integrate classroom content with direct application of a variety of anesthesia techniques in the provision of anesthesia care to all patient populations and risk categories. The education of nurse anesthetists also includes experiences in pain management, emergency resuscitation, intensive care experience, and postanesthesia care. Curricula vary widely in programs throughout the country within the confines of accreditation standards and resources of the local community.

Current standards and guidelines for nurse anesthesia programs require, at minimum, the following academic coursework:

- Professional aspects of nurse anesthesia practice—45 hours
- Advanced anatomy, physiology, and pathophysiology—135 hours
- Chemistry and physics related to anesthesia—45 hours
- Advanced pharmacology—90 hours
- Principles of anesthesia practice—90 hours
- Clinical and literature review conferences—45 hours

Most nurse anesthesia programs exceed these minimum requirements, and many programs require some additional course work such as methods of scientific inquiry, statistics, and nursing or educational theory. In addition, many programs require that the student participate actively in ongoing or original research that culminates in research project presentations or formal thesis defenses.

The clinical curriculum requirements of a nurse anesthesia program mandates that each student administer a minimum of 450 anesthetics to patients, representing at least 800 hours of anesthesia time. To meet this requirement, students provide these services under the supervision of a qualified clinical instructor, which includes CRNAs or anesthesiologists. Requirements further specify that each student's anesthesia experiences include (1) the major anesthesia techniques and monitoring modalities in current use and (2) patients whose concomitant medical interventions are representative of the broad spectrum of medical specialty procedures used today.

Admission to nurse anesthesia programs requires graduation from an approved school of nursing, a baccalaureate in nursing or other appropriate bachelor's degree, current licensure as a registered nurse, and a minimum of 1 year of professional nursing experience in an acute care setting. It should be noted that some programs require several years of experience postlicensure as a registered nurse.

Most applicants have acquired extensive clinical backgrounds as professional nurses in such settings as coronary, respiratory, postanesthesia, and surgical intensive care units; emergency rooms; or as members of a trauma or cardiac surgical team. Applicants to nurse anesthesia programs have demonstrated records of professional work and a high level of clinical competence.

ACCREDITATION OF EDUCATIONAL PROGRAMS

The AANA Council on Accreditation of Nurse Anesthesia Educational Programs is the body responsible for promulgating, publishing, and assessing compliance of programs with the *Standards and Guidelines for*

Programs of Nurse Anesthesia.[5] From 1952 to 1975, the AANA was the accrediting body for all nurse anesthesia programs. However, in 1975 the Department of Health Education and Welfare required that the accrediting body be separated from the parent professional organization. Consequently, in 1975 the AANA Council on Accreditation (COA) of Nurse Anesthesia Education Programs was formed. This council was developed and functions as an independent entity from the AANA; however, it remains within the corporate structure of the parent organization.

The COA, multidisciplinary in composition, is itself recognized (accredited) by the United States Department of Education and the Council on Postsecondary Education Accreditation (COPA) as the sole accrediting authority for nurse anesthesia programs. Recognition from these agencies is important not only because it validates the quality of the educational programming to the public but also because it ensures eligibility for federal grant funding and student financial aid.

The COA requires that each program undergo a systematic self-study and on-site evaluation at least every 6 years. The purpose of this exercise and visit is to document that each accredited program is in compliance with the standards of the council as it seeks to improve the overall conduct of the clinical and academic curriculum. Twice a year, the COA publishes a list of the accredited nurse anesthesia educational programs, which is available from the offices of the AANA.

CERTIFICATION OF NURSE ANESTHETISTS

In 1933, at the first Meeting of the NANA, the concept of developing certification examinations was a predominant topic of discussion. Educational leaders promoted the importance of a mechanism that would provide surgeons' official documentation of a nurse anesthetist's knowledge level and minimum clinical compentencies by requiring them to pass an examination. The purpose of gaining approval from a certification body would be to safeguard the interests of the surgeon, hospital, and public.

The AANA Council on Certification of Nurse Anesthetists (CCNA) is charged with protecting and serving the public by assuring that individuals who are credentialed have met predetermined qualifications or standards for providing nurse anesthesia services. The purposes of the CCNA are to formulate and adopt requirements for admission to the certification examination for certification of registered nurse anesthetists; formulate and adopt the administration of the certification examination; determine candidate eligibility for the examination; and evaluate the candidates' performance on the examination and grant initial certification.[6]

The certification process was introduced by the AANA in 1945. In 1975, the AANA recognized the CCNA as an autonomous, multidisciplinary body existing under the corporate structure of the AANA in a fashion similar to the COA. The CCNA is an autonomous entity having the functions to certify, protect, and benefit the public in regard to documenting competencies and granting a recognized credential (CRNA). Credentials are recognized as a different entity from that of licensure. State licensure provides the legal credential for the practice of professional nursing, whereas certification indicates compliance with the professional standard for practice in the nurse anesthesia specialty. The certification credential for nurse anesthetists has been continually recognized through proceedings involving malpractice litigation, selected State Nurse Practice Acts, and state and federal regulations. It is the responsibility of the CCNA to certify registered nurses anesthetists who have fulfilled educational and other criteria for the practice of nurse anesthesia.

Each graduate of a nurse anesthesia program must successfully pass the national certification examination before he or she can be certified as a CRNA. To be eligible to take the certification examination, the applicant must (1) hold a current, valid state license to practice as a registered professional nurse, (2) be a graduate of a nurse anesthesia educational program that is accredited by the COA, (3) submit a completed application form, and (4) provide a notarized transcript from the nurse anesthesia program documenting the applicant's academic and clinical experience.

The purpose of the certification examination is to measure the knowledge, skills, and abilities required of an entry-level nurse anesthesia provider. The CCNA maintains responsibility for the examination content and the test specifications, maintains an item bank of test questions, approves an individual's application to take the examination, and determines the passing score. Content validity for the examination is documented through a job analysis, which is linked with the knowledge and skill statements of practitioners. The examination is prepared and administered in conjunction with a nationally recognized testing agency in higher education.[7]

COUNCIL ON RECERTIFICATION

In the late 1960s, the AANA recognized the importance of documenting to the public evidence of continued professional excellence for CRNAs. In 1969, a bylaw change was adopted stating that members had to demonstrate clinical and didactic experiences reflecting their skills in practice. This bylaw was approved and made continuing education an optional program. However, in 1976 members amended the bylaws to make continuing education mandatory for all CRNAs. This bylaw was approved and implemented in August 1978.

As the Council on Recertification of Nurse Anesthetists became more involved in the profession, the duties and responsibilities of the council also expanded. With this potential growth in activity and responsibility to the public, the council sought an autonomous relationship with the AANA. In 1983 the Council on Recertification became the third autonomous body within the AANA.

The Council on Recertification of Nurse Anesthetists seeks to advance the quality of anesthesia care provided to patients. The council particularly focuses its efforts on making sure that nurse anesthetists maintain their skills and keep current with contemporary scientific and technologic developments. The council provides objective criteria designed to determine whether an individual nurse anesthetist is properly licensed, engages in practice to maintain an adequate level of skill, has obtained continuing education credit sufficient to keep current, and has avoided mental, physical, and other problems that could interfere with the practice of anesthesia. The council also serves the role of approving continuing education programs that meet criteria for approval for continuing education credit. The recertification period for the CRNA is 2 years and renewable. Recertification signifies that the nurse anesthetist has undergone updates, both clinical and/or didactic, from an approved continuing education activity for the purpose of improving practice, and is not known to have developed any impairment that could interfere with his or her ability to provide anesthesia.

The purposes of the Council of Recertification of Nurse Anesthetists are to:

1. Recertify qualified CRNAs on a biennial basis.
2. Formulate and adopt criteria for recertification.
3. Formulate and adopt criteria for approval of continuing education programs and offerings.
4. Formulate and adopt criteria for delegating to recognized continuing education agencies the authority to approve programs.
5. Develop and maintain mechanisms to provide a hearing and appellate review on adverse decisions.
6. Develop and maintain a mechanism for the investigation and final resolution, by the council, of charges brought against a CRNA holding recertification.
7. Make recommendations to the AANA board of directors, councils, and committees to conform with the stated purposes of the Council on Recertification of Registered Nurse Anesthetists.

To meet the criteria for full recertification candidates must have (1) initial certification, (2) current licensure as a registered nurse with no restrictions, (3) completed 40 hours of continuing education in a 2-year period, (4) substantial engagement in a practice of anesthesia, (5) no mental or physical condition that may cause or interfere with practice, (6) no convictions of a felony nor be under indictment, and (7) not been subject to any documented allegations of misconduct, incompetent practice, or unethical behavior.[8]

SUMMARY

The discipline of nurse anesthesia is one of the oldest advanced nurse practice professions. The public image and visibility of CRNAs as leaders in the field of nursing and health care services in general stems directly from their commitment to clinical excellence. For years, the profession has grown stronger and continues on an upward course in terms of professional credibility and market demand. This is only possible because of our rich history of collective participation by all members and practitioners toward the goals of accountability, cost efficiency, integrity, and vision. Welcome to this futuristic, dynamic, and demanding profession!

REFERENCES

1. Membership Survey. American Association of Nurse Anesthetists, Park Ridge, IL, 1992.
2. Study of Nurse Anesthetist Manpower Needs. Department of Health and Human Services, Public Health Service, National Institutes of Health, National Center of Nursing Research, Washington, DC, 1990.
3. Thatcher, VS: History of Anesthesia, with Emphasis on the Nurse Specialist. JB Lippincott, Philadelphia, 1953.
4. Bankert, M: Watchful Care: A History of America's Nurse Anesthetists. Continuum, New York, 1989.
5. *Standards and Guidelines for Programs of Nurse Anesthesia.* Council on Accreditation, American Association of Nurse Anesthetists, Park Ridge, IL, 1990.
6. Council on Certification Bylaws. The American Association of Nurse Anesthetists, Park Ridge, IL, 1991.
7. Certification Examination for Nurse Anesthetist 1992: Candidate Handbook. Council on Certification of Nurse Anesthetists, Park Ridge, IL, 1992.
8. Council on Recertification of Nurse Anesthetists. Criteria for Recertification. Council on Recertification of Nurse Anesthetists. Park Ridge, IL, 1992.

2

Professional Roles of the Certified Registered Nurse Anesthetist

Wynne R. Waugaman

OUTLINE

OBJECTIVES

On completing this chapter, the reader will be able to:

1. Compare and contrast educational diversity of nurse anesthetists.
2. Describe the factors that differentiate graduate education in nurse anesthesia from undergraduate study.
3. Define professional socialization.
4. Discuss the dimensions or categories of variables associated with the professional socialization of nurse anesthetists.
5. Identify two factors that facilitate the socialization of nurse anesthesia students into the profession.
6. Discuss the emerging professional roles of nurse anesthetists beyond the scope of traditional clinical practice.

The circumstances under which a person enters a profession are highly predictive of the way that person will view the profession for the rest of his or her life. Nurses seek a career in nurse anesthesia for many reasons. Some identify a need for increased autonomy as their impetus, whereas others seek more challenges in their work setting and view nurse anesthesia as a means of expanding their knowledge base in nursing. No matter what the reason, students entering this profession have a more profound awareness of their chosen career than do most other professional students. The integration of nursing preparation and socialization into new advanced practice roles impacts tremendously on career preparation for professional roles in practice, management, academics, and research.

NURSE ANESTHESIA AS A CLINICAL SPECIALTY

Although nurse anesthesia is considered the oldest nursing specialty, feelings of collegiality have not always existed between nurses and nurse anesthetists. Following World War II, when many nurse anesthesia educational programs were being established, a political decision by the American Nurses Association (ANA) not to establish a section within its organization for nurse anesthetists led to a schism between generic nursing and the specialty of nurse anesthesia. In addition, the growth of anesthesiology as a medical specialty led many nurses to believe that nurse anesthesia would be replaced by physician anesthesia within a short time.[1] This philosophy precluded the recognition of nurse anesthesia as an advanced nursing specialty in many schools and colleges of nursing for many years.

This split between nurse anesthesia and the nursing educational community at large may have served as the stimulus for the diversity of educational degrees in nurse anesthesia. We have witnessed the movement of programs toward higher education with the planned mandatory requirement that all programs offer a graduate degree by 1998. Programs have evolved from the certificate, to the baccalaureate, to the master's degree level. Some also offer their curricula in a doctoral framework, combining the nurse anesthesia curriculum within a nursing doctoral degree. Yet, the quest for the appropriate degree continues. To date, we have been unable to agree whether educational programs should culminate in a master of science in nursing degree or another appropriate master's degree, for example, master of science in nurse anesthesia.

Depaolis-Lutzo[2] identified 36 factors influencing the operation of nurse anesthesia educational programs, which she categorized as financial, recruitment, political, philosophic, psychologic, practice, and educational. Although some factors were attributed as critical to program closures in the early 1980s, recruitment and political issues were named as primary factors influencing the operation of the educational programs. The trend toward master's degree education coupled with the high cost of nurse anesthesia education has complicated the movement of nurse anesthesia educational programs from hospital-based programs to collegiate-based affiliations. In addition, nurse anesthesia educators must face numerous political issues. Primary among these is access to the clinical component of the educational program. Because this is often controlled by anesthesiologists, their support is vital to the continued existence of programs. With the move toward graduate education, program directors must also establish an academic relationship with a department, school, or college within a university. It is essential that the basic program philosophy be compatible with the newly sought academic affiliation so that support for educational goals is ensured. Therefore, factors such as educational philosophy, geographic proximity, type of academic affiliation, and clinical access influence the collegiate affiliation sought by the program.

Educators in nurse anesthesia are proud of the educational diversity of CRNA practitioners although the value of this diversity has never been quantified in terms of an academic power base or educational credibility.[3] Educational diversity among graduate degree offerings in nurse anesthesia stems from several sources. First, the variety of academic relationships established by the first graduate programs in the 1970s was probably based on convenience and on the attitude of academic administrators or deans who were willing to take a risk on a unique clinical program with small student enrollment. Second, differing educational philosophies of program faculty or the organizational structure of the university may have ultimately dictated the selection. The first four graduate programs in nurse anesthesia all had different academic affiliations: medicine, nursing, allied health, and education.[3] These visionary programs probably had no intention of being a model for educational diversity, yet they remain the classic models for nurse anesthesia education. Nurse anesthetists must evaluate whether the maintenance of this educational diversity should be a goal for the future.

The question often posed in the educational community is whether we are helping or hurting ourselves by not aligning completely with nursing. The answer requires that one consider the consequences of such an action carefully given our current economic and political climate.[3] Most educational leaders agree that if unity is feasible or desirable, it can best be achieved through education.[4] From an educational perspective, the discipline of nurse anesthesia would be much enhanced by forming alliances with a firmly entrenched academic discipline other than medicine. For some, nursing seems a likely and obvious source. For others, the basic sciences or allied health fields offer an equally credible alliance with less intradisciplinary conflict.

From a political standpoint, federal lobbying efforts of CRNAs may be more effective if done in conjunction with general nursing. Although the AANA maintains a highly effective lobbying effort in Washington, D.C., and the AANA maintains many cooperative activities with the ANA, added strength in terms of sheer numbers may be desirable since nurses are the largest group of health professionals in the country. Conversely, our nursing colleagues will have to be educated about, and become more sensitive to the needs of, our nursing specialty just as they would about others, such as midwifery or pediatric nurse specialists. Arguably, a case can be made for either position. We must look forward to our future and to those factors that will likely benefit the specialty, in both the short and long term, in order to confirm a rational position.

The benefits of our past and current associations with other disciplines cannot and should not be ignored. Professional unity is as valuable as diversity, but diversity may be the antithesis of empowerment. This issue is of paramount importance because the professional strength and the recognition of nurse anesthetists, as primary providers of anesthesia services, must be firmly established as we prepare for the next century of practice.

THE NATURE OF GRADUATE EDUCATION IN NURSE ANESTHESIA

Often students entering nurse anesthesia programs undergo a tremendous adjustment to graduate-level curricula. For many students, sitting in a classroom each day for one or more academic terms, when they have been accustomed to active clinical practice in an intensive care setting, is at best difficult. Some students may have been away from the academic setting for a decade or more and must develop new study habits to ensure success as graduate students. For a variety of reasons, a nurse anesthesia educational program is unlike any other form of higher education most students have been exposed to. It is certainly unlike undergraduate education. This reality may be even further compounded by the type of graduate program selected and its particular educational emphasis or faculty orientation.

Graduate education in nurse anesthesia demands that students be self-motivated, independent thinkers. Pedagogic teaching styles, whereby teachers impart knowledge to passive students, do not exist. Specialist education requires that students take primary responsibility for learning, developing skills of critical thinking, and integration of theory into practice. Nurse anesthetists must learn to apply a scientific or theoretic basis to their clinical practice in order to make rational, independent judgments and decisions relative to patient care problems.

Instruction involves small group discussions, student presentations, scientific writing, and a vast amount of reading from books and journal literature. Student nurse anesthetists are well versed in methods of inductive and deductive reasoning, and analytical skills are honed through the conduct of research. Although the practice of anesthesia would appear to the uninformed to be purely task-oriented, skill-intensive work, the art and science of practice requires the integration of many skills: cognitive, analytic, and behavioral.

Above all, independent thinking and self-motivation are essential to the practice of nurse anesthesia. Nurse anesthetists must be capable of making independent judgments and implementing anesthesia care within the anesthesia care team and in independent practice where CRNAs are part of an interdisciplinary or interprofessional team.

SELECTION OF A NURSE ANESTHESIA PROGRAM

Students entering a graduate program in nurse anesthesia should consider what their long-term career goals are in order to select the degree offering that will best prepare them to meet these goals. Nurses hoping to pursue a career in scientific research may select a nurse anesthesia program offering a basic science degree to better prepare them for doctoral work in the basic sciences. Graduate education within nursing appears to offer more career options for aspiring nurse anesthetists who may be interested in pursuing faculty appointments within schools or colleges of nursing.[4] While it may not have been true in the past, nursing education is now more prepared to fully embrace nurse anesthesia education. In fact, many nurse educators want to facilitate nurse anesthesia in reclaiming its nursing heritage.[4] Regardless of the type of program selected, all students should conduct a careful assessment of the quality and credentials of faculty, scope of laboratory services, clinical affiliations, and abilities to practice contemporary anesthesia in a setting that does not restrict practice unduly.

Anecdotally, there is a trend toward the requirement of the MSN degree for all nursing specialties including clinical nurse specialists, nurse practitioners, and nurse anesthetists. Although this issue has been presented before, the National Council on State Boards of Nursing has reintroduced this concept for consideration by state boards of nursing as a requirement for licensure in specialty nursing practice. If this credentialing requirement is adopted for nurse specialists, it may influence the types of academic degrees offered by nurse anesthesia educational programs.

PROFESSIONAL SOCIALIZATION: FROM NURSE TO NURSE ANESTHETIST

Sociologically, the development of a profession involves more than acquiring a distinct body of knowledge.[5] It involves the realization that professionals are part of an ethical and moral community. Members have social links not only to their patients and colleagues in the profession but also to groups with whom their activities and skills must interface. The legitimacy of their professional contribution must be acknowledged inclusively by all groups with whom they work, as well as by other professions.[5] Professions hold autonomy as an ideal. The ability to function freely and independently has been used both for and against groups of professionals. An occupation that lacks autonomy has no mechanism established for self-direction, and more than likely will not have the sufficient resources available to develop those networks necessary for members of the occupation to acquire prestige and socioeconomic rewards.[6]

Etzioni[7] described occupations such as teaching, social work, and nursing as "semi-professions." Overall, these professions historically seemed to have less control over their own work through educational standards, licensing, and legislation. The autonomy of these groups is changing but still does not appear to be equal with some of the classic or "traditional" professions. The reader is referred to Chapter 3 for a more detailed discussion of professionalization.

What happens during the nurse anesthesia program to transform a nurse into a nurse anesthetist? The transformation process that occurs is professional socialization. Professional socialization, the process of developing skills, knowledge, professional behavior, and career commitment, occurs concurrently with the educational process, that is, the clinical and academic educational program.[8] On completion of this process, the individual is accorded membership with rights, privileges, and status as a publicly identified member of the group.[9] It is reported that not only does the socialization process adjust students to their educational roles but also that, unlike adjustments to specific situations, it persists across status transitions and situational changes.[10] Simpson[10] regards professional socialization as a directional change or pattern of changes persisting across lifelong changes and transitions. That is, socialization is time and space multidimensional. It consists of three analytically distinct dimensions or categories of variables: education or the imparting of occupational knowledge and skills, development of occupational orientations, and forming personal relatedness to the occupation (Table 2-1). According to Simpson, the first two of these dimensions are mainly cognitive; the third is motivational. These dimensions encompass occupational knowledge and skills in addition to occupational orientations such as collegialism, working within the hospital organizational structure, and views concerning leadership and authority.[10] Socialization also enables the student nurse anesthetist to form personal relatedness to the field through developing career commitment and self-identification as a nurse anesthetist.[8]

The professional socialization process has been studied in a variety of professions. Are students really socialized to assume a professional role or are they shaped both by intent and by unplanned circumstances of their academic environment? Two opposing views of professional socialization were developed from studies of the socialization of medical students by Merton[11] and Becker.[12] The pattern of socialization described by Merton focuses on professional education itself and the acquisition of the professional role during this process. This pattern considers attitudes, values, and outlooks as well as the skills and knowledge that comprise the professional role. This pattern of behavior takes motivation for granted and sees the students as being "inducted into a role."[11]

The pattern of socialization espoused by Becker[12] views the school as the social organism or social system. This pattern centers on motivation, identities, and commitments. Social control appears to be a matter of power. Behavioral options increase power, whereas constraints on behavior reduce it. These constraints put pressure on students to limit their ability to act in accordance with their goals[12] in order to achieve a sense of well-being and comfort.[13] This view of socialization sees learning as situational; previous ways of dealing with problems are unlikely to be adaptable when the conditions change.[12]

The main difference between these two views of professional socialization rests on the question of social control of behavior, its place, and its effects on the orientations and behavior of the student and the professional.[10] The model proposed by Merton[11] pictures a profession as a group with a unity of purpose, with social control arising from shared outlooks and mutual interests. The professional school is conceived as both a part and an instrument of the professions, charged with the responsibility of inducting students into it in a way that ensures its continuity of structure. Students learn the

TABLE 2–1

THE DIMENSIONS OF SOCIALIZATION*

Dimension	Definition
Education	The imparting of occupational knowledge and skill in nurse anesthesia
Cognitive occupational orientations	
Cognitive orientations to the occupational role	Orientation to the functions of a nurse anesthetist
Cognitive orientations to a place in the occupation	Expresses the interests of the professional organization and the professional position within anesthesia and the health care industry
Relatedness to the professional role	The individual is related to the profession of nurse anesthesia in three ways: status identification through socioeconomic rewards, personal attraction to the profession, and career commitment to nurse anesthesia

*Adapted from Waugaman[8] and Simpson.[10]

accepted behaviors and professional moral and ethical values that guide them as professionals to act in ways that are consistent with the professional role. Becker,[12] in contrast, does not believe that a professional product is produced during professional education. The view of socialization proposed by Simpson,[10] differentiation of dimensions of the socialization process as previously described, seems to overcome the oversocialized view of the professional product implicit in Merton's model[11] as well as the limitations of the model of social control proposed by Becker.[12]

The socialization process is dynamic. A person's view of the work role may shift to fit the circumstances and demands of a particular work situation without any effect on job commitment.[10] On the other hand, with changing family situations, social roles, and social orientations, commitment to the job itself may decline while views of the work role and the occupation of nurse anesthesia remain stable.[8] This is the ever-changing face of professional socialization. Professional roles adapt to meet the necessary situation.

Early exposure to clinical practicum and learning the work of the profession facilitates all aspects of socialization in nurse anesthesia. The emphasis in nurse anesthesia education on practical experience during the curriculum enables students to visualize their professional roles with a high degree of realism from early in the program. Role modeling by nurse and physician anesthetists throughout the educational program is a valuable tool of professional socialization.[8] The mentoring role is especially important in the helping professions because of the interdependent working conditions among these professionals. The interdependent working conditions impact tremendously on both the intraprofessional and interprofessional team process.

Educational program content, design, and faculty/practitioner/mentor role models all play a vital role in the professional socialization of nurse anesthetists.[8] All of these factors influence the degree to which students are socialized into the profession, and the continuation of the socialization process influences the degree of professional career commitment as people mature from nurses to nurse anesthetists.[8] Interprofessional education is a component of the socialization process, because professions do not operate in a vacuum. Nurse anesthetists must be socialized to interact and communicate in collaboration with other health care providers with whom they interface. The intraprofessional team a nurse anesthetist may participate in is the anesthesia care team. The team may consist of nurse anesthetists, physician anesthetists, student nurse anesthetists, anesthesiology residents, and anesthesia technicians. Each provider may have a defined individual role as well as a team role. The goal of this team is to provide optimal anesthesia care to the patient. Team membership may change depending on the type of case or particular needs of a given patient. Nurse anesthetists may also be part of an interprofessional team that may include but not be limited to surgeons, medical specialists, nurses, respiratory therapists, and pharmacists. Problem solving for a specific patient is the common professional goal. Each professional brings to the team not only his or her own set of professional norms and values but also knowledge, expertise, skills, and autonomy. Although certain aspects of professionalism such as peer review of work appear equal among all disciplines, in the team process, not all professionals within a bureaucracy may be permitted to function at the same optimum level of professional autonomy.[14] Health care team roles may be changing, but more often than not if a physician is part of the team, he or she will be the leader or "superconsultant."[15–17] These interprofessional and intraprofessional team roles will evolve as changes in the health care delivery system occur. Nurses have been assuming more leadership roles as professional practice has expanded and the health care delivery emphasis shifts toward wellness and prevention. The professional socialization of nurse anesthetists will continue to grow as professional roles among all nursing specialties expand and as the changing health care environment makes new professional demands on us all.

EMERGING PROFESSIONAL ROLES

Excellence in clinical practice is the primary goal of graduating nurse anesthetists.

This reputation of outstanding clinical performance in the provision of quality anesthesia care has long been characteristic of nurse anesthesia practice. Expanded clinical roles now involve numerous areas of specialty practice such as obstetrics, pediatrics, cardiovascular, and neurosurgery. Since nurse anesthesia clinical practice is no longer confined to the traditional hospital surgical suite, many nurse anesthetists practice in ambulatory surgical settings in hospitals, clinics, or physician's offices. Nurse anesthetists in these settings may specialize in providing anesthesia for plastic surgery, ophthalmic surgery, or oral surgery. Pain management has become a new focus for some nurse anesthetists, involving departmental staffing, management, and consulting on patients who present with acute or chronic pain disorders.

Medical economics will continue to impact on nurse anesthesia practice in all settings as we enter the next century. Applicants to nurse anesthesia programs must consider more factors than whether the individual will be prepared as an excellent clinical practitioner. A solid foundation in clinical practice is essential, but nurse anesthesia practice today requires many other skills beyond those needed for the operating room or obstetric suite. Nurse anesthetists must be prepared to assume a variety of other professional roles and responsibilities.

One avenue of employment for nurse anesthetists is pharmaceutic or manufacturing companies and a host of public and private agencies that deal with health care products and services. The unique educational background and clinical expertise of CRNAs makes them particularly well suited to positions in education, marketing, or sales with companies that manufacture and sell anesthesia equipment, devices, and pharmaceutic agents and adjuncts used in anesthesia practice. Some nurse anesthetists have assumed positions as advisors to public and private agencies such as the Food and Drug Administration (FDA) or the American Society of Testing and Measurement (ASTM). These professional contributions by nurse anesthetists also enhance public awareness and our professional image.

Entrepreneurial businesses have been developed by nurse anesthetists. Some CRNAs have become successful as educational conference or seminar providers, whereas others have developed and marketed computer software. Locum tenens or CRNA placement agencies have been successfully developed by CRNAs. A wide variety of skills and experiences not only in clinical practice but also in education, business, and management are beneficial to CRNAs seeking these career options.

The field of administration has been embraced by nurse anesthetists who serve as departmental managers, chief nurse anesthetists, or directors of clinical service. Departmental administration will be discussed in Chapter 20. Nurse anesthetists have also assumed positions in educational administration. These professional opportunities include deanships or other academic administrative roles, department or division chairs, and program directorships. Administrative positions in nurse anesthesia are seldom purely office jobs. Administrators often participate in a variety of professional roles including teaching and clinical practice. Nurse anesthesia administrators in higher education must be well versed not only in accreditation and certification requirements in nurse anesthesia but also in graduate school and university policies and guidelines as well as public and case law that impacts on higher education.

CRNAs who become faculty members assume the responsibility for educating the next generation of nurse anesthetists to continue the profession's tradition of excellence, serving as role models to student nurse anesthetists. Unlike faculty in other disciplines, such as primary and secondary education and nursing, CRNA faculty provide students with a realistic view of their future professional roles.[18] This is in part because students work under the direction of and in collaboration with nurse anesthetists in the clinical setting throughout the educational program, thereby allowing students to assume and feel committed to the nurse anesthetist role early in their educational process. Faculty in nurse anesthesia educational programs may teach both in the classroom and in the clinical area or they may teach in only one of these areas. Some programs afford faculty the opportunity to be course coordinators or to assume the responsibility for the instruction of an entire course or course sequence. In addition to teaching, many faculty members also serve as academic advisors to student nurse anesthetists.

Students must recognize their obligation to the generation of nurse anesthetists that come after them and accept the responsibility to give back to the profession some of what they have received. This is best accomplished by assuming an active role in nurse anesthesia education as a clinical and/or classroom instructor, a faculty advisor, a seminar leader, or a clinical preceptor. The best way to alleviate the current CRNA faculty shortage is for new graduates to provide their special expertise in educational activities to those who will be providing anesthesia in the future.

The role of a CRNA faculty member may also include active participation in bench or clinical research. The type of research engaged in is usually directly related to the educational background of the researcher. Those CRNAs with doctoral degrees in the basic sciences more than likely will carry out their research in a basic science laboratory, often using an animal model. Some CRNAs prefer applied research that involves testing and evaluation of clinical theories and modes of practice and therapy. Clinical studies may include those using anesthesia equipment or clinical trials of pharmaceutic agents or other relevant clinical applications. CRNAs who have doctoral degrees in behavioral sciences or education may prefer to conduct research that evaluates educational models and theories applied to nurse anesthesia practice or professional behavioral adjustments such as socialization. The recent movement of nurse anesthesia programs into the graduate framework has introduced research into the curricula of many programs. Research is no longer reserved for students earning the PhD because some outstanding research and publications have evolved from master's degree projects among nurse anesthesia graduate students as well as from practicing CRNAs. Credible research conducted by nurse anesthetists is extremely important to our professional development and acceptance among other established professions.

Professions are often measured by their scholarly works and their peer-reviewed publications, and not exclusively by the quality of their clinical practice.[19] Nurse anesthesia, although the oldest nursing specialty, unfortunately has the smallest number of publications, both textbooks and journals, when compared with other nursing specialties. Nurse anesthetists have been practicing their art for nearly 100 years, yet we have been content to sit back and allow physician colleagues to become the anesthesia experts by writing the majority of the textbooks and journals in the field.[19] CRNAs have a professional obligation to share knowledge with professional colleagues so that others can benefit from these experiences. One of the most effective means to transmit this information is through publication. This dissemination of knowledge is a link to the next generation, our legacy.

Publications include much more than original research. Clinical case reports of unusual or interesting situations should be published, and topical reviews of the literature can be valuable resources in clinical practice. Each and every CRNA is capable of publishing one article, case report, book review, editorial, or other professional contribution. Publishing is a measure of professionalism.[20] CRNAs have a professional responsibility to peers and future generations of nurse anesthetists to publish their work. Without published scholarly works in the field, nurse anesthetists would be unable to evaluate the quality of anesthesia care because what and how nurse anesthesia is practiced is based on what has been read and learned.[19] Nurse anesthetists must accept the challenge to become active participants in the dissemination of professional knowledge through publication.

REFERENCES

1. Gunn, IP: The history of nurse anesthesia education: Highlights and influences. National Commission on Nurse Anesthesia Education Report and Monographs. American Association of Nurse Anesthetists, Park Ridge, IL, 1990, p 198.
2. DePaolis-Lutzo, MV: Factors influencing nurse anesthesia educational programs: 1982–87. National Commission on Nurse Anesthesia Education Education Report and Monographs. American Association of Nurse Anesthetists, Park Ridge, IL, 1990, p 49.
3. Waugaman, WR: Nurse anesthesia: The practice of nursing, medicine, or something else. Nurse Anesthesia 2:157–159, 1991.
4. Fitzpatrick, JJ: Point: MSN is the appropriate aca-

demic credential for nurse anesthetists. Nurse Anesthesia 2:160–162, 1991.
5. Katz, FE: Nurses. In Etzioni, A (ed): The Semiprofessionals and Their Organizations. The Free Press, New York, 1969.
6. Brutvan, EL: Intro-role conflict: A result of naive attempts toward professionalization. J Allied Health 14:3–11, 1985.
7. Etzioni, A (ed): The Semi-Professions and Their Organizations. The Free Press, New York, 1969.
8. Waugaman, WR: From nurse to nurse anesthetist. In Waugaman, WR, Rigor, BM, Katz, LE, Bradshaw, HW, and Garde, JF (eds): Principles and Practice of Nurse Anesthesia. Appleton & Lange, East Norwalk, CT, 1988, p 3.
9. Mizrahi, T: Getting Rid of Patients: Contradictions in the Socialization of Physicians. Rutgers University Press, New Brunswick, NJ, 1986.
10. Simpson, IH: From Student to Nurse. Cambridge University Press, New York, 1979.
11. Merton, RK, Reader, GG, and Kendall, P, (eds): The Student-Physician. Harvard University Press, Cambridge, MA, 1957.
12. Becker, HS, Geer, B, Hughes, EC, and Strauss, AL: Boys in White. University of Chicago Press, Chicago, 1961.
13. Olesen, VL and Whittaker, EW: The Silent Dialogue. Jossey-Bass, San Francisco, 1968.
14. Lurie, EE: Nurse practitioners: Issues in professional socialization. J Health Soc Behav 22:31, 1981.
15. Brody, S: A diagnostic and treatment center for the aging: A program of preplacement intervention. Gerontologist 16:47, 1976.
16. Schuman, J, Ostfeld, A, and Willard, H: Discharge planning in an acute hospital. Arch Phys Med Rehab 57:343, 1976.
17. Zola, J and Miller, S: The erosion of medicine from within. In Friedson, E (ed): The Professions and their Prospects. Sage, Beverly Hills, CA, 1973.
18. Cohen, H: Authoritarianism and dependency: Problems in nursing socialization. In Flynn, B and Miller, M (eds): Current Perspective in Nursing: Social Issues and Trends. CV Mosby, St. Louis, 1980.
19. Waugaman, WR: Why publish? AANA J 59:457, 1991.
20. Waugaman, WR: Publication as a measure of professionalism. Nurse Anesthesia 3:1, 1992.

3

Committing to Professional Involvement

Scot D. Foster

OUTLINE

OBJECTIVES

On completing this chapter, the reader will be able to:

1. Understand the functional definition of professionalism within the context of its historical development and application to the practice of nurse anesthesia.
2. Recount the major characteristics of professional behavior.
3. Construct a meaningful "professional profile" from a range of professionally related activities, within the context of personal talent and capability inventories.
4. Describe various leadership styles and factors that influence leadership behavior based on follower competence.

UNDERSTANDING THE IMPLIED AND EXPLICIT DEFINITIONS OF PROFESSIONALISM

For Certified Registered Nurse Anesthetists (CRNAs) who have spent the greater part of their professional careers as educators, it has become increasingly clear that success of the educational endeavor for student nurse anesthetists hinges directly on the accomplishment of two distinct objectives. The first is generally the easier of the two and requisite to clinical practice; that is, to equip students with the skills and abilities to conduct and manage a safe and competent anesthetic. The second objective is equally vital but oftentimes far more difficult to achieve: *to instill in students a clear and functional understanding of the tenets of professionalism as they apply to personal behavior and a commitment to become involved in professionally related activities both in and outside the operating room.* To reemphasize, the reader should anticipate that the substantive portions of this text deal with the concepts of professionalism within both personal and occupational contexts.

The difficulty in meeting the educational challenge described above stems from a variety of sources. The primary reason is probably that the concept of "professionalism" is not an easy one to understand, because the term has been applied so broadly and indiscriminately that a clear conceptual picture is often hard to formulate. In addition, there are very few cogent descriptions of professional behavior or scales by which it can be measured. This is due, in large part, to the fact that those persons considered "of professional status" or likely to teach or transmit knowledge about it to others, lack clear definitions themselves of the term or effective methodologies that would aid in the transfer of such information to students. Students rely heavily on role modeling to aid in their understanding of the principles of professionalism. To complicate matters, students too often find that assuming professional roles is hampered because so many of those who are considered members of a profession neither consistently project professional behavior nor involve themselves in the broad range of occupationally related activities that encompass *committed, professional involvement.* The emerging professional is often reminded, through personal experiences or events recounted by the popular media, of countless abuses of professional authority by many occupational groups, including those outside health care. These experiences undoubtedly serve to devalue the principles of professionalism to the degree that it is often reserved for self-serving means. Yet, professionalism in its ideal form remains the single characteristic of anesthesia practice that will spell success or failure of the CRNA in the workplace and for the profession of nurse anesthetists at large. Clinical competence alone is not sufficient to secure the continued successes of nurse anesthetists as leaders in health care.

As the reader may have already surmised from earlier chapters, the profession of nurse anesthesia is substantially different from many other professions, given the numbers of CRNAs who have chosen to join the professional association, the American Association of Nurse Anesthetists (AANA). Although membership is not required for clinical practice, most CRNAs readily acknowledge the benefits of membership. The success of CRNAs as an effective force in the marketplace and a leader in the continuing development of nurse specialty practice attests to the commitment the majority of CRNAs have to sustain the visibility of nurse anesthetists as leaders in the provision of anesthesia care. This fact alone provides ample justification for the importance of this chapter if future generations of CRNAs are to enjoy the substantial benefits of specialty nursing practice in anesthesiology.

This chapter is introduced by a short chronology of the development of the professional occupations from a historical perspective. With the foundation laid, the author describes, in more contemporary terms, the definitions and responsibilities of a professional practitioner. This definition is followed by a discussion of what constitutes appropriate professional behavior and methods for developing a personal "commitment profile" enumerating a variety of potential activities the student or CRNA practitioner can undertake to further refine his or her professional development. The chapter concludes with a discussion of leadership and the role it plays in professional development.

Historical Evolution of the Professions

As one might expect, the professions derived largely from those who sought to teach or "to profess." Originally, this meant to take the vows of a religious order, but by the 17th century, the definition of the word was secularized to mean "that process of achieving due qualification."[1] From this concept developed the notion that persons claiming membership in the professions "profess to know better than others the nature of certain matters and to know better than their clients what ails them or their affairs."[1] The origins of professionalism were initially associated with the clergy; however, the professions slowly became secularized and separately organized when religion was no longer a predominant social force. The professions became more formally associated with the universities of medieval Europe but still could be characterized as mere training schools for what would be later termed the traditional professions of law, medicine, and theology.

Most commonly, professional occupations were learned through apprenticeships or short training courses. Since both theory and practice had always been considered dual components of the learned professions, the advent of apprenticeships put renewed emphasis on the practice component. The professional candidates placed themselves under the able tutelage of ministers, lawyers, or doctors and hoped by observation and imitation to be subsequently admitted to professional status. In the American colonies, early professional education came primarily from the great European universities for lack of colonial faculties or organized professional schools. Slowly the American colonists began to develop their own system of higher education, from which would eventually emerge the professional school. This effort was greatly aided by the establishment of professorial chairs and special professorships in traditional academic disciplines. Proprietary schools (staffed by teaching practitioners) were also developed during this time and helped to provide greater numbers of professionals. The instruction and overall quality of many of these schools were dubious at best. They did, however, provide employment for what many considered a proliferation of doctors and lawyers so ill trained that they could not find gainful employment elsewhere. Proprietary schools did contribute in small part to the development of professional education by emphasizing didactic instruction and relying less on apprentice-type learning "by experience." However, the actual contributions of proprietary schools to the theoretic base of the professions remains a point of historic contention.

It was not until after the Civil War that the scope and sophistication of professional schools began to develop fully. Medical practice drew increasing respectability from the incorporation of scientific principles of research gleaned largely from European physicians. Curricula became more comprehensive and were based on new developments in chemistry and biology that would form a solid scientific base for the conduct of physicians' professional work. Lawyers would come to value the need for more balanced educational approaches incorporating longer, more formalized internships under qualified mentors. Even professional faculty in schools of theology were beginning to incorporate some of the newer modes of scholarship adapted from the German models of professional education. These activities ushered the movement of professional schools into the university setting, away from the more disorganized and oftentimes ethically barren proprietary schools. The occupations of engineering and certain of the social science and health care fields (e.g., nursing) were becoming recognized and accepted as professions subsequent to the move of those disciplines into more formal educational frameworks. Also, due to the diverse missions of emerging types of institutions of higher education, the land grant institutions (eventually state universities) began to recognize agriculture and home economics as professional occupations. With the advent of state examinations and regulatory authorities, accreditation mechanisms, and performance standards development, professional schools became more firmly entrenched as vital social service providers.

To this day, most professional schools, despite their unquestionable value to society, enjoy no better than a tenuous relationship to the larger, more traditional university of which they are often a part. The reasons are many, and only a few will be mentioned. The primary source of conflict is that health education necessarily incorporates substantial numbers of clinical work hours for students in order to prepare them for practice. Traditionally, most doctoral degree–granting, research-based universities aspire to more "lofty goals" involving movement from the level of practice experience to the theoretic realm in which empiric research and pursuit of knowledge is the preeminent goal. To quote Brusbacher and Willis[2]:

> . . . it has been argued that concern with the practical is concern with the specific and routine. Professional study, if it is to remain worthy of higher learning and not be anti-intellectual, must consist of general principles and fundamental propositions. Since professional education is more prone to succumb to practical exigencies, some were prepared to separate it altogether from the university, if need be, to preserve the integrity of the graduate school as a place for pure research.

Although most of these arguments have been put to rest in favor of a more cooperative relationship between the academic and clinical disciplines, vestiges of the conflict remain. It is exactly for need of this balance between the theoretic and practical that schools of nurse anesthesia are increasingly choosing to move into the graduate framework of colleges and universities.

Nurse anesthesia programs that grant academic degrees on completion of graduation requirements may, in fact, be one of the best examples of problems associated with the move of nontraditional clinical disciplines into institutions of higher education. First, professional schools are expensive to run, staff, and capitalize with required learning resources. This necessarily takes up a large portion of the total university or hospital budget, directing resources away from the traditional academic disciplines or other missions of the institution. Medical and specialty nursing faculty usually receive, on average, much larger salaries for their work than do faculty in nonhealth care disciplines, independent of faculty rank. This causes obvious friction. As major cuts in health care reimbursement continue to occur, hospitals and large medical centers associated with major universities find it increasingly difficult to maintain a wide variety of costly educational programs, yet the traditional academic institution is ill equipped to accommodate clinically based programs. The problem then becomes one of who, within the medical/academic complex, is to be responsible for the conduct of professional educational programs in health care.

This issue of an appropriate "academic domicile" may continue to plague nurse anesthetists in a university setting for years to come. Since the majority of schools housed within universities are not a major part of a recognized, traditional academic discipline such as nursing or medicine, its power structure and authority within the university-based organization may be weak and only casually recognized. The issue of establishing a proper academic affiliation or separate academic identity will continue to be problematic and make it difficult for CRNAs to secure a permanent place for themselves in the university academic, clinical, and administrative organizational structure. This problem will be resolved only when more CRNAs are prepared academically at the master's and doctoral levels, allowing them to compete credibly with other mainstream faculty. CRNAs must be prepared to become full partners in academic policymaking, governance, administration, and research, all of which will better prepare them to negotiate more permanent and credible recognition for CRNAs in the university setting.

Defining the Responsibilities of Professionalism

Before discussing professional behavior or related activities, it is vital that the student nurse anesthetist understand, and the practitioner be reminded, that our abilities to practice anesthesia within the scope of what we term a "professional capacity" is not a right that was afforded us unconditionally. In its most global connotation, the professions (traditionally medicine, law, and theology) were recognized as occupational groups that over time had gained the recognition and trust of the public for services that were highly valued by society.

Consequently, professional recognition was an earned right granted solely and exclusively by the public in exchange for certain services and conduct (see Historical Evolution of the Professions, earlier). As such, society retains the right to deny recognition of any professional service provider at any time when those services no longer meet the needs, expectations, or standards of the public. Too often CRNAs are under the mistaken notion that their rights to practice are provided directly by statute or some particular licensing or regulatory body. Remember first that these bodies are merely social conventions designed to facilitate the sanctions of the public at large. Although this notion on its face may appear of little importance, it should remind us that we practice anesthesia because we have earned the confidence and trust of the public. If the quality, scope, and vigilance attendant to our work fails, so may our ability to claim professional status.

Chief among the responsibilities for which the public holds the CRNA responsible (in exchange for the designation, benefits, and prerogatives of professional practice) is for professional activities to benefit the public, not the profession. That is, the primary goal of any profession should be public service. For instance, in cases in which a professional organization comes to value their pecuniary interest over that of the public to afford such services, it is likely the profession will risk extinction.

Many scholars have described what they believe constitutes the rights and responsibilities of the professional practitioner in much more comprehensive terms than the example provided earlier regarding public service.[3] There is some degree of difficulty encountered in these definitions because of the evolving and changing nature of social values placed on services. Further, most authors agree there is a need for a description of professionalism that uses multiple criteria. The most critical features of this definition, with which most sociologists concur, include skill and competence acquired by rigorous clinical training, research-based theoretic education, and an ethical code of behavior. Table 3-1 provides a comprehensive listing of professional attributes.

Nearly all professional societies have made available to their members a code of ethics, that is, a code of "right" behaviors based on a set of values or principles that the profession reveres. The AANA has a code of ethics that was written as a guide for CRNAs to use in professional dealings with patients, colleagues, and institutions for whom they work, as well as other external agencies with whom CRNAs must deal (Appendix 1). Although these codes are often cited as requisite for any professional disci-

TABLE 3–1

CRITERIA FOR QUALIFICATIONS AS A PROFESSION

1. The professional is engaged in a full-time occupation that comprises his or her principal source of income. Professionals have a strong motivation or calling to the occupation manifested by a lifetime commitment.
2. The professional possesses a specialized body of knowledge and skills acquired during a prolonged period of formal education and training.
3. The professional makes decisions on behalf of a client by means of a clearly defined, yet broad foundation of theoretic knowledge and expertise in clinical application.
4. The professional has a service orientation. This service implies diagnostic skill, competent application of general knowledge to the special needs of the client, and an absence of self-interest or self-promotion.
5. The professional's service to the client is assumed to be based on the objective needs of the client and independent of the particular sentiments that the profession may have about the client. The professional promises a "detached" diagnosis and is expected to withhold moral judgement about the client's revelations or diagnosis.
6. The professional demands autonomy in actions and judgment. He or she subscribes to standards judged by a panel of peers. Legal protection is sought through political influence.
7. Professional associations are formed that define criteria of admission, educational standards, licensing, entry examinations, and areas of jurisdiction for the profession. Ultimately, the professional association's function is to protect the autonomy of the profession; it develops reasonable strong forms of self-government by setting rules or standards for the profession.

*Adapted from Schein.[3]

pline, there are often difficulties with interpretation and application to real-life situations. Consequently, CRNAs will be faced with many questions and problems attendant on professional practice for which there are no clear or obvious answers. The CRNA then must rely on substantial measures of personal maturity, introspection, critical analysis of issues, elucidation of personal values, and keen problem-solving skills.

Pellegrino[4] provides another persuasive and perhaps more humanistic perspective of what constitutes a professional. He states that the philosophic grounding of a true profession lies in the special kind of interpersonal relationship it requires between its practitioners and those who seek its assistance. Components of his approach include (1) the need for health care providers to understand that patients exist in a special and compromised state of vulnerability; (2) the understanding by health care providers that the patient needs the professions address are of the most sensitive kind, centering on the most personal things a human being must confront—mortality, freedom, human values, and rights; (3) the understanding that the health care provider must always uphold the values of dignity and privacy; and (4) the realization that patients trust that the health care provider will use knowledge only in their best interest. Pellegrino[4] concludes his remarks with the following admonishment:

> To be a professional is to make a promise to hope, to keep that promise, and to do so in the best interests of patients. It is to accept the trust the patient must place in us as a moral imperative, one that the ethos of the marketplace or competition does not expect us, in our society, to honor. The special nature of the helping and healing professions is rooted in the fact that people become ill and need to trust others to help them restore health.

Abuses of Professionalism

It should be evident to even the most naive observer of the professional scene that the traditional privileges and social status of the professions have been slowly eroded over the past 30 to 40 years. Whether the discipline be law, medicine, religion, or nursing, one can cite numerous examples that have accounted for the downturn in public esteem the professions once enjoyed. The reasons are many and a discussion of them could fill an entire textbook. Suffice it to say that most of the problems have been brought to bear by professionals who have abused the privileges afforded them. In the field of health care, the reasons for the decline in public esteem are generally attributable to decreasing sensitivity of providers to public need; resistance on the part of medicine to allow patients decision-making authority; crass commercialism; increasing costs for decreased health care services; failure to remove incompetent practitioners; and favoring professional interests over those of the public. Unfortunately, for those who maintain a commitment to service, public scrutiny and criticism will be a likely companion for decades to come.

As a result of these abuses, adverse public opinion has been reasonably effective in initiating needed changes in medical policy and in the conduct of its practitioners as well as the general system of health care delivery, although most readily admit that the greatest work is yet to be accomplished. Among those changes was the emergence of a patient's bill of rights, which delineates rights and expectations the patient may legally have in actions associated with their care. Many hospitals, at the patient's behest, provide other mechanisms that protect the rights of self-determination, including putting the physician-patient relationship on a contractual basis (a specific service for a specific fee) or declaring a patient's rights to confidentiality, disclosure, and informed consent. State and federal legislative agendas abound with examples that the public is beginning to reassert its authority to control professional activities that it determines not to be in its best interest. Those include caps on certain legal fees in medical malpractice cases, support for competition with physicians by non-physician providers (such as CRNAs) to provide the public with rights of choice of provider at lesser cost, easier access to medications without prescriptions, less bureaucratic red tape to gain access to life-saving drugs that have not received final Food and Drug Administration (FDA) approval, establishment of a federal data bank on the status of provider competence, and of course the substantial fee reductions to physicians (especially anesthesiologists) distributed through federal aid programs such as Medicare and Medicaid.

The trend appears obvious. The health care professions, in general, may be moving away from the traditional concept of professionalism as forces of the competitive marketplace require that it compete in the same manner as those engaged in the trades or crafts. Undoubtedly, a redefinition of professionalism will emerge that will, it is hoped, retain the best of the old with new emphasis on the moral obligations of professionals to service and ethical conduct. Traditional prerogatives such as high pay and prestige will undoubtedly *not* be the centerpiece of this new social construct without tight social controls on its development and function. This more egalitarian shift in public attitude and perspective about health care practitioners will hopefully provide a window of opportunity for professionals such as nurse anesthetists to reverse this damaging trend with a recommitment to traditional professional values that wisely incorporate the changing norms of contemporary society.

EXHIBITING PROFESSIONAL BEHAVIORS

Student Commitment to Educational Integrity

Among the most critical of all professional behaviors for the student nurse anesthetist is the commitment to academic integrity. This term implies that a student is resolved to pledge all of his or her intellectual resources to the process of learning. Students should enter an educational program as informed consumers; that is, they should be clear as to their motivations and capabilities for pursuing a career in nurse anesthesia; they have made a studied analysis of their educational needs in relation to program resources; and they have placed acquisition of certification as a priority in their lives. During the course of the program, faculty measure a student's commitment to academic integrity in a variety of ways: optimal classroom preparation and study, meeting deadlines, well-executed planning and organizational skills, self-motivated inquiry, self-discipline, and exceeding minimal performance standards, both in the classroom and the clinical area.

Sustaining Professional Behaviors in Clinical Practice

Few CRNAs would argue the fact that nurse anesthetists have earned their substantial reputation and practice authority based on two achievements: first, their high-level competence, service, and quality of care to patients; second, their active participation in professional activities required to secure their practice rights, public exposure, academic credibility, and clinical acumen. Our profession is where it is today because of the dedication and commitment made by pioneers who gave of all their professional resources to secure these benefits for today's generation of practicing CRNAs.[5] It is the responsibility of our generation to make similar efforts for the one that will follow.

In short, it is not enough for us to prepare ourselves and our students as competent clinicians. On a daily basis, competent clinicians who do not go the extra mile in maintaining their rights and privileges as CRNAs, because they lack either the skills or the desire to do so, are abused, denigrated, and left largely unappreciated. This is especially ironic considering the fact that the skills required of the specialist in anesthesiology are usually highly prized and valued by employers. This is supported by the recent federal government study that has called for existing educational programs to triple their output of graduates in order to meet projected anesthesia human resources needs by the year 2010.[6]

Practicing CRNAs, as well as student nurse anesthetists, must enhance their professional image by becoming facile in reading, understanding issues, promoting discussion, gaining consensus, identifying and analyzing trends, and devising and promoting policy. They must understand measures of quality in performance of their clinical duties, collect data to verify their competence, and gain sufficient theoretic knowledge to justify their decisions and choices. They must gain appreciation and skills for speaking publicly, writing, researching, questioning, negotiating, debating, lobbying, risking new ideas, and abandoning outdated ones. They must explore their potentials as educators, clinicians, investigators, politicians, philanthropists, and visionaries—none of these roles to the exclusion of the others. Above all, they must care for things and people beyond themselves. Nurse anesthesia is a profession of giving both to patients and colleagues even though we increasingly find ourselves in a marketplace and social system that is often characterized by ambiguity, indifference, and intolerance. Clinical skills alone are not sufficient to maintain marketplace strength and consumer credibility. Today's CRNAs must be well schooled in the area of professional commitment. They must develop an informed appreciation of, and active participation in, activities that will serve to enhance their professional standing among colleagues, employers, and the public.

ASSESSING AND PLANNING A COMMITMENT PROFILE

The old adage "you only get out of things what you put into them" has never been more true or had more applicability to health care professionals than it does today. CRNAs have long cherished their ability to practice with relative autonomy, to conduct patient care activities in ways they believe are most appropriate, and to participate fully in the health care system as respected, primary care providers. However, these privileges have neither been without cost nor will they be available in future without active participation by all CRNAs in activities that strengthen their public image, political acumen, clinical and academic credibility, and public service. Students and practitioners alike should periodically evaluate their commitment to such activities according to where their talents and interests lie, such that the scope of their professional life becomes a balance between taking advantage of professional prerogatives and "giving back" to the profession. These activities can be conveniently grouped into four primary areas: clinical service to the community, teaching and research, political advocacy, and establishing interdisciplinary networks.

Clinical Service to the Community

Perhaps the most important of all characteristics that might fit into a commitment profile are those activities CRNAs undertake to maintain and advance their clinical skills for the benefit of patient care. In 1978, the profession of nurse anesthesia realized the need to demonstrate to the public its desire to keep abreast of the newest clinical and patient care advances by mandating that all CRNAs achieve 40 hours of continuing education every 2 years for recertification. These recertification functions are administered by the Council on Recertification, an autonomous body under the corporate structure of the AANA. Nurse anesthesia was the first nursing specialty group to adopt mandatory continuing education, thus fulfilling an obligation to the community to provide the most competent service possible.

CRNAs have a long history of providing clinically related services to the community beyond those that take place in a typical operating room. Among them are sponsorship of health-related physical assessment seminars or fairs; teaching in publicly sponsored/funded cardiopulmonary resuscitation (CPR) classes; staffing immunization clinics; providing missionary or volunteer work in federal government or private ventures to foreign countries that provide emergency, palliative, or corrective surgical procedures for underprivileged pediatric populations; and serving as staff anesthetists to international health care organizations like the Red Cross, Project Hope, Project Ibis, and many others. In addition to the valuable service provided by CRNAs because of their nursing and anesthesia backgrounds, participation in these efforts provides valuable public relations exposure for the profession.

Teaching and Research

The concept of teaching others is critical not only for the continuation of a particular health profession but also for the continuation of societal values, norms, traditions, and cultures. Civilized society has long valued the concept of education as a means to cultivate products and service, enhance the style of living, secure a competent work force, and thus ensure a productive society and thriving economy. The profession of nurse anesthesia is no different; rather, it is a microcosm of society at large. All CRNAs must become teachers in ways that promote a more enlightened client base, as well as a competent and well-educated cadre of health care providers. Teaching, therefore, will naturally encompass CRNA interchanges with patients, student nurse anesthetists, physician residents, other nurses, and a host of providers in ancillary health care fields. Most often teaching responsibilities fall on those CRNAs traditionally associated with education, that is, faculty actively involved in directing or teaching in formal educational programs. They often hold specific academic degrees or academic appointments. However, teaching responsibilities must become much broader and must be shared by all professional nurse anesthetists in every practice setting.

There should be no CRNA in any practice setting who cannot provide to a student nurse anesthetist some teaching-related service. These services may come in various forms, but all have immense value in the preparation of the next generation of CRNAs. It should be remembered that the growth of programs of nurse anesthesia throughout this country is singularly dependent on students' access to clinical sites where they can gain clinical experiences. Without this critical access, schools will not be able to supply sufficient human resources, not to mention the unfortunate circumstance when the public is not afforded benefits of anesthesia provided by CRNAs. That fact has tremendous ramifications for the future of the profession; if there are too few CRNAs available to provide services, the public will demand from other professional groups that service be available. If adequate numbers of CRNAs are not available, society will shift the mantle of professionalism to occupational groups who can most readily provide anesthesia services.

For some CRNAs, participation in education and teaching may include an invitation to a student to observe or actually practice in a hospital, outpatient, surgical office, or other clinical environment in which the CRNA acts as a formal instructor or mentor. Many CRNAs serve as affiliate coordinators for established programs of nurse anesthesia where the number of rotating students per year may range from a few to several dozen. Other CRNAs provide clinical supervision of students as clinical preceptors in advanced or specialty areas of clinical practice where supervision and instruction is quite close and intensive due to the acuity of the patient. Many CRNAs provide an invaluable service to schools by regularly providing guest lectures on topics related to their particular area of interest or clinical expertise. Lecture services are often provided not only to CRNA colleagues and students, but also to other health care providers via morbidity and mortality conferences, in-services, or speaking at state, national, or international professional meetings.

Closely tied to the area of teaching is the arena of research. CRNAs are beginning to emerge as credible and effective researchers who have established substantial publication records in a variety of well-known and respected peer-reviewed scientific journals. This movement is due in large part to the fact that more than 70 percent of all nurse anesthesia educational programs are at the graduate level where curricula include both didactic and practical experiences for students in research laboratories and clinical research environments. In addition, the number of doctorally prepared CRNAs is rapidly increasing, which further promotes the production of scientific papers and competent mentorship of others in research activities. As testament to the expansion of CRNAs into research roles, the profession of nurse anesthesia has witnessed the development of four scientific journals within the last 5 years whose editors and editorial boards are CRNAs.

The involvement of CRNAs in research is often intimidating for the novice, yet this activity is a requisite responsibility of any professional group. From earlier discussions of professionalism, recall that a professional group is responsible for the development of a scientific base on which practice principles can be founded. Clinical anesthesia services will fail to grow if not substantiated and expanded by well-conducted, clinically applicable research. CRNAs participate in research at many levels. Several are engaged in full-time basic research in established clinical laboratories at universities, private pharmaceutical firms, or federal government agencies. For CRNAs in academic centers, research is often a mandated activity for promotion and tenure. Most CRNAs who are involved in research are in contact with students during their formal educational program, helping them to identify potential areas of inquiry, mounting investigations of current literature, and collecting data in operating room environments.

Political Advocacy

Perhaps the greatest legacy of the profession of nurse anesthesia has been its record of legislative activities undertaken to secure practice rights and privileges for all CRNAs. Many CRNAs have developed substantial skills in elucidating clear legislative goals and priorities and translating them into positive changes in social policy affecting health care. Countless numbers of CRNAs participate daily in a variety of activities supporting these efforts. These may include—but certainly are not limited to—working with bureaucratic agency staff in state governments, such as insurance commissioners, heads of state health regulatory agencies and boards; and with congressional representatives and support staff both at the state and federal level. Most state organizations of CRNAs retain professional lobbying firms whose activities they direct to achieve legislative or policy goals.

Again, virtually every CRNA can and should play an effective role in promoting advocacy measures that will ensure optimal patient care through effective health care policy. Depending on the unique talents, aptitude, and interest of individual CRNAs in advocacy activities, each can find a niche. For some it will be insightful analysis of how potential legislation will effect practice, or establishing internal communication networks among CRNAs to quickly notify and mobilize the anesthesia community to call or write legislators about certain issues. Other CRNAs will participate in on-site lobbying efforts with congressional staff or will write position papers, potential legislation, or letters. Still other CRNAs will engage in public speaking to promote a particular position. Some of the most effective CRNAs are those who have, over the years, established productive interpersonal relationships with governmental or regulatory officials. In those roles they have spent many hours educating others about CRNAs, how they work, what they do, services they provide, and how they can be used most effectively in the general schemata of health care delivery.

In sum, CRNAs cannot afford the luxury of nonparticipation in activities that secure their abilities to practice and the public's right to choose the type of practitioner they want. It is incumbent on each CRNA to examine closely his or her ability to participate fully in the process of decision making as it relates to public policy.

Interdisciplinary Networks

Much of the work of professional organizations and occupational groups depends on collaborative efforts between a variety of related disciplines in order to bring about effective change. Policy formulation, especially legislative in nature, is rarely influenced substantially by a single professional group; rather, its achievement is greatly enhanced when groups work together for a common goal.

CRNAs have long realized this and have worked to establish effective liaisons with other professional groups, whether it be on a formal or informal basis. There are many day-to-day activities that CRNAs can become involved in that will promote interdisciplinary efforts. On a local level, CRNAs are often involved in hospital committee work, on which a wide variety of disciplines are represented. These committees often deal with issues of provider credentialing, quality assurance or continuous quality improvement, patient care standards, operating room policy, medical staff issues, continuing education, academic standards, equipment procurement, pharmacy acquisitions, and many others. Participation on each is important in establishing the reputation of CRNAs as decision makers and active and valued participants in health care provision.

On a more formal basis, CRNAs are often involved through their state or national professional organizations in a variety of interdisciplinary efforts. Within those roles, they serve as representatives to other specialized nursing groups or as consultants to a wide variety of governmental, military, and academic institutions for which they help develop policy, promote special projects or programs, or advance legislative agendas. CRNA consultants are used by the surgeon general, federal equipment standards boards, pharmaceutical houses, boards of registered nursing, peer review committees, accreditation teams involved in approving a variety of educational programs, and by law firms as expert witnesses; as management consultants to institutions developing anesthesia departments and to state academic boards of regents; and in countless other roles.

The professional commitment profile of a CRNA, beyond the traditional activities of providing clinical service, should be a lifelong project based on a clear assessment of personal abilities and talents. The profile will necessarily change over time to accommodate activities that require more skill and dedication of time, yet there are tremendous personal and professional rewards in achieving goals that promote the welfare of all involved. Inherent in all these activities is the dimension of public relations. For too many years, CRNAs have been relegated to the operating room and have suffered immeasurable harm for lack of public exposure. It is, after all, inconceivable that CRNAs provide over half of all anesthetics in this country yet still lack sufficient influence in the political arena. CRNAs must emerge from their traditional roles and assume a much more active stance in regard to professional activities that combine their considerable talents in patient care and professional advocacy.

ASSUMING LEADERSHIP ROLES

Throughout this chapter, special emphasis has been placed on the need to develop and maintain values that enhance professional growth and maturity. As has been discussed, there are many venues for participation, most of which call for some element of leadership skills. CRNAs often begin their anesthesia careers as recognized nursing leaders and authorities in clinical care, yet find it difficult to translate those skills into the areas of advocacy beyond those afforded the patient in a clinical setting. Subsequently, most CRNAs have to learn the basics of leadership only when they are confronted with obstacles in their professional life that require aggressive action and leadership skills to effect a solution. This is an arduous task and one that is not learned easily; yet without competent leadership, little personal or professional success will be realized.

The following section is a cursory discussion of leadership skills as they relate to the CRNA in professional practice. Acknowledging that the literature is replete with leadership paradigms and discussions of what constitutes an effective leader, it is best left to those experts to delve into a more comprehensive study of the topic. This discussion will be reserved for review of leadership roles many CRNAs assume during their professional careers and the basic behavioral characteristics inherent to effective leaders.

The Character of Leaders

Walter Lippmann stated, "the final test of a leader is that he leaves behind him in other men the conviction and the will to carry on." Much in that same vein, contemporary management and leadership theorists subscribe to the view that leadership is the process of influencing others to subscribe to your own or your organization's values and goals. Leadership *style* constitutes a pattern or constellation of personal behaviors used to influence the behaviors of others. These personal behaviors must of course take into consideration not only how you view yourself but also how others view you. That is, to effectively influence others, you must have both a substantial insight and understanding of self and an equally valid perspective of how others view your behavior and values and the importance they attach to them. If that perception is not clear, others will most likely act on their own accord, independent of your leadership.

Most early leadership theorists subscribed to the idea that leadership styles existed on a continuum; one end was exemplified by sociologist Max Weber, whose leadership theory consisted of *directing* the follower's activities in terms of task accomplishment, within an authoritative context. That is, employees or followers were told what to do, when and how to do it, and were directed via one-way communication down the organizational hierarchy. Emphasis was given to structure, tight supervision, and control. On the other end of the continuum is the *supportive behaviorist*, whose leadership style consists of two-way communication up and down the hierarchy. Supportive leaders provide encouragement, facilitate interaction, and involve followers in the decision-making process. This model valued personal praise, facilitation, and listening. Most leaders fall someplace in between, depending on the circumstance and the people with whom they are dealing. In fact, most good leaders are able to adjust their leadership styles fluidly to accommodate the unique requirements of the situation. Figure 3-1 provides a graphic representation of the four basic leadership styles for problem solving and decision making based on the concepts of the continuum between *supportive behavior* and *directive behavior*.[7] Note in that diagram that S1 (style 1), *directing*, implies that the leader takes sole responsibility for direction,

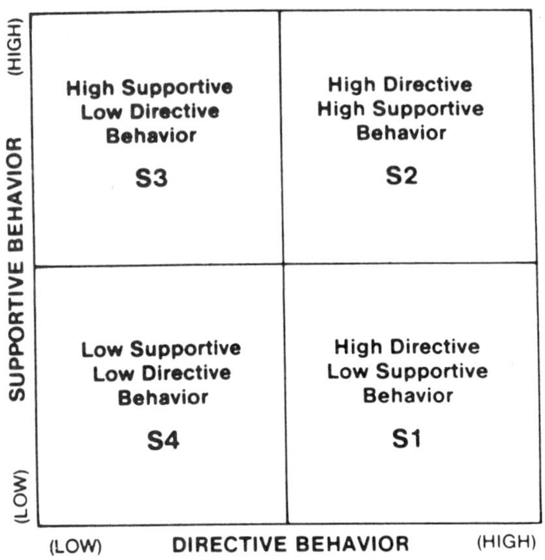

Figure 3–1. The Four Basic Leadership Styles as Types of Problem-solving and Decision-making Processes. This paradigm lists leadership behaviors that are prototypic of the four basic leadership styles. S1 = Directing, S2 = Coaching, S3 = Supporting, and S4 = Delegating. (From Blanchard KH, A Situational Approach to Managing People. Blanchard Training and Development, Inc., 1985. Reprinted with permission.)

decision making, and communication. S2, *coaching*, implies that the leader maintains decision-making authority but accommodates input from followers and listens to their ideas. S3, *supporting*, calls for low directive behavior by the leader, and the follower assumes much more control of the decision-making process. Style 4, *delegating*, occurs when followers are essentially autonomous to manage operations or decisions according to organizational goals and priorities.

Blanchard[7] maintains that *situational leadership*, the ability to change leadership styles appropriately and effectively, is based largely on the development or competence of followers. He subscribes to the idea that leaders should be able to adjust their degree of leadership authority according to the need followers have for supervision or autonomy coupled with evidence of their proven commitment to the organization. He designates the developmental level of followers accordingly: D1—low competence and high commitment, D2—some competence and low commitment, D3—high competence and variable commitment, and D4—high competence and high commitment. Figure 3-2 superimposes the variable of follower development (via commitment and competence) on the grid of leadership styles discussed earlier. As the follower demonstrates increasing levels of commitment and competence in organizational tasks, leadership styles must necessarily change. For instance, in graphic D1, followers have a high commitment but lack competence, so leaders need to provide direction. Since D3 followers have competence but variable commitment, leaders have to rely on supportive leadership styles.

Leaders need to develop many other behavioral characteristics. Among the most important are the abilities to listen, set priorities, manage change, support and motivate others, exercise control, manage crises, delegate tasks, make decisions, solve problems, take risks, promote collaboration, develop trust and commitment from others, become responsible and accurate in speech and written information, and above all, demonstrate personal integrity. All these attributes must be grounded in a personality profile in which the leader deals well with ambiguity and intolerance from others less

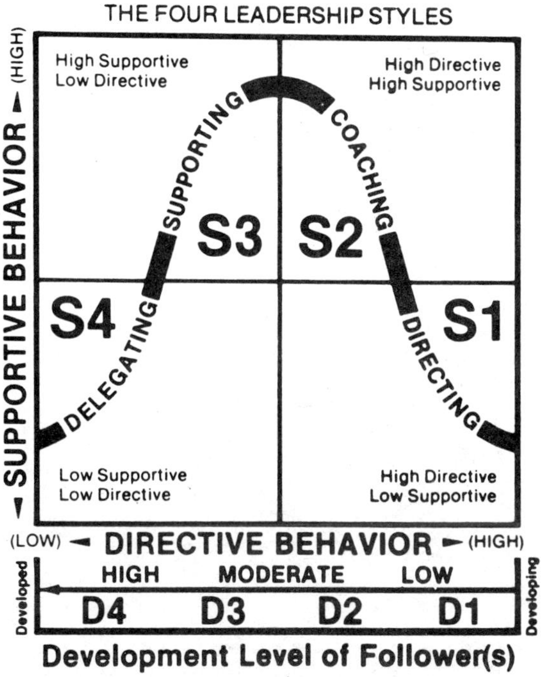

Figure 3–2. Situational leadership. Superimposed are the developmental levels of followers (D1–D4), which correspond to the amount of directive behavior required of the leader in decision-making and problem-solving activities. (From Blanchard KH, A Situational Approach to Managing People. Blanchard Training and Development, Inc., 1985. Reprinted with permission.

capable of leadership and has the ability to make keen and studied judgments via contemplation of potential outcomes and futuristic perspectives.

CRNAs are often called to leadership positions both within their own work environments and professional state and national organizations. Many serve as members of state committees, on boards of directors, and as officers of their professional group. Since more and more political and legislative issues relating to health care are determined at the state level, these leaders are increasingly relied on for resolution of issues that profoundly effect nurse anesthesia practice. For some individuals, leadership positions will become available at a national level within the AANA, as staff executives, committee and council members, board members, and officers. A great responsibility rests with those individuals to manage and guide the affairs of nurse anesthetists from a national perspective. Leadership has no rank and few perks that do not exact a high price in terms of commitment and dedication to organizational values.

SUMMARY

Since 1931, when the professional organization was first formed, the foundations of its development rested firmly on the belief that the survival of nurse anesthesia would require uncommon commitments to excellence. As one can readily appreciate, professional responsibilities incorporate a wide range of activities to which all CRNAs must commit their energies, not only for the care of patients but for their own well-being.

REFERENCES

1. Stein, HD and Kristenson, AL: The professional schools and the university: The case of social work. Council on Social Work Education, 1970, p 2.
2. Brubacher, JS and Willis, R: Higher Education in Transition: A History of American Colleges and Universities, ed 3. Harper & Row, New York, 1976.
3. Schein, EH: Professional Education: Some New Directions. McGraw-Hill, New York, 1972.
4. Pellegrino, ED: What is a profession. J Allied Health 168, 1983.
5. Bankert, M: Watchful Care: A History of American's Nurse Anesthetists. Continuum, New York, 1989.
6. Manpower Needs Assessment. Health Economics Research, Inc., Boston, 1990.
7. Blanchard, K: A Situational Approach to Managing People. Blanchard Training and Development, New York, 1985. Adapted from Hersey, P and Blanchard K: Management of Organizational Behavior: Utilizing Human Resources, ed 4. Prentice-Hall, Englewood Cliffs, NJ, 1982.

4

The American Association of Nurse Anesthetists: The Role of the Professional Organization

John F. Garde
Scot D. Foster

OUTLINE

OBJECTIVES

On completing this chapter the reader will be able to:

1. Describe the role of professional associations in relation to their goals of providing membership support services as well as their accountability functions to the public sector.
2. Recount the historical development of the AANA.
3. Describe the philosophy and objectives of the AANA.
4. Describe the structure and function of the organizational entities of the AANA Executive Office.
5. List the comprehensive services available to CRNA members.

It has been claimed by many that, since the inception of nurse anesthesia more than 100 years ago, our collective strength and influence in the health care arena today has been largely the result of two factors: first and foremost, the quality of anesthesia services provided by Certified Registered Nurse Anesthetists (CRNAs) and second, the strength of the professional association of CRNAs, the American Association of Nurse Anesthetists (AANA). Given birth and guided by such towering and legendary figures of the discipline as Agatha Hodgins, Hilda Salomon, Adeline Curtis, Gertrude Fife, Alice Magaw, and Helen Lamb, the AANA has evolved into a professional organization of substantial influence. This chapter charts that growth since 1931 and acquaints the anesthesia student with the organizational structure of the AANA, the role members will play in its continued development, and the services derived from active participation in association business.

A PHILOSOPHIC PERSPECTIVE

Professional organizations, regardless of the discipline with which they are associated, play a unique and demanding role in society. Often the roles they assume are complex, multifaceted, and seemingly contradictory; yet they have become the necessary vehicle by which professional health care providers are able to promote their interests, interface with the public, maintain relationships with external health care agencies, and effectively influence health policy in both state and federal legislatures.

There are several basic tenets that every student of nurse anesthesia should come to appreciate about professional organizations. First, organizations are devised and established by members for the pursuit of collective goals that will serve the self-interest of the provider. Organizations such as the AANA would not exist if not for the support and mandate of its members; therefore, organizational goals should be based largely on the basic tenets, philosophies, and values of its membership. Second (and herein lies a conceptual conflict), professional organizations cannot exist apart from the underlying fabric of social norms and values. As stated in Chapter 3, professions exist only at the behest of society; that is, they are given the rights and privileges of practice because they remain accountable to the public. Consequently, professional organizations are required to "walk a fine line" that represents a balance between member and consumer interest. It is largely this ambiguity that, if not managed with great aplomb, dooms professions to reputations characterized by overriding self-interest, which will eventually lead to public skepticism and disregard. As an example, witness the current attitudes of society in relation to the legal and medical professions. In the past several decades, both have suffered immeasurable detriment in the eyes of the public because this balance has not been maintained. One obvious result of this situation is the extent to which the public (via legislative action) is exerting much more control over medicine in terms of reimbursement and peer review activities. When a profession fails its public responsibility, the public will usually demand, and obtain, change.

Some have claimed that it is exactly this problem that underlies the notion that the real goals of professional organizations are inherently in conflict with the greater good of society and as such should be abolished. However, for all the rationale that would support this argument, few alternatives have been suggested to adequately substitute the work of professional organizations. The fact still remains that a strong, visionary professional association is one of the best means of securing the rights and privileges of practice for its members. It is with this concept in mind that all CRNAs are admonished to appreciate this delicate balance and maintain it credibly and truthfully.

The AANA remains unique in several respects when compared with other professional organizations. The AANA was among the first nursing specialty professional organization to be recognized within nursing. Few other professional specialty organizations in nursing can claim its tenure, experience, or stature. The AANA also claims the active membership of nearly 96 percent of all CRNAs in the country. This fact is unparalleled in any other professional organization of health care providers or among disciplines external to health care. Given the fact that CRNAs are not required to join the professional organization to practice, it would appear obvious that the vast majority of CRNAs value highly the role and productivity of the AANA.

Finally, the success of the AANA may be predicated on the unique relationship between its members, the executive office, and its elected leadership. Decision making relative to AANA business is encouraged at every level. Each individual member has direct access to communication to its elected state or national leaders and exercises direct voting privileges; that is, membership sentiment is not funneled through a delegate system in which individual opinions may be diluted or distilled into a group or consensus opinion. CRNAs remain singularly individual in their ability to participate and to be heard on issues that affect their practice or pique their concern or interest.

HISTORICAL DEVELOPMENT

In 1926, the first meeting of the Lakeside alumnae group of nurse anesthetists was held in Cleveland, Ohio. There, Agatha Hodgins announced her vision of establishing a national association of nurse anesthetists. Prior to this time, a few states had had varying success with establishing small groups of CRNAs in which to discuss difficult cases, yet none were organized to the extent that they could claim a national following.

Although Hodgins maintained the philosophy that nurse anesthesia should not be considered a part of nursing service, but rather a part of general hospital service, on several occasions she approached the American Nurses Association (ANA) in regard to nurse anesthetists being recognized within that group. However, the ANA failed to approve the proposition, and required more study. Headstrong and tiring of inattention by the ANA, Hodgins called CRNAs around the country to convene at Western Reserve University "for the purpose of considering the organization of the nurse anesthetists group." Forty-four CRNAs from 12 states agreed to form the National Association of Nurse Anesthetists (NANA) and to continue their efforts to affiliate with the ANA.

Over the next several years, Hodgins again attempted affiliation with the ANA but to no avail. Their board of directors finally rejected the proposal of the NANA, stating that affiliate membership could be accomplished through regular, established channels at the state level. Few of the association's early leaders were surprised at this outcome, none less than Hodgins, who by now was in ill health and left a small, fledgling organization still without the national recognition she fervently sought.

By 1933, the NANA had still not convened its first national meeting and suffered from general disarray organizationally. However, Gertrude Fife, the recently elected president of the organization, was encouraged by John Mannix, a department of anesthesia administrator, to seek recognition from the American Hospital Association. Given the fact that this group readily recognized the value of nurse anesthetists to their hospitals, the AHA invited NANA to present their first national meeting in conjunction with them. Fife stated, "We were going to put on the first convention. Who was going to make out the program? We had very little time. And Mannix said that we had to meet . . . we had to put that convention on. And, consequently, Helen Lamb and Walter Powell came to Cleveland and we made out the program over my kitchen . . . my dining room table. The three of us."[1] And so was born a renewed, vibrant, and committed organization of nurse anesthetists in Milwaukee, Wisconsin, September 13–15, 1933. By the close of the first annual meeting of the NANA, Gertrude Fife, the newly elected second president of the association, declared, "I feel that we are making history and that we are laying the foundation for a fine organization that will be a great benefit to the future of the work."

After this meeting, Fife was faced with the first and most important issue facing nurse anesthetists—education. She then called for a committee to investigate all schools of nurse anesthesia with the object of creating a list of "accredited" schools. Additionally, she called for "the establishment of national board examinations for nurse anesthetists." With this agenda set for the NANA in 1933, the members continued to move forward. In 1939, the organization's name was changed to the American Association of Nurse Anesthetists.

In 1955, the Commissioner of Education recognized the AANA as the national accrediting authority of nurse anesthesia education. This was a major milestone for the AANA as it afforded accredited programs and/or their students eligibility for such federal funds as might be available through a variety of legislative programs.

PHILOSOPHY AND OBJECTIVES

The philosophy of the AANA is simple and direct. The bylaws and standing rules of the AANA state, "The members of this professional association are dedicated to the precept that its members are committed to the advancement of the education standards and practices, which will advance the art and science of anesthesiology and thereby support and enhance quality patient care."

Since the founding of the association, its objectives have changed very little from those presented at the first annual meeting in Milwaukee, Wisconsin. As required by law in the state of Illinois, the objectives appear in the original certificate of incorporation of the AANA notarized October 11, 1939 and filed with Edward J. Hughes, then Secretary of State of Illinois, on October 17, 1939. The certificate is renewed annually. The objectives were amended at the AANA 1978 Annual Meeting to read as follows:

1 To promote continual high-quality patient care.

2 To advance the science and art of anesthesiology.

3 To develop and promote educational standards in the field of nurse anesthesia.

4 To develop and promote standards of practice in the field of nurse anesthesia.

5 To facilitate effective cooperation between nurse anesthetists, anesthesiologists, and other members of the medical professions, the nursing profession, hospitals, and agencies representing a community of interest in nurse anesthesia.

6 To publish scientific journals, bulletins, and other publications pertinent to the objectives of the Association.

7 To maintain informational and statistical data for reference and assistance in matters pertaining to the profession or its practice.

8 To provide opportunities for continuing education in anesthesia.

9 To provide members with direction pertaining to governmental policy, legislation, or judicial decisions of importance to anesthesia.

THE RESPONSIBILITIES AND QUALIFICATIONS OF MEMBERSHIP

The ability for CRNAs to become involved in the workings of their professional association is not without cost and responsibility. First and foremost is the responsibility of each CRNA to carefully assess the extent and veracity of her or his professional commitment by making the decision whether or not to become an active, dues-paying member. This decision should be based largely on careful study of what the professional association can provide to the member by way of services and the extent to which the individual CRNA shares the values and objectives promoted by the membership at large. Too, active membership implies that all CRNAs who become involved in association activities become sufficiently conversant with current issues so that they can effectively engage in discussions and decision-making activities that will advance the cause of the profession's goals and objectives. As students will soon realize, most CRNAs have little problem voicing their opinions; however, as with any professional organization, the quality of those decisions is predicated largely on an informed position, one that not only serves the individual member but also recognizes the needs and priorities of colleagues.

There are five categories of active membership:

1 Active Certified—Individuals who have been granted initial certification by the Council on Certification of Nurse Anesthetists. Once certified, membership is automatic for the remainder of said fiscal year and then only until the individual is eligible for membership as an active recertified member.

2 Active Recertified—Individuals who are currently recertified by the Council on Recertification of Nurse Anesthetists.

3 Active Nonrecertified—individuals who are required to be recertified but are not currently recertified and desire to enjoy the rights and privileges of active membership. Individuals who are actively practicing anesthesia may not remain in this category of membership for a period to exceed 2 years or one recertification period following the date of expiration of their recertification. Individuals who are not actively practicing anesthesia may remain in this category. Upon recertification, active nonrecertified members shall become active recertified members provided they have met all criteria for recertification.

4 Life—This is a closed category of membership comprised of individuals who have held this category of membership since August 31, 1976 and will do so for the remainder of their lifetime. Life members shall be granted the category of active membership for which they qualify. Life members shall be exempt from payment of dues.

5 Emeritus—Individuals who have held active membership for a minimum of 25 years and who desire to enjoy the privileges of active membership but have retired from the practice of anesthesia.

Qualifications for active membership are graduation from an approved school of nursing, possession of a current license as a registered professional nurse, graduation from an accredited program in nurse anesthesia, successful completion of the certification examination, and compliance with association guidelines, standards, or other qualifications set forth in the bylaws of the association. Students who are enrolled in accredited programs of nurse anesthesia are eligible for student associate membership at a fraction of the cost of full membership.

Current dues for membership in the AANA are $300 per year, of which approximately one third is allocated to the state association in which the CRNA resides. Membership in the AANA constitutes automatic recognition of membership of the CRNA in his or her respective state organization. The privileges and rights of members will be addressed in a later section of this chapter.

ORGANIZATIONAL STRUCTURE AND FUNCTION

Incorporation Status and Association Bylaws

The AANA was incorporated on October 17, 1939 in the state of Illinois and designated as a tax exempt organization by Subsection 501(C)(6) of the Internal Revenue Service. AANA's Education and Research foundation was incorporated on July 15, 1981 and designated as a tax exempt organization by Subsection 501(C)(3) of the Internal Revenue Code.

The AANA bylaws are essentially the AANA's working constitution and dictate how the association functionally operates. The bylaws currently consist of 23 articles that in turn have a number of important subheadings, called "sections," that further detail important facts about the association and its policies. The articles address areas such as the different classes of membership available, decision-making procedures, the responsibilities of the AANA's elected officials, and configurations of committees and function of their members.

Proposed amendments to the bylaws of the AANA must be submitted in writing by five active members to the executive director not less than 90 days prior to the next annual meeting. The proposed amendments must be referred to the Bylaws Committee for review and recommendations and then are forwarded to the membership at least 30 days prior to the annual meeting. Amendments to the bylaws may be adopted by an affirmative vote of two thirds of those members present and voting at a business meeting. Many of the Articles of Incorporation will be discussed in this chapter.

The National Headquarters

The AANA executive office moved from Cleveland to Chicago in 1937. After being situated in downtown Chicago, the AANA Executive Office (national headquarters), moved in 1980 to 216 Higgins Road in Park

Ridge, Illinois, a northwest suburb of Chicago. However, in 1992, due to limited space, expanding staff, and increased member services, the AANA purchased a 43,000-square-foot building at 222 S. Prospect Avenue, in the downtown area of Park Ridge (Figure 4-1). This new building nearly tripled the size of the AANA's national headquarters, allowing the housing of all member services and subsidiaries at one site, including a new learning center from which monthly continuing education seminars will be available to members on a variety of clinical and professional topics.

Due to the increased attention given to federal-level issues affecting nurse anesthetists, the AANA recognized a need to have continuous representation in Washington, D.C. In 1991, the AANA established a federal affairs office to increase nurse anesthetists' visibility nationally and to deal with relevant practice issues. Currently, the Washington, D.C. office has two lobbyists and a director of federal government affairs working on behalf of members, relative to a wide variety of federal issues that impact CRNA practice.

Departmental Organization

The AANA executive office consists of approximately 65 professional and clerical staff. The organization of the association is composed of the following departments, each with its own director, who reports to the executive director of the association. These include the executive unit, education, continuing education, membership and finance, practice, state government affairs, federal government affairs, public relations/publications, meetings and programs, quality assurance, and risk management and information systems (Figure 4-2). Within each of these major departments are member service sections. The executive staff serve in many capacities, including staff functions to each of the standing and ad hoc committees of the association.

The executive director remains responsible for the administrative functions of the national office and reports directly to the elected AANA Board of Directors. The executive director, a position created by President Richards in 1948, is responsible for keeping minutes of all AANA meetings, attending meetings of the Board of Directors and the Executive Committee, and any other activities designated by the president. The executive director has no voting privileges on the board of directors. He or she provides advice and guidance on policy formulation, maintains professional AANA staff, negotiates and renews necessary service contracts for the AANA, oversees all financial decisions for the national office at the direction

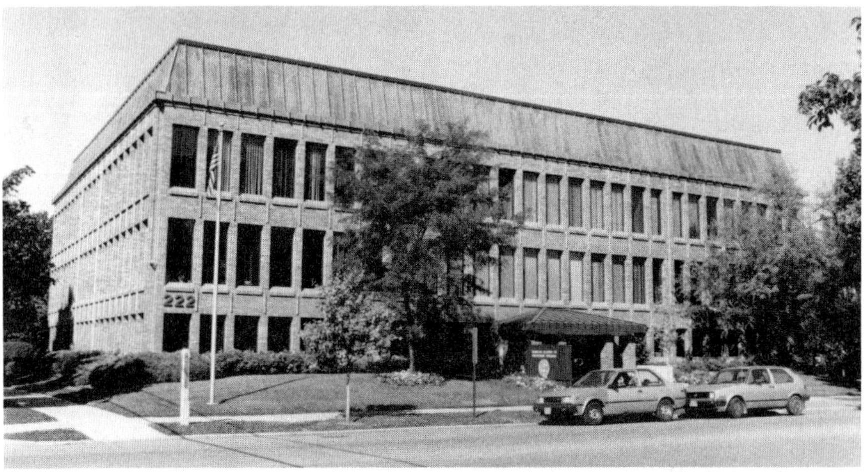

Figure 4–1. The AANA national headquarters in Park Ridge, Illinois, contains more than 60,000 sq ft of space and houses nearly 60 professional staff who maintain day-to-day operations of the association and its subsidiaries. Among the unique and important functions of this office are ongoing, in-house continuing education activities for all CRNAs to keep abreast of the latest trends in clinical practice and technology.

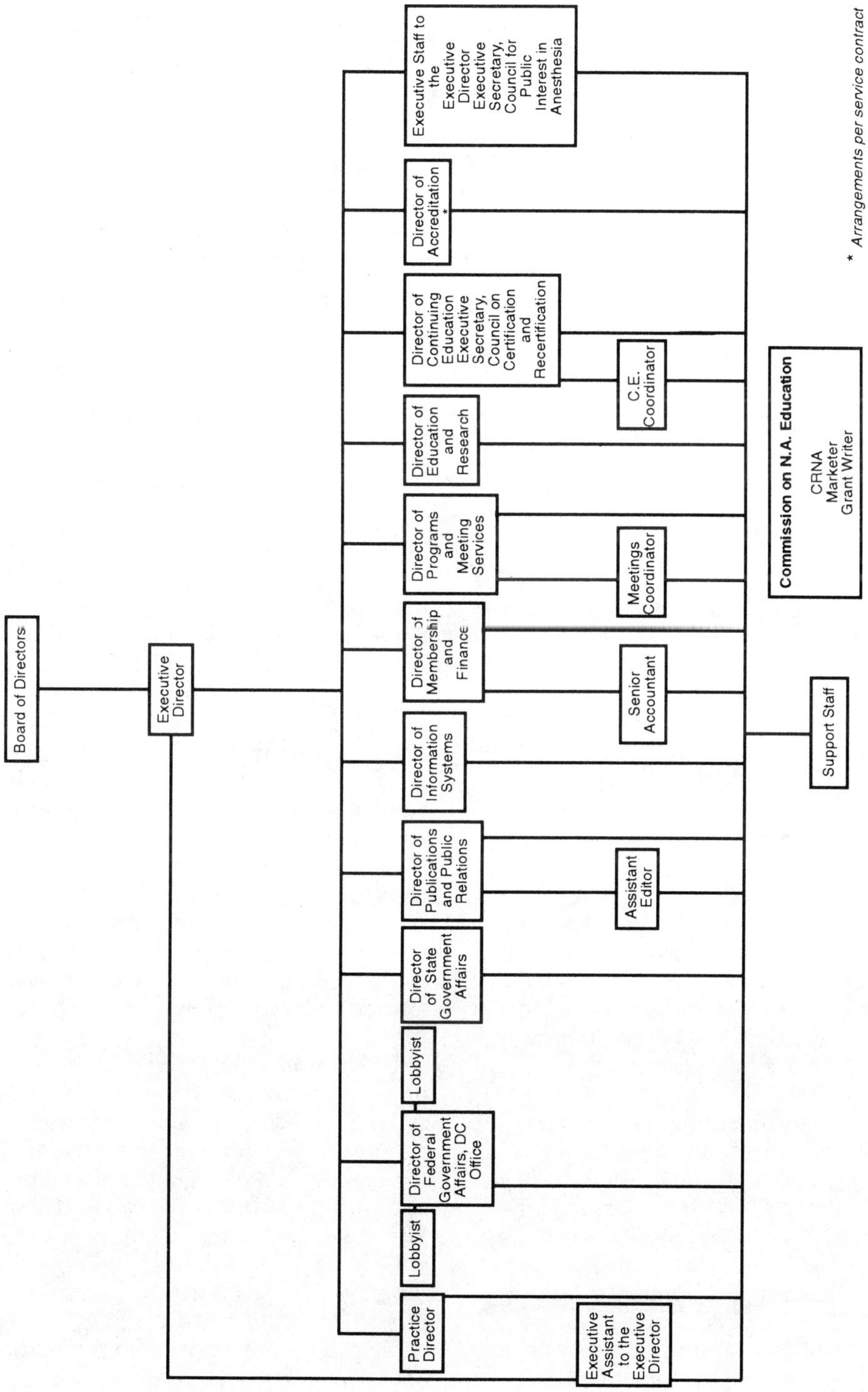

Figure 4–2. AANA organizational chart—executive office structure.

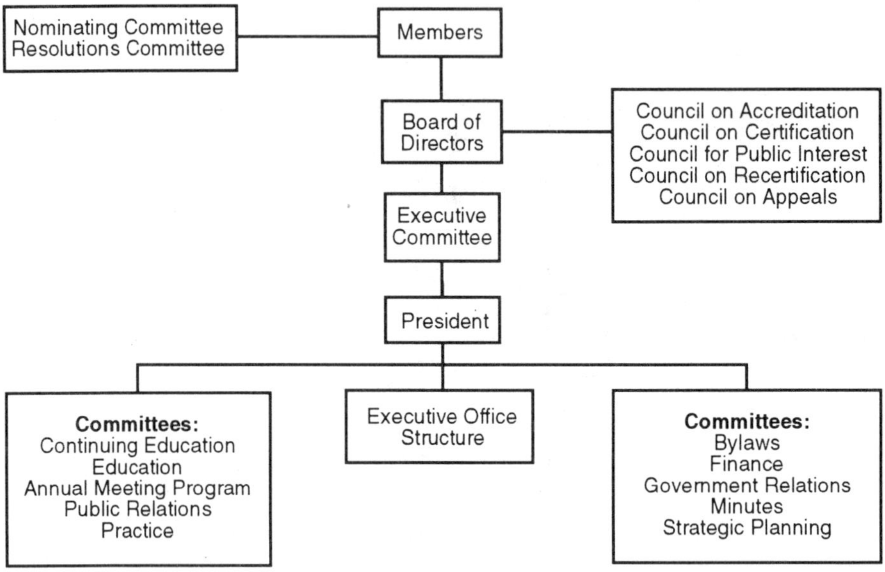

Figure 4–3. AANA organizational chart—communities of interest.

of the board, and provides leadership to educational, legal, and legislative entities of the AANA, as well as serving as a representative of the AANA to external organizations.

Council Configurations and Relationships

Within the AANA bylaws, there are provisions that have allowed establishment of four separate councils that function independently of the AANA executive office: the Council on Certification, the Council on Recertification, the Council on Accreditation of Educational Programs of Nurse Anesthesia, and the Council for Public Interest in Nurse Anesthesia (Figure 4-3). These councils are solely responsible for their own internal affairs, including the election of officers and the direction of financial activities. Membership on these councils includes CRNAs, students, physicians, and the laity, according to their own internal set of bylaws. They have been established to ensure the public that certification, recertification, accreditation, and public interest functions of the discipline of nurse anesthesia are separate from and not unduly influenced by the national professional association (refer to discussions of philosophy in earlier sections of this chapter). Most professional health care organizations of similar type to the AANA have made provisions within their operational bylaws to establish these necessary bodies, which, although supported financially in part or whole by the professional organization, do not interfere with their basic functions. The reader should remember that it is not necessary for a CRNA to be an AANA member. This council configuration allows CRNAs who choose not to join the professional association to still receive benefit of certification or recertification services. Communication between the AANA and the councils takes place through a formal liaison committee of council chairs and association officers to facilitate discussion of issues of mutual concern.

The Council on Accreditation of Educational Programs of Nurse Anesthesia (COA) consists of 11 individuals representing the community of interest involved in the accreditation process of educational programs and promulgation of educational standards. The purpose of the COA is to formulate and/or adopt standards, guidelines, procedures, and criteria for the accreditation of nurse anesthesia educational programs, subject to review and comment by the board of directors of the AANA as well as the communities of interest in nurse anesthesia at large. They are the body solely responsible for ensuring to the public that educational programs of nurse anesthesia comply with a set of minimum performance standards. The COA is itself accredited (recognized) by the Council on Postsecondary Accreditation and the U.S. Department of Accreditation as the sole agency empowered with the right to confer accreditation status to member programs.

The Council on Certification of Nurse Anesthetists consists of 11 individuals representing the community of interest involved in the process of certification of nurse anesthetists. The purpose of this council is to formulate and adopt requirements, guidelines, and prerequisites for certification and for eligibility to take the certification examination. The council is also responsible for administering each qualifying examination and evaluating the candidate's performance. The council grants initial certification to those candidates who successfully complete the certifying examination and who meet the other criteria for eligibility.

The Council on Recertification of Nurse Anesthetists consists of nine individuals representing the community of interest involved in the process of recertification of nurse anesthetist practitioners. Its purpose is to formulate and adopt criteria for eligibility for recertification of CRNAs based on participation in approved continuing education activities and other recognized activities conducive to professional proficiency. The council is also responsible for formulating and adopting criteria for approval of continuing education programs and offerings.

In response to increasing interactions between the communities of interest in anesthesia, the general public, and health care organizations, the AANA board of directors in 1974 appointed an Ad Hoc Council on Nurse Anesthesia Practice. In 1975, the Council was officially established and named the Council on Nurse Anesthesia Practice. In 1988, it was renamed the Council for Public Interest in Anesthesia and charged with the responsibility of monitoring issues that affect the public interest in matters regarding nurse anesthesia practice. Few other professional health care organizations have addressed the issue of public accountability in the manner of referring such issues to an autonomous body. This action again serves to ensure that public interest issues are not subordinated to the self-interest of the professional organization.

Subsidiaries

The AANA owns two subsidiaries that provide a source of nondues revenue for the association as well as services to the general membership. These subsidiaries are AANA Publishing, Inc. and Anesthesia Professional Liability Services, commonly referred to as "A Plus."

AANA Publishing, Inc. is the publishing company for the *AANA Journal*, the official publication of the AANA. The *AANA Journal* disseminates original research, information on current issues, and serves as a source of information for persons interested in the art and science of anesthesia and the role and functions of the nurse anesthetist.

A Plus was incorporated in 1988 as the AANA-owned insurance policy carrier for professional liability programs for CRNAs. A Plus currently provides approximately 2500 CRNAs with different lines of professional liability insurance. The A Plus office consists of nine employees, including a director of insurance services. All A Plus insurance agents are appropriately licensed and undergo continuing education to maintain their positions.

Under the subsidiary of A Plus, the AANA has also recently introduced a new continuous-quality improvement program designed for hospitals and anesthesia providers nationwide. The program, entitled "Anesthesia Quality Plus," was developed to continuously monitor the quality of patient care through a computerized data information system based on patient outcomes. The program has been designed to meet and exceed the Joint Commission on Accreditation of Health Care Organizations (JCAHO) guidelines for quality improvement (see Chapter 16).

THE ELECTED LEADERSHIP

Titles and Role of Elected Leadership

The affairs of the AANA are handled by an elected Board of Directors. The board consists of the president, president-elect, vice-president, treasurer, and seven regional directors. Officers serve for 1 year and directors serve for a 2-year term. To be eligible to serve as a director, an individual must have served at least one term as an officer or director of a state association and must have been active in state or AANA affairs. A nominating committee presents a slate of candidates for the Board of Directors at the Assembly of States meeting, prior to the annual business meeting. All CRNA members are allowed to vote for all officers and directors regardless of the region for which the candidate is running.

The Board of Directors is the administrative authority of the AANA. It receives and considers the reports of committees and directs the president to prepare an annual report that is submitted to the membership of the AANA reviewing the work of the preceding year. The Board of Directors assumes many other responsibilities on behalf of the AANA, including the handling of contracts and all budgetary and related financial matters, record keeping, maintaining procedural policies, promoting position statements, promulgating clinical standards, managing the association standing committees, and maintaining a liaison with a myriad of external governmental and professional agencies. An executive committee of the Board of Directors is composed of the president, president-elect, vice-president, and treasurer. The Executive Committee manages the affairs of the AANA between meetings of the board of directors.

Committee Configurations

The appointed committees of the AANA include the Annual Meeting Program, Bylaws, Continuing Education, Education, Finance, Government Relations, Strategic Planning, Minutes, Practice, and Public Relations. Committee members are appointed by the president with approval of the board of directors. All committees consist of at least three active members to be appointed for a 1-year term by the president, who shall designate their chairperson subject to the approval of the Board of Directors. The committees conduct their business at the direction of the president via written charges of responsibility submitted to them on an annual basis.

The elected committees of the association are the Nominating Committee and the Resolutions Committee. Election of these two committees is by mailed ballot, in conjunction with the election of officers and directors. The Nominating Committee is responsible for slating and determining eligibility of candidates for office for the AANA board of directors and elected committees. Members of the Resolution Committee submit resolutions (a resolution is a written "main motion" that contains subject matter potentially having significant impact on the policies of the AANA) to the executive director of the AANA, signed by at least five active members no less than 90 days prior to an annual meeting. At the annual meeting, the Resolutions Committee holds an open hearing at which time all submitted resolutions may be discussed. The Board of Directors is responsible for implementing any resolutions approved by the general membership.

CONDUCTING THE BUSINESS OF THE ASSOCIATION

In addition to the daily activities of maintaining the national office, the business of the association is conducted largely via primary meetings of different membership segments of the association. These include the Assembly of School Faculty, Assembly of States, Government Relations Workshop, and the Annual Meeting. All members are invited to attend and fully participate in these activities.

Assembly of School Faculty

The Assembly of School Faculty takes place twice a year, once in February and again in conjunction with the annual meeting. Participants generally include program directors, associate directors, physician and CRNA faculty, PhD faculty, educational advisors, students, and other interested individuals. Participants of the assembly discuss affairs pertinent to the conduct of programs including current issues, standards, legal implications, legislative trends, clinical practice, teaching/instruction, and research. The meeting is conducted by the Education Committee of the AANA.

Assembly of States

There are two Assembly of States meetings held each year, one in the spring and one in the fall. Attendees of these meetings include the AANA Board of Directors, members of the standing AANA committees, officers and board members of affiliated state associations, and other interested members. Traditionally, the site of the fall Assembly of States meeting rotates to a different city in the seven AANA regions each year, and the spring Assembly of States meeting is held in Chicago. Assemblies usually take place over an extended weekend and are held to disseminate information on current issues affecting practice and other programming to assist state organizations in the conduct of their business. Both the Assembly of School Faculty and Assembly of States meeting provide ample open forums during which any member may speak to issues of his or her concern. Additionally, the AANA board of directors usually meets in conjunction with these meetings to further facilitate communication between all segments of association membership.

Government Relations Workshop

Each year, the AANA hosts a Government Relations Workshop in the Washington, D.C. area, primarily to provide guidance to CRNAs on how to effect improved relationships with elected officials of government as they relate to promoting the AANA's legislative agenda. This meeting also provides an opportunity for participants to take a rare behind-the-scenes look at the legislative process and learn firsthand about federal legislative activities. Guest speakers for the workshop are selected on the basis of their expertise in federal and legislative health care issues.

Topics discussed include national health care reform, Medicare reimbursement for anesthesia services, and federal policies and law affecting health care cost, access, and quality as well as current issues affecting practice patterns of CRNAs. Many of the CRNAs attending the meeting convene personally with their members of Congress on the final day of the conference to discuss their positions on varied topics or proposed legislation. Much of the Government Relations Workshop is given to preparing the CRNA on the issues and how to best deal with congressional members and staff during these meetings.

Annual Meeting

One of the most popular meetings the AANA holds is its annual meeting, which typically lasts for approximately 1 week in early to mid-August in a city representing a different AANA region each year. Attendance at this meeting continually increases. Nearly 3000 members and more than 750 students attend. Members cite many benefits of attending an annual meeting, such as earning continuing education credits from more than 100 scientific sessions, networking with fellow CRNAs, seeing the latest in technology and equipment, hearing nationally and internationally known speakers, and sharing ideas and positions with colleagues and the leadership of the nurse anesthesia profession. The meeting includes an entire day of activities for students, among which are the National College Bowl, student luncheon, and numerous other activities; the student program is managed by the AANA Education Committee and its elected student representative. In addition, the meeting includes the AANA general business session, opening ceremonies, numerous business hearings, scientific sessions, workshops (Figure 4-4), focus sessions concentrating on special issues, exhibits, receptions, and the glittering annual banquet.

STATE ORGANIZATIONS

State Office Organizational Configuration

State associations are formed by AANA members who live and work in a particular state and are recognized by the AANA board of directors as a duly incorporated entity. State associations are responsible for organizing their own committees, electing state officers, and handling their own financial affairs. States are supported financially by the AANA through portions of annual membership dues paid to the national association. Officers and

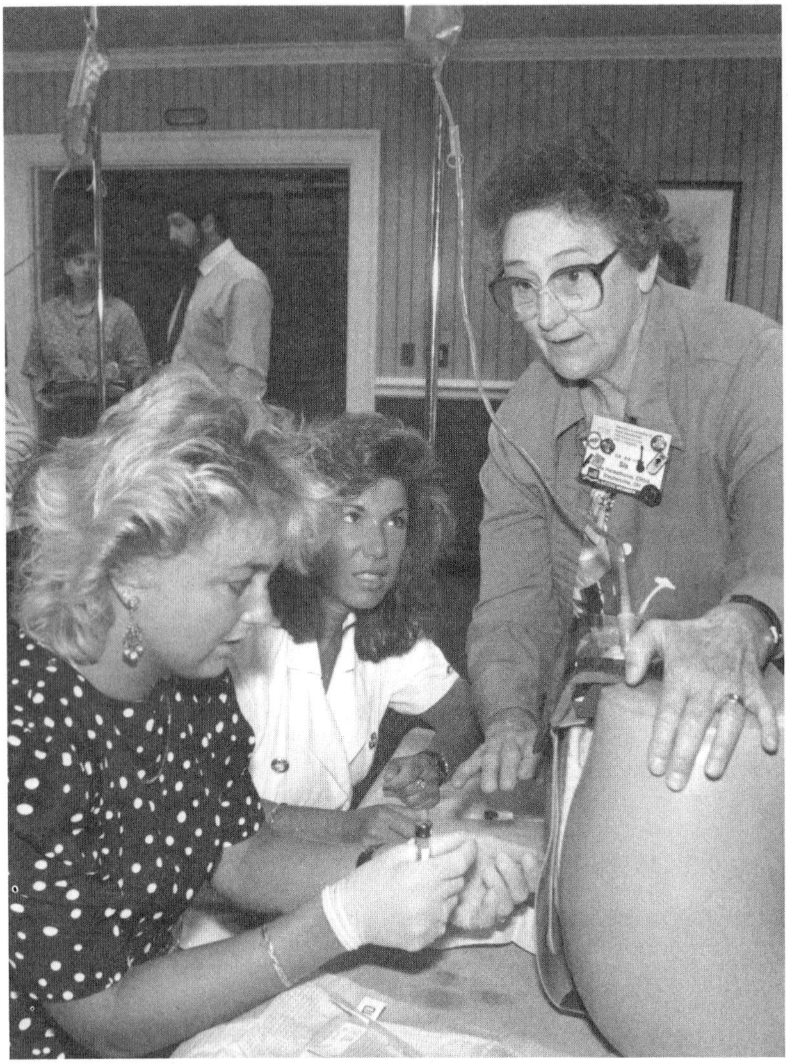

Figure 4–4. One of the most popular scientific sessions of the AANA annual meeting are those involving hands-on workshops in the area of regional blocks.

board configurations of state associations are similar to the national organization.

CRNAs at the state level deal with many of the local issues that impact on CRNA access to hospitals and other health care institutions, clinical privileges, and ability to receive adequate reimbursement. Activity of the state association is dependent largely on the volunteer effort of CRNAs and is of primary importance to the profession, as most of the legislative activity affecting CRNAs is conducted at the state level. Participation by CRNAs in their state association is usually considered the point of entry into activities and offices at the national level.

Relationship to the American Association of Nurse Anesthetists

Members from each state association maintain contact with the national office by providing them annually with a list of its officers, committee members, and current bylaws. Officers and members of individual state associations often contact executive office staff, seeking advice and counsel on issues related to practice, government affairs, education, public relations, and membership. In addition, a complete library located in the AANA executive office and staffed by a full-time librarian/archivist

TABLE 4–1

BENEFITS AND SERVICES PROVIDED TO AANA MEMBERS

Practice Issues

1. Valuable employment and salary information on a nationwide basis as a result of an annual membership survey.
2. Consultation services in employment practice matters.
3. Assistance with regulatory and accreditation issues.
4. National representation with external health agencies that impact nurse anesthesia practice.
5. Development of guidelines and standards for practice.
6. Preparation of numerous practice monographs.
7. Legal commentary on practice and quality of care issues.
8. Information and assistance on numerous practice settings.
9. Assistance in obtaining equitable reimbursement from third-party insurers.
10. Professional Practice Manual development and updates. Manual includes the following documents:
    a. Guidelines for Nurse Anesthesia Practice
    b. Qualifications and Capabilities of CRNAs
    c. Professional and Legal Issues
    d. Guidelines for Infection Control
    e. Informed Consent
    f. Implementing QA Programs in Anesthesia
    g. Risk Management Guide
    h. AANA Position Statements
    i. Code of Ethics
    j. Documenting Standard of Care: Anesthesia Record
    k. Anesthesia Outcome by Provider Studies
11. Expert witness referral program.
12. Anesthesia department consultation referrals.
13. AANA hotline for chemically impaired professionals, dial 1-800-654-5167.

Governmental Representation

1. National representation on governmental issues through the AANA Washington, D.C. office.
2. Broad legal interpretation of events that impact the profession.
3. AANA government relations hotline, dial 1-800-423-0625.
4. Assistance with Medicare carriers in obtaining equitable reimbursement.
5. State legislative/regulatory tracking service.
6. Analysis of state legislation/regulations for state associations.
7. Legislative updates in each *AANA NewsBulletin* and *AANA Journal.*
8. Political Action Committee furthering nurse anesthesia causes.

Publications

1. Bimonthly *AANA Journal* containing the latest in scientific and educational advancements.
2. Monthly *AANA NewsBulletin* carrying timely information of health care policy and issues facing nurse anesthetists.
3. Bimonthly *Anesthesia Quality Plus Newsletter* discussing quality assurance/risk management policies.
4. *NewsBulletin* classified advertisements listing open positions and professionals seeking new positions.
5. Calendar of continuing education program events.
6. Annual *AANA Journal* correspondence course for six CE credits.

Public Awareness

1. Professional recognition and identity.
2. National public relations campaign focused on educating general public on the role of nurse anesthetists.
3. National campaign to purchasers of anesthesia services, expanding employment possibilities for nurse anesthetists.
4. Development of patient information brochures for use by CRNAs in practice.

Meetings

1. Reduced registration fees for AANA events.
2. AANA Annual Meeting representing the single largest gathering of CRNAs, colleagues, and past classmates each year.
3. Assembly of States, two meetings each year focused on state association management and national issues.
4. Assembly of School Faculty, two meetings each year targeted specifically to educators.
5. Government relations workshop, held in Washington, D.C., to focus on and use the lobbying efforts of CRNAs on health care issues.

Education

1. Recruits nurses into the profession through exhibits, speaking engagements, and printed material.
2. Standards and guidelines for educating CRNAs.
3. Secures funding from governmental sources for nurse anesthesia programs and students.
4. Offers numerous national professional and educational workshops, seminars, and meetings.
5. Maintains continuing education records for easy submission to the Council on Recertification.
6. Identifies sources and procures funding for research.
7. Offers faculty development programs.

Continued

TABLE 4–1

BENEFITS AND SERVICES PROVIDED TO AANA MEMBERS—*CONTINUED*

8. Offers fellowship programs for CRNAs obtaining further education.
9. Consultative services to potential new nurse anesthesia programs sites.
10. Reviews and approves of continuing education programs.
11. Provides school transcripts.
12. Provides consultation for research activities.

Member Services

1. Group insurance programs that include health, life, and income protection through David L. Jelinek Agency, insured through ITT Hartford.
2. Credit card program through Maryland Bank.
3. Partial payment of biennial recertification fee.
4. AANA-owned professional liability insurance agency dedicated solely to malpractice insurance for nurse anesthetists nationwide.
5. Maintain database of CRNAs appropriately credentialed to obtain Medicare reimbursement from HCFA.
6. Emergency student loan program for nurse anesthesia students and CRNAs furthering their education.
7. Financially support Council on Accreditation of Nurse Anesthesia.
8. Educational Programs and Council on Public Interest in Anesthesia.
9. Professional liability insurance dividend program.

Quality Assurance

1. Assist practices in establishing quality assurance programs.
2. Developed computerized continuous quality improvement information system meeting all JCAHO requirements.
3. Computerized patient satisfaction software.
4. Quality assurance workshops.
5. Developing database of anesthesia cases to assist research.

serves as a central repository of information for state associations when devising position statements, conducting research, or proposing legislative language.

MEMBERSHIP SERVICES

There are many reasons to become a member of the AANA or to renew one's membership. Table 4-1 provides a listing of the benefits CRNAs enjoy through active participation in the AANA. Membership services are conducted and promoted through the Department of Membership and Finance of the AANA, whose staff are available to any CRNA seeking counsel or information.

SUMMARY

As the entire health care field continues to grow, so does the AANA, thanks to its loyal members, who continue to serve with the dedication, enthusiasm, and perseverance characteristic of its founding members. The AANA is indeed a unique organization in that it has the support of 96 percent of the nation's CRNAs. Unlike some professional organizations, the AANA allows each member a voice in its decision-making procedures through regular meetings and open sessions of the Board of Directors. We believe each CRNA has something of importance to contribute to the AANA, and the diversity among its members is a vital factor in the AANA's continued growth and success. To meet the challenges of the future, we must continue to remain an informed and unified organization that serves all its members and extends its promise of quality and caring service to the public.

REFERENCE

1. Bankert, M: Watchful Care: A History of America's Nurse Anesthetists. Continuum, New York, 1989.

TWO

The Rights and Responsibilities of Professional Practice

5

Governmental Regulation of Nurse Anesthesia Practice

Mitchell H. Tobin

OUTLINE

OBJECTIVES

On completing this chapter, the reader will be able to:

1. Describe the historical development of formal state regulation of nursing practice.
2. Discuss the methods states use to regulate nurse anesthetist practice.
3. Describe the statutes and regulations that can affect nurse anesthetist practice.
4. Discuss how state statutes and regulations can affect nurse anesthetist practice.

The author wishes to acknowledge the assistance of Karen P. O'Neill in compiling the numerical summaries in the section of the chapter regarding state statutory and regulatory requirements concerning nurse anesthetists. Ms. O'Neill is a student at DePaul University College of Law in Chicago and is a legal assistant at the Chicago law firm of Sidney and Austin.

HISTORICAL BACKGROUND

Formal state regulation of nursing practice in the United States is so entrenched that it is easy to assume it always existed. State laws and regulations concerning nursing, however, are a 20th century phenomenon. To understand why and how nurse anesthetists are formally recognized in states today, it is necessary to first explore the development of state regulation of medicine, then nursing.

Spurred by the efforts of the American Medical Association, Texas passed the first modern medical practice act in 1873.[1] The enactment of this state law was significant, because it heralded the beginning of an era in which physicians would have to obtain a license to practice medicine. The legitimacy of compulsory licensure for physicians did not go unchallenged. There were those who did not believe government had the right to require health care professionals to be licensed to practice. The United States Supreme Court, however, put the issue to rest in the 1889 case of *Dent v. West Virginia*.[2]

In *Dent*, the Supreme Court upheld the constitutionality of the West Virginia Medical Practice Act. In doing so, the court relied on the Tenth Amendment to the U.S. Constitution, which states that "The powers not delegated to the Untied States by the Constitution, nor prohibited by it to the States, are reserved to the States respectively, or to the people." The Tenth Amendment is the source of the states' "police power," or right to regulate the public health, welfare, and safety. As *Dent* confirmed, states have the authority as part of their police power to regulate and license health care professionals.

Following the *Dent* decision in 1889, states moved quickly to adopt compulsory licensure laws for physicians. By 1905, 39 states had enacted medical practice laws that required physicians to obtain a license before practicing medicine.[3]

Medical licensure led the way for formal state regulation of nursing. As Bullough[3] has noted, because organized medicine had already fought the battle concerning the legitimacy of state licensing laws, nursing's path was easier. Further, medicine's efforts in state legislatures constituted a guide for the political actions necessary for adoption of state nursing laws. (Basic state regulatory terms such as "laws" are explained in Box 5–1.)

The fact that widespread medical licensure preceded nursing's efforts, however, also had negative implications. Physician medical practice laws defined the practice of medicine broadly. As Bullough[3] stated:

> The authors of the early registration laws and those who worked on subsequent revisions in the early twentieth century assumed that medicine was the only health profession, and the language they used in the registration statutes often reflected that assumption. This meant that nursing and the other health professions had to consciously avoid that area previously carved out by medicine or, if they intruded therein, had to be prepared to face a battle. The nursing profession, as a result, avoided challenging the position of medicine. Only recently have things begun to change.

THE DEVELOPMENT OF NURSING LICENSURE

With medical licensure well established, the stage was set for formal state regulation of nursing. Bullough[3] identified three primary phases in the development of nursing regulation in the United States:

1903 to 1938. Enactment of nurse registration acts in numerous states

1938 to 1971. State legislatures began defining the scope of nursing practice

1971 to present. Increasing state recognition of the expanded roles and advanced practice specialties (such as nurse anesthesia) of registered nurses (RNs)

First Phase

In 1903, North Carolina enacted the first nurse registration act in the United States.[3] The act provided that, beginning in 1904, only persons that the North Carolina Board of Examiners certified could be listed as registered nurses (RNs).[3] By 1923, similar laws had been passed in all states and the District of Columbia.[4]

BOX 5–1
BASIC STATE REGULATORY TERMS

Throughout this chapter, terms such as statutes, laws, regulations, and the like are used. It is important to understand these terms, because they represent the building blocks states use to recognize nursing professionals. The following section defines some of the more common terms you will encounter in this area.

Jurisdiction

A *jurisdiction* is a geographic area having the power to adopt, implement, and enforce laws. All states are jurisdictions as are entities such as the District of Columbia, Puerto Rico, and the Virgin Islands.

Statutes

Statutes are also known as laws. Statutes are enacted, that is, passed, by state legislatures. The level of specificity of statutes varies. They are often general, leaving the specifics to administrative regulations. Every state has a primary law governing nursing practice. The law is usually called the "nurse practice act," "nursing practice act," or a similar designation.

Regulations

Regulations are also frequently referred to as "rules." *Regulations* are specific written policies adopted by an administrative agency. States typically have a law that sets forth the procedures state administrative agencies must follow to adopt regulations. Commonly, an administrative agency must publish a regulation, accept written comments, and hold hearings before the regulation can be finalized.

State administrative agencies derive their rule-making authority from an enabling law. An *enabling law* is one in which the state legislature delegates to an administrative agency the authority to adopt regulations to implement the law's purposes. The NPA in every state is an enabling statute in that it commonly authorizes the state board of nursing or similarly named entity to adopt regulations to implement the NPA's provisions. In a few jurisdictions, board of nursing rules sometimes must be either jointly promulgated or adopted with the state board of medicine.

Once finalized, regulations generally have the force of law. To be valid, however, regulations must be consistent with the enabling statute under whose authority they were adopted. To the extent a regulation is inconsistent with an enabling law, the law will control. Regulations often contain a severance or savings clause that states that to the extent any particular provision of the regulations proves invalid, the remainder of the regulations will still be in effect.

Greenlaw[4] has identified four weaknesses that characterized these laws.

1 These laws were title protection or "certification" laws in nature. The laws regulated the titles "registered nurse" and "RN" rather than the practice of nursing itself. Nurses who had not registered with the state as "registered nurses" could still practice as long as they did not refer to themselves as registered nurses or use the title RN.

2 The nursing boards created to implement registration laws often had physician members as well as nurses. As late as 1938, 17 state nursing boards still included at least one physician.

3 The registration laws required minimal educational requirements. As of 1938, 19 states did not require graduation from high school as a prerequisite of nursing registration.

4 Nursing practice was not defined in the registration laws. Registered nurses were defined exclusively by their qualifications rather than the functions they performed.

Second Phase

In 1938, New York passed the first mandatory nursing licensure law.[3] As Hadley[5] points out, the law contained two attributes that became the hallmark of all modern nursing statutes—a definition of what constitutes nursing practice and a prohibition against unauthorized practice. As Bullough[3] states:

> [I]t was necessary to specify the scope of practice of the occupation that was being protected against encroachment. The older nursing laws made it illegal for an unauthorized person to use the title "registered nurse," but not illegal for such a person to practice nursing. Once the new mandatory laws made it illegal for an unauthorized person to practice nursing, a definition of the scope of practice had to be written into those laws.

The New York definition of the practice of nursing became a model for many other states. The New York statute defined "the practice of nursing" as follows[3]:

> A person practices nursing within the meaning of this article who for compensation or personal profit (a) performs any professional service requiring the application of principles of nursing based on biological, physical and social sciences, such as responsible supervision of a patient requiring skill in observation of symptoms and reactions and the accurate recording of the facts, and carrying out of treatments and medications as prescribed by a licensed physician, and the application of such nursing procedures as involve understanding of cause and effect in order to safeguard life and health of a patient and others; or (b) performs such duties as are required in the physical care of a patient and in carrying out of medical orders as prescribed by a licensed physician, requiring an understanding of nursing but not requiring the professional service as outlined in (a).

The New York definition did not refer to specialty nursing practice per se or identify specific specialties such as nurse anesthesia. Such formal recognition of advanced practice would not emerge in the states for quite some time to come.

By 1946, 10 states had adopted a definition of nursing.[3] In 1955, while the trend to define nursing practice and adopt mandatory licensure laws continued to gain momentum, the American Nurses Association (ANA) adopted a model definition of nursing.[3] Like the seminal New York law of 1938, the ANA model definition did not refer to specialty nursing or identify specific specialties such as nurse anesthesia. The ANA's model definition of nursing practice stated that[3]:

> The practice of professional nursing means the performance for compensation of any acts in the observation, care, and counsel of the ill, injured, or infirm, or in the maintenance of health or prevention of illness of others, or in the supervision and teaching of other personnel, or the administration of medications and treatments as prescribed by a licensed physician or dentist; requiring substantial specialized judgment and skill and based on knowledge and application of the principles of biological, physical, and social science. The foregoing shall not be deemed to include acts of diagnosis or prescription of therapeutic or corrective measures.

The ANA's definition of nursing practice became the new model for state nurse practice acts. Fifteen states adopted the definition verbatim, and six states adopted the language with slight modifications.[3] Bullough criticizes the definition's specific exclusion from nursing practice of "acts of diagnosis or prescription of therapeutic or corrective measures." The fascinating thing about the disclaimer is that it was made not by the American Medical Association but by the ANA. Although a reasonable assumption might be that the nurses believed the disclaimer necessary to avoid medical opposition to the new practice acts, there is little evidence of overt pressure by physicians. In effect, organized nursing surrendered without any battle over boundaries.[3]

Greenlaw[4] notes that the disclaimer was troublesome for nurses who were already practicing independently. She also notes that the disclaimer failed to take into account that many nurses were currently performing acts constituting diagnosis and treatment. To reconcile discrepancies between the definition of nursing and existing practice, joint statements were sometimes adopted by nursing, hospital, and medical organizations and associations. The joint statements typically specified activities qualified nurses could perform in certain settings. Interestingly, the joint statements were usually considered authoritative even though they were not legislatively authorized.[4]

Third Phase

The third and current phase of state regulation of nursing involved an increasing recognition of the role of RNs such as Certified Registered Nurse Anesthetists (CRNAs) practicing in an advanced or expanded role. Bullough[3] noted that factors influencing this growing formal recognition for nursing specialties were discussed and encouraged by a special committee appointed by the Secretary of the U.S. Department of Health, Education and Welfare in 1971. The special committee's report supported an extended scope of function for registered nurses. Bullough[3] stated that in "response to that request and to those forces that stimulated it, the state nurse practice acts began to change."

Some of the factors Bullough noted that influenced the growth of specialty nursing included upgrading of educational standards, increased complexity of practice because of developments in science and technology, and an aging population that required competent and affordable care. As Bullough[3] pointed out, the women's movement was also a factor, because it helped reduce the sexual stereotyping that classified medicine as men's work and nursing as women's work. More men entered nursing specialties such as nurse anesthesia, and nurses in general assumed functions previously performed exclusively by physicians.

Another significant impetus for the third phase of nursing practice legislation was the ANA's amending of its model nursing definition in 1970. The ANA definition now stated that a professional nurse may also perform such additional acts, under emergency or other special conditions, which may include special training, as are recognized by the medical and nursing professions as proper to be performed by a professional nurse under such conditions, even though such acts might otherwise be considered diagnosis and prescription.[4]

The reference to "additional acts" performed "under emergency or other special conditions" marked a recognition, albeit somewhat oblique, that RNs with advanced education (such as CRNAs) existed and were practicing. The ANA's choice of language was unfortunate, however. The definition required that the additional acts be ones recognized by both the "medical and nursing professions." This implied that nursing could not legitimately be the sole arbiter of appropriate advanced nursing practice and needed medicine's consent to do so. The ANA's language choice is representative of nursing's struggle through the years for self-governance.

The ANA's current model nursing practice act deletes both the reference to "additional acts" and the requirement that such acts be ones recognized by both the medical and nursing professions. The ANA's model act now defines "professional nursing practice" in part as follows[6]:

> [P]rofessional nursing practice encompasses the full scope of nursing practice and includes all its specialties and consists of application of nursing theory to the development, implementation, and evaluation of plans of nursing care for individuals, families, and communities. Professional nursing practice requires substantial knowledge of nursing theory and related scientific, behavioral, and humanistic disciplines. Professional nursing practice includes, but is not limited to. . . .(8 section 201 [d])

The ANA's model definition of nursing practice, therefore, now contains an explicit reference to nursing's "specialties." It has been the ANA's longstanding philosophy, however, that nurse practice acts should not refer to specific areas of specialized nursing practice, for example, nurse anesthesia. In the comments section to its model nursing practice act, the ANA states that nursing practice acts[6]

> should not provide for recognition of particular clinical specialists in nursing or require certification or other recognition or credentialing beyond the minimum qualifications established for licensure. Standards for specialized areas of practice and the certification of individuals as competent to practice in specialized areas is the domain of the professional association (p. 9).

The ANA believes that the scope of nursing practice should be defined by nursing organizations rather than by state legislatures. Further, the ANA believes that nurse practice acts "should not require certification or other recognition for practice beyond the minimum qualifications established for licensure"[6] (p. 5). The ANA states that it should be the job of professional associations "to establish the scope and desirable qualifications required for specialized areas of practice, and to certify individuals as competent to engage in specific areas of nursing practice"[6] (p. 5).

As Bullough[3] notes, the ANA has argued that nursing should emulate the medical model of licensure: grant all practitioners a broad scope of practice in state law and leave specific regulation of specialties to professional organizations. The ANA's position is reflected both in the document containing its model nurse practice act and in its 1980 document entitled "Nursing: A Social Policy Statement."[7]

Despite the ANA's position, the trend in recent years has been for states to increasingly grant specific recognition to identifiable nursing specialists such as CRNAs, nurse-midwives, and nurse practitioners. Later in this chapter we explore this phenomenon in detail as it relates to CRNAs.

Most nursing specialties have applauded the trend toward specific recognition in state nurse practice acts or board of nursing regulations, as opposed to exclusive reliance on broad definitions of nursing. As Greenlaw[4] states, "Nurses relying upon broad statutory language do not always feel confident that their practice will go unchallenged by physicians and, indeed, challenges have occurred."

In addition, states continue to defer in great measure to professional organizations regarding certification of specialties, as well as accreditation of educational programs. Greenlaw[4] points out that:

> In the mid-1970s, when the states began to recognize advanced nursing practice through statutory and regulatory provisions, the states also began to require that nurses in advanced practice obtain certification by the appropriate national nursing specialty organizations. While this practice goes against the position of the American Nurses' Association that professional organizations, and not the state, should regulate the nursing specialties, it can be viewed as a reasonable compromise between the authority of the state and the function of the professional association. The state is not usurping the functions of the professional associations; rather, the state, exercising its power to safeguard the public, is giving statutory recognition, or deferring, to the role of the professional associations.

Mandatory Licensure—Is It Necessary?

Mandatory licensure of RNs and physicians is so well established that its necessity might seem a given. This is not the case, however, as many commentators have debated whether mandatory licensure per se should be eliminated.

Licensure is the most restrictive type of state-granted credential. Mandatory licensure laws require individuals to obtain a license before practicing a specified profession. The scope of practice of the profession is commonly defined. Persons who do not possess the requisite license may neither use the title of the profession (e.g., RN) nor practice the profession as it is defined. In this sense, mandatory licensure laws protect both titles and practice. Unauthorized practice is commonly punishable by sanctions handed down by the state administrative board that oversees the profession (e.g., the board of nursing). Depending on the specifics of state law, sanctions may include letters of reprimand, license suspension or revocation, fines, and other appropriate penalties. Criminal sanctions may also apply.

The primary rationale for mandatory licensure laws is the protection of the public's health and welfare. It has been stated often that the purpose of licensing laws is to protect the public and not individual professions. As Clayton[1] points out, it has been argued that patients are unable to obtain sufficient information to adequately judge health care practitioner competence. Further, patients arguably do not possess the knowledge to accurately gauge the risks to their health of inadequate health care. Patient "informed consent" is arguably a myth in many instances. Clayton[1] states:

> By setting minimum standards for the qualifications and training required of health care personnel, licensure laws attempt to control the quality of health care. Competent health care is, in turn, more likely to preserve the health and well being of patients and to save society the costs of unnecessary injuries and deaths that may result from bad medical care (p. 16-6).

Despite its purported benefits, mandatory licensure has been criticized. Commentators have questioned whether it actually improves patient care and have expressed concerns about its economic impact. Clayton states that by granting a monopoly over the practice of a profession to those individuals who meet state-defined standards, the state thereby outlaws competition by other individuals who might also deliver good medical care even though they cannot satisfy the criteria required for licensure. State licensing boards have been accused of being slow to accept changes in technology, prone to establishing professional practice standards that bear little relationship to an applicant's actual ability to take care of patients, and overly protective of licensed professionals' vested interest in maintaining their own privileged status. State disciplinary and licensure bodies are also criticized for having little success in controlling professionals who, though licensed, either do not practice competently or practice in an unethical fashion. Licensure, it has been argued, contributes to high health care costs and reduces innovation and consumer choice. Alternatives to licensure, such as a voluntary accreditation system or a complete abolition of licensure, have been suggested.[1]

Gunn[9] has also discussed the criticisms of mandatory licensure. She points out that some have argued for allowing institutions such as hospitals to assume the responsibility for screening health care professionals and eliminate the government's involvement. Gunn states, however, that opponents of institutional licensure have cited the possibility that institutions may sacrifice quality to assure fiscal soundness and profits, thereby engaging in marginal or unsafe care. Other major concerns about institutional licensure include the fear that there would be no consistency of health care standards or qualifications of providers, such as educational requirements; decreased geographic mobility for providers; and no way for consumers to make truly informed choices about their care.

At least in part because of criticism of the proliferation of mandatory licensure, some states now require groups seeking passage of mandatory licensure legislation to demonstrate why licensure, rather than registration, certification, or no regulation, is necessary.[1] Despite the criticisms of mandatory licensure, no state has eliminated licensure for either RNs or physicians.

STATE RECOGNITION AND REGULATION OF NURSE ANESTHESIA PRACTICE

As with RNs in general, formal state recognition of nurse anesthetists followed well-established practice. It is important to bear in mind that CRNA practice was widely regarded as legal and legitimate long before states formally regulated the profession. For the most part, formal state recognition and regulation of CRNAs has ratified existing practice rather than reshaping the parameters of the profession.

On a day-to-day basis, institutional policies and procedures usually have a greater impact on nurse anesthesia practice than state statutes and regulations. An example of this practical reality is regional anesthesia practice. No state laws or regulations prohibit CRNAs from administering regional anesthesia; some hospitals, however, have institutional policies prohibiting CRNAs from administering regional anesthesia.

This example demonstrates another facet of state laws and regulations. Merely because a particular activity may be legal under state law does not compel institutions to permit practitioners to engage in the activity. In other words, employers such as hospitals and private anesthesiologist groups have wide latitude to impose policies more restrictive than state law. Employer policies may not violate antitrust, civil rights, and other types of laws potentially applicable to the workplace, but such laws often provide less protection than the unwary employee suspects.

Although institutional and employer policies often have a more immediate impact on practice than state law, this does not mean state statutes and regulations are irrelevant. First, state nurse practice acts and board of nursing regulations often specify qualifications CRNAs must possess in order to practice. Second, while state statutes and regulations usually do not restrict actual practice in significant ways, the potential for such restrictions always exists. CRNAs must always be vigilant concerning proposed legislation or regulations that affect practice. In addition, CRNAs must be alert to statutory or regulatory proposals to mandate anesthesiologist supervision. Currently, many states require that CRNAs be "supervised" by a "licensed physician." No state, however, specifically requires in either its nurse practice act or board of nursing regulations that the supervising physician be an anesthesiologist.

The supervision issue is a subject of continuing debate between state nurse anesthetist associations and their anesthesiologist counterparts. Anesthesiologist societies continually insist that CRNAs are technicians who must be supervised by anesthesiologists to ensure quality care. The American Association of Nurse Anesthetists (AANA) disagrees, however, and opposes any statutory or regulatory proposal to require that CRNAs be supervised by anesthesiologists. It is important to preserve the right of CRNAs to choose the practice situation in which they are most comfortable. Once anesthesiologist supervision is mandated in a statute or regulation, that choice is lost or seriously compromised, particularly for those who would like to be self-employed.

Significance of Nonnursing Statutes and Regulations

To the extent CRNAs are specifically regulated in a state's statutes and regulations, the most significant provisions concerning the type and manner of nurse anesthetist recognition usually appear in a state's nurse practice act or board of nursing regulations.

There are other state statutes and regulations, however, that can affect nurse anesthesia practice, albeit in less obvious ways. For example, every state has hospital licensing regulations commonly promulgated and adopted by the state department of health. Hospitals must comply with these regulations to receive a license to provide patient care.

Hospital licensing regulations frequently contain provisions concerning anesthesia. Although the provisions are often brief, they sometimes are significant. For example, some hospital licensing regulations require that CRNAs perform anesthesia under the supervision of a physician. Suppose such a provision appeared in the hospital licensing regulations of a state that did not specifically require physician supervision in its nurse practice act or board of nursing regulations. A hospital would nevertheless have to require physician supervision of CRNAs in order to comply with the state's hospital licensing requirements; to do otherwise would jeopardize the hospital's state license.

This also demonstrates that CRNAs and state nurse anesthetist associations cannot afford to restrict their attention to proposals to amend state nursing statutes and regulations. An anesthesiologist supervision requirement in a state's hospital licensing regulations has as much potential for damage as would one found in a state's nurse practice act or board of nursing regulations.

There is considerable reason to believe that CRNAs are potentially more vulnerable to restrictions in state facility licensing regulations than in board of nursing regulations. Boards of nursing are typically much less inclined to entertain proposals to restrict CRNA practice than are state departments of health that regulate hospitals and ambulatory surgery centers. Departments of health are less likely than nursing boards to understand the nature of nurse anesthesia practice.

The preceding discussion illustrates that there are state statutes and regulations other than nurse practice acts and board of nursing regulations that can affect CRNAs. Individual states sometimes use different names for the various statutes, regulations, and regulatory agencies that can affect CRNAs, but most states have at least the generic equivalent of the following:

1 *Nurse Practice Act.*
2 *Board of nursing regulations.* In some states, these are jointly developed or

approved with the state board of medicine.

3 *Medical Practice Act/board of medicine regulations.* The medical practice act or its generic equivalent is the state law setting forth the scope of practice for physicians.

4 *Hospital licensing statute and regulations.* Although many states do not have a hospital licensing statute, virtually every state has hospital licensing regulations. As noted previously, these regulations are commonly promulgated and adopted by a state's department of health.

5 *Ambulatory surgery center (ASC) licensing statute and regulations.* Although relatively few states have an ASC licensing law, many states have ASC regulations. As with hospital licensing regulations, ASC regulations are usually promulgated and adopted by a state's department of health.

6 *Trauma center statute or regulations.* Only a handful of states have specific statutes or regulations concerning trauma centers. Those that do tend to emulate the guidelines of the American College of Surgeons (ACS). The ACS guidelines are troublesome in a number of respects. For example, the ACS guidelines for Level I trauma centers do not mention CRNAs in the provisions concerning anesthesia, raising the question of whether the guidelines contemplate use of CRNAs in such facilities. To the extent, therefore, that state regulation of trauma centers increases, CRNAs will have to work to prevent widespread adoption of the objectionable features of the ACS guidelines.

7 *Dental Practice Act/board of dentistry regulations.* These statutes and regulations are often relevant because they frequently contain specific provisions concerning anesthesia. It is very common for states to require dentists who use anesthesia in the office to have advanced anesthesia education and training and obtain a special permit, even if the dentist uses a CRNA to administer the anesthesia.

The AANA believes that dentists who use CRNAs or anesthesiologists to administer anesthesia should be exempted from advanced anesthesia education and training requirements. While a handful of states have such exemptions, it appears that most do not. CRNAs who work with dentists, therefore, particularly in dental offices, should make sure that such dentists meet any applicable state requirements. In addition to requirements concerning who may administer anesthesia in the dental office, there are often equipment requirements as well.

A final caveat concerning CRNAs and dentists is relevant. As noted previously, state-imposed supervision requirements concerning CRNAs vary. States having supervision requirements sometimes specifically state that CRNAs can work under dentist supervision. Other states, however, merely state that CRNAs must practice under the supervision of a licensed physician. Taken literally, this would preclude CRNAs from working with dentists absent physician supervision. In some states, however, it may be possible to argue that the term "licensed physician" in the context of CRNA supervision was intended to include dentists as well as medical doctors. This is a legally intricate argument that can be made only after careful research.

8 *Podiatry statute or regulations.* In some states, podiatrist practice is addressed in a statute or regulations specific to podiatrists. In other states, podiatry provisions are found as sections of the medical practice act or board of medicine regulations. Like dentists, whether podiatrists may supervise nurse anesthetists in the absence of a licensed medical doctor depends on state law.

In addition, questions sometimes occur concerning the range of services a podiatrist can order a CRNA to perform. For example, podiatry statutes often restrict podiatrists from administering any type of anesthesia other than local. While a podiatrist clearly could not personally administer regional anesthesia, would a nurse anesthetist working with a podiatrist be precluded from administering regional anesthesia as well? This is a difficult legal question, the answer to which will, again, depend on interpretation of a particular state's laws and regulations.

9 *Pharmacy/drug statutes or regulations.* States usually have statutes and regulations that address various aspects of drug use. The statutes and regulations often distinguish between controlled and noncontrolled substances. In addition, states commonly have statutes governing pharmacies and regulations adopted by the board of pharmacy. State statutes and regulations governing drug use can affect nurse anesthetists, particularly if questions are raised concerning whether a nurse anesthetist is properly handling drugs or has the authority to engage in certain practices.

10 *Attorney general opinions.* Attorney general opinions are not statutes or regulations, but they are mentioned here because of their link to statutes and regulations. Each state has an attorney general whose function as the state's chief legal officer is in part to give legal interpretations concerning state laws or regulations. For example, a state administrative entity such as a board of nursing might ask an attorney general to render an opinion concerning whether an adopted regulation is legal or whether the agency has exceeded the scope of its statutory authority. In addition, a board of nursing could ask an attorney general whether a specific activity of a nurse was permitted or prohibited by state law.

An attorney general opinion is not binding in the manner of a court's decision but often carries great weight. For this reason, to the extent the legality of an aspect of CRNA practice is in dispute in a state, CRNAs must carefully consider whether to seek an attorney general opinion for clarification.

State Recognition of Nurse Anesthesia Practice

Few states formally recognized nurse anesthetists in state statutes and regulations until the 1970s. That decade marked the beginning of an era of increased formal and specific state recognition of nursing specialties. State statutory and regulatory recognition of nurse anesthetists quickly grew throughout the decade.

Currently, all 50 states mention nurse anesthetists in at least one state statute or regulation. Puerto Rico does not appear to specifically refer to nurse anesthetists. The Puerto Rico nurse practice act, however, mentions nurses practicing in a "specialized area," which at least implicitly recognizes nurse anesthesia practice. The Virgin Islands mentions nurse anesthetists in board of nursing regulations. Finally, the District of Columbia recognizes nurse anesthetists in both its statute governing health occupations and in Department of Consumer and Regulatory Affairs regulations.

Although it is clear that the legitimacy of nurse anesthesia as a profession is widely accepted, the manner, type, and frequency of statutory and regulatory recognition of CRNA practice varies considerably. State statutes and regulations sometimes refer to nurse anesthetists as a type of "advanced registered nurse practitioner," or "advanced practitioner of nursing," or as nurses practicing in an "expanded role" or "specialty area." States use such categories to describe nurses such as CRNAs who have qualifications beyond those required of RNs. In some states, CRNAs are named both specifically as a discrete nursing specialty and more generally as one of several specialties that fall within a broader generic category such as "advanced registered nurse practitioner." In addition, some states have general statutory or regulatory provisions that apply to all specialty nurses and additional provisions that apply specifically to individual specialists such as nurse anesthetists.

As Table 5–1 indicates, nurse anesthetists are specifically mentioned in all 50 states. The figures in Table 5–1 are estimates based on the AANA's review of pertinent state laws and regulations. In many states, nurse anesthetists are mentioned in statutes and regulations other than nurse practice acts or board of nursing rules or regulations. Table 5–1, however, does not attempt to categorize every statutory and regulatory reference to nurse anesthetists. Rather, the table's

TABLE 5–1

STATE STATUTORY/REGULATORY SOURCES OF RECOGNITION

Sources of Recognition	Number of States
NPA Only	4
SBON R&R Only	15
NPA and SBON R&R	21
MPA	2
Department of Health	9

NPA = Nurse Practice Act; SBON R&R = State Board of Nursing rules or regulations; MPA = Medical Practice Act.

purpose is to demonstrate that nurse anesthetists are recognized in every state, even if there is not a specific reference in the nurse practice act or board of nursing rules or regulations. The following is an explanation of each of the table's categories.

Nurse Practice Act Only

Approximately four states explicitly mention nurse anesthetists in the Nurse Practice Act (NPA) but not in board of nursing regulations.

State Board of Nursing Regulations or Rules Only

Approximately 15 states (and the Virgin Islands) explicitly mention nurse anesthetists in state board of nursing regulations or rules (SBON R&R) but not in the nurse practice act.

Nurse Practice Act and State Board of Nursing Regulations or Rules

Approximately 21 states explicitly mention nurse anesthetists in both the NPA and SBON R&R.

Taking the above three categories together, 40 states explicitly mention nurse anesthetists in either the nurse practice act or board of nursing rules or regulations. This is dramatic evidence of the rapid growth of formal state recognition of nurse anesthesia as a specialty during the 1970s and beyond.

Medical Practice Act

Two states (Ohio and Indiana) recognize nurse anesthesia in the Medical Practice Act (MPA) as an exception to the unauthorized practice of medicine. This is an antiquated approach at best. Ohio also mentions nurse anesthetists in its NPA and is included in the "NPA only" category of Table 5–1, in addition to the MPA category. This accounts for the 51-state total for all categories combined in Table 5–1.

Department of Health

Approximately nine states that do not recognize nurse anesthetists in NPAs, SBON R&R, or MPAs, nevertheless explicitly mention nurse anesthetists in state department of health facility licensing regulations. In two of these states—Oregon and North Carolina—there is explicit recognition from the boards of nursing but not in regulations per se. In Oregon, the board of nursing recognized CRNAs in a 1990 position statement the board adopted to acknowledge the legitimacy of CRNA practice. In North Carolina, the board of nursing recognizes nurse anesthetists in formal "interpretations" that constitute "Category V" of the board's nursing practice interpretations.

Methods of State Regulation of Nurse Anesthesia Practice

Every state requires that RNs apply for and receive a state-issued license before practicing. Although licensure is the uniform method of state recognition of RNs, there is no such consistency concerning the way states recognize specialty nurses such as nurse anesthetists.

It does not appear that any state deems the mere possession of a license as an RN sufficient authority to administer anesthesia. In every state, there appears to be statutory or regulatory language of some sort that enables only certain RNs to practice nurse anesthesia. States vary widely, however, in the specific method of regulation they use to authorize nurse anesthesia practice. Some states require RNs to obtain a specialty license in addition to the RN license before they can practice nurse anesthesia. Other states require nurse anesthetists to register, obtain a certificate, or to apply for "recognition," "authorization," or "approval" to practice. Finally, some states do not specify a specific method or process by which they authorize nurses to administer anesthesia. These states, however, generally state qualifications needed to practice as a nurse anesthetist.

Commentators frequently refer to licensure as the only method of state regulation that protects both a profession's practice and title, because licensure is the only method that ensures that unauthorized persons do not practice a profession. Other methods of state regulation of professions such as recognition, certification, and registration are often thought of as forms of title protection only. In other words, these methods are sometimes thought to merely prohibit individuals who do not possess certain qualifications from using a protected title, such as CRNA. Individuals who do not use the protected title may still supposedly practice the profession.

A close examination of the state statutes and regulations in which nurse anesthetists are recognized, however, reveals the potential danger of relying on classic definitions of licensure, registration, and the like. There is no substitute for examining these terms as they are actually used in a particular state and evaluating their substantive effect.

In contrast to the definitions sometimes used by commentators, methods of regulation sometimes thought of as "title protection" only often appear to be something more than that as they are actually used in state laws and regulations governing nurse anesthesia practice. For example, in many states in which recognition is the method of regulating nurse anesthesia practice, it is clear that nurses may not administer anesthetics unless they possess certain state-delineated qualifications. This is the case regardless of whether the nurse is called a nurse anesthetist or a CRNA. In these states, recognition is actually being implemented in a way that resembles licensure in the sense that both the practice *and* title of a profession are being protected.

The practical reality is that regardless of what a state calls its particular method of regulating nurse anesthesia practice, the goal of the method is usually the same: to allow and authorize only those nurses with certain qualifications to administer anesthesia. Table 5–2 summarizes the methods states use to authorize nurse anesthesia practice. The figures in the table are estimates based on the AANA's review of pertinent state laws and regulations.

TABLE 5–2

STATE METHODS OR TYPES OF RECOGNITION FOR NURSE ANESTHETISTS

Method/Type of Recognition	Number of States
Licensure	7
Certification	11
Authorization or Approval	10
Registration or Recognition	7
Method Not Specified	15

Data from Clayton, JE,[1] and *Dent v. West Virginia,* 129 US 114 (1889).

Combining all categories but the last (method not specified), Table 5–2 shows that approximately 35 states explicitly mention a specific process in which nurse anesthetists participate before practicing as CRNAs. These state mechanisms are uniformly described in state NPAs, or, more commonly, SBON R&R.

The mechanisms summarized in Table 5–2 are in addition to whatever state procedures nurse anesthetists must comply with to obtain their RN licenses. As noted previously, every state requires that RNs obtain an RN license before practicing. Because nurse anesthetists are RNs as well as a kind of nursing specialist, nurse anesthetists in every state must at least have an RN license to practice.

While the ostensible purpose of formal state processes for CRNA recognition is to ensure that only qualified RNs administer anesthesia, the practical importance of these state requirements is diminished by a key factor. Most hospitals require that, apart from students and new graduates, nurse anesthetists be graduates of an accredited nurse anesthesia educational program and be certified by the AANA's Council on Certification of Nurse Anesthetists. Apart from quality of care considerations, hospitals are motivated by liability concerns. Regardless of whether states required CRNAs to possess certain qualifications, most nurse anesthetists would ultimately be forced to pass the AANA council's certification examination if they wished to continue to practice.

The following is an explanation of each of the categories in Table 5–2.

Licensure

Approximately seven states require that nurse anesthetists obtain a state license in addition to licensure as an RN. The nature of the additional license varies. In some states, the additional license is as a CRNA. In others, the license is a more general license, such as an advanced registered nurse practitioner. States that require additional licensure do not necessarily delineate stricter qualifications for practice than states that do not require additional licensure. In no way, then, are CRNAs who receive additional licensure better qualified than those who do not.

An example of this method of recognition is Arkansas. In Arkansas, RNs are granted a license as an RN practicing in the expanded role of CRNA after providing proof of completion of a nurse anesthesia educational program that meets the standards of the Council on Accreditation of Nurse Anesthesia Educational Programs or other nationally recognized accrediting body. The applicant must also provide documentation demonstrating current certification from the Council on Certification of Nurse Anesthetists or recertification from the Council on Recertification of Nurse Anesthetists or other nationally recognized certifying body.

Certification

Approximately 11 states, the District of Columbia, and the Virgin Islands require that nurse anesthetists apply for and receive certification as a CRNA or in a particular kind of general specialty nurse category, for example, advanced registered nurse practitioner. The certification is not a license. Further, the certification is issued by the state and should not be confused with the certification conferred by the AANA's Council on Certification of Nurse Anesthetists on passage of the council's examination. The state certification is granted after the CRNA provides evidence that he or she possesses certain qualifications.

In South Dakota, for example, an applicant for certification as a CRNA must provide written evidence to the board of nursing that the applicant has completed an approved program of nurse anesthesia that has been accredited by the Council on Accreditation of Nurse Anesthesia Educational Programs. The applicant must also provide written evidence that he or she has passed a board-approved examination that has been validated and scored in accordance with generally accepted testing procedures. To renew certification, the applicant must show evidence of meeting the recertification requirements of the Council on Recertification of Nurse Anesthetists.

Authorization or Approval

Approximately 10 states require that nurse anesthetists formally apply for and receive "approval" or "authorization" to practice. In Alabama, for example, CRNAs apply to the board of nursing for approval to practice. The CRNA must submit documentation that he or she has graduated from a school of anesthesia accredited by the Council on Accreditation of Nurse Anesthesia Educational Programs and has been certified by the Council on Certification of Nurse Anesthetists or recertified by the Council on Recertification of Nurse Anesthetists. The board of nursing then notifies the CRNA that he or she has been approved to practice and endorses the CRNA's registered nurse license card with the letters "CRNA."

Registration or Recognition

Approximately seven states, after receipt of appropriate documentation concerning qualifications, formally recognize or register nurse anesthetists. The documentation required is typically similar to documentation required in states that approve, authorize, or certify nurse anesthetists to practice. After receiving such documentation, Montana, for example, recognizes that a specialty nurse such as a CRNA may practice in his or her area of specialty. The board of nursing lists the area of specialty on the nurse's RN license.

Method Not Specified

The remaining 15 states and Puerto Rico do not delineate a specific method or process by which they authorize nurses to administer anesthesia. Many of these states nevertheless state qualifications needed to practice as a nurse anesthetist. In Arizona, for example, the NPA merely states that a licensed RN may administer anesthetics if the nurse has completed a nationally accredited program in the science of anesthesia. Arizona, therefore, does not delineate a specific process, such as authorization or approval, that nurse anesthetists must observe to practice. To legally practice in Arizona, however, nurse anesthetists must possess the requisite qualification, that is, completion of a nationally accredited nurse anesthesia educational program.

QUALIFICATIONS NEEDED TO PRACTICE

As discussed previously, regardless of whether a state has a specific process by which nurse anesthetists are recognized (e.g., licensure, authorization, or approval), most states specify qualifications nurse anesthetists must possess to practice. Such requirements are generally delineated in nurse practice acts or board of nursing rules or regulations. The requirements specified, however, vary.

Before practicing in a state, it is prudent for a nurse anesthetist to obtain copies of the state's nurse practice act and board of nursing rules or regulations. These documents are commonly available from the board of nursing either at no charge or for a minimal fee. In addition, when contacting a board of nursing for these documents, it is advisable to ask whether there are any particular forms or applications that must be completed to practice as a nurse anesthetist. Remember, too, that regardless of any requirements a nurse anesthetist must meet to practice as a nurse anesthetist in a particular state, he or she must also comply with any requirements for practice as an RN.

The most common qualifications that states specify a nurse anesthetist must possess to practice concern education, certification, and recertification. Many states also address new graduate practice. In addition, a number of states delineate nurse anesthetist scope of practice. Each of these subjects will be discussed later.

Education

Approximately 44 states require nurse anesthetists to have graduated from a nurse anesthesia educational program in order to practice. The approximately six remaining states do not specifically require graduation from a nurse anesthesia educational program. Of the 44 states that require graduation from a nurse anesthesia educational program, approximately 35 states (and the District of Columbia, Puerto Rico, and the Virgin Islands) require nurse anesthetists to have graduated from an *accredited* program. Approximately 9 of the 44 states require graduation from a nurse anesthesia educational program but either do not specifically refer to accreditation or have ambiguous language concerning whether the program must be accredited. In practice, the omission of a specific requirement that the nurse anesthesia educational program be "accredited" is not meaningful, because all existing programs are in fact presently accredited.

The specific language states use to require graduation from a nurse anesthesia educational program varies. Many states require that a nurse anesthetist graduate from a program accredited by the AANA's Council on Accreditation of Nurse Anesthesia Educational Programs. Some states do not specifically refer to the AANA's council but instead require graduation from a program that is nationally recognized or nationally accredited. These states sometimes add the caveat that the national accrediting body must be approved by the board of nursing. Language of this sort is in effect a requirement that one graduate from a program accredited by the AANA's council, since there is no other national entity that accredits nurse anesthesia educational programs. In addition, in states that require that the national accrediting body must be approved by the board of nursing, no state with such a requirement has failed to approve the AANA's council as the appropriate accrediting body.

Certification

Approximately 40 states (and the District of Columbia, Puerto Rico, and the Virgin Islands) require nurse anesthetists to be certified to practice. As is discussed in the next section of this chapter, however, some of these states exempt new graduates from the certification requirement for varying periods of time. Approximately 10 states do not specifically require nurse anesthetists to be certified to practice, but nurse anesthetists must bear in mind that many individual institutions will require certification even if a particular state does not.

As with state educational requirements, the language of certification requirements varies; the manner in which certification requirements vary tends to parallel language variations in educational requirements. For example, just as many states require graduation from a program accredited by the AANA's Council on Accreditation of Nurse Anesthesia Educational Programs, many states require that a nurse anesthetist be certified by the AANA's Council on Certification of Nurse Anesthetists. Some states do not specifically refer to the AANA's certification council but instead require certification from a nationally recognized or national certifying body. These states sometimes also require that the national certifying body must be approved by or acceptable to the board of nursing. This is in effect a requirement that one be certified by the AANA's council, since there is no other national entity that certifies nurse anesthetists. In addition, in states that require that the national certifying body must be approved by the board of nursing, no state with such a requirement has failed to approve the AANA's council as the appropriate certifying body.

Recertification

Approximately 37 states (and the District of Columbia and Puerto Rico) require nurse anesthetists to maintain certification, that is, to be recertified at appropriate intervals. The Virgin Islands Board of Nurse Licensure rules are somewhat ambiguous concerning whether recertification is required, merely stating that CRNAs shall be "afforded every opportunity" to maintain their certification status.

The comments in the preceding section of this chapter regarding variation in language used to require certification apply to recertification as well. In other words, some states specifically require that nurse anesthetists be recertified by the AANA's Council on Recertification of Nurse Anesthetists, but other states merely refer to a "nationally recognized" or "national" recertifying body. The recertifying body sometimes must be approved or accepted by the board of nursing. In such states, the AANA's recertification council has uniformly been the entity approved or accepted. Again, bear in mind that regardless of state requirements, most institutions will require that nurse anesthetists maintain certification.

New Graduates

New graduates of nurse anesthesia educational programs are not certified at the time of graduation; that is, they have not yet taken and passed the AANA's Council on Certification of Nurse Anesthetists' examination. Consequently, in states that require nurse anesthetists to be certified, the question arises as to whether new graduates are allowed to practice for a period of time following graduation but prior to certification.

In approximately 29 states (and the District of Columbia and Puerto Rico), there are explicit provisions in the NPA or SBON R&R regarding new graduate practice. Of the 29 states, approximately 19 permit new graduates to practice while they are awaiting results of the first certification examination they have taken. In these states, however, a new graduate who fails the examination must stop practicing until he or she passes the examination. Approximately 5 states permit new graduates to practice for up to 1 year; commonly, this allows such graduates two opportunities to pass the certification examination. Finally, approximately 5 states permit new graduates to practice for more than 1 year while awaiting results of the certification examination. Of these 5 states, 4 permit new graduates to practice for up to 18 months, whereas 1 appears to allow new graduates to practice for up to 2 years if supervised by a CRNA or a board-certified anesthesiologist.

The remaining 21 states (and the Virgin Islands) do not have explicit new graduate provisions in the NPA or SBON R&R. This does not necessarily mean, however, that new graduates in such states may not practice. At least 10 of the 21 states clearly do not require certification as a prerequisite to practice. In the approximately 11 remaining states, in which certification appears to be required, a state board of nursing may or may not feel that the requirement can be interpreted to permit new graduate practice for a period of time. To find out the definitive status of new graduate practice in any particular state, a nurse anesthetist should contact the applicable board of nursing.

Scope of Practice

There is little uniformity concerning how states regulate nurse anesthetist scope of practice. Some states define nurse anesthetist scope of practice broadly. Others define scope of practice by delineating a "laundry list" of permitted activities. Still other states merely state that nurse anesthetists must practice in accordance with the AANA's guidelines for practice. Finally, the majority of states do not specifically address or define nurse anesthetists' scope of practice.

Every state, although not always explicitly, permits nurse anesthetists to administer local, regional, and general anesthesia. As a practical matter, therefore, nurse anesthetists are not prohibited by state law from engaging in the common anesthesia practices they were educated to perform in nurse anesthesia educational programs. State law, of course, can change; nurse anesthetists, therefore, must always be alert to any proposals to change state statutes or regulations to restrict their scope of practice.

While state laws and regulations are generally not an impediment to nurse anesthetists providing the full range of anesthesia services for which they are qualified, the same cannot be said for institutional policies. Institutions sometimes do not permit CRNAs to perform all of the functions permitted by state law. Some institutions, for example, do not permit CRNAs to administer regional anesthesia. Even in states with a broad state-defined scope of practice, CRNAs must still be prepared to address scope of practice issues at the institutional level. This is because institutions are generally free to define scope of practice more restrictively than does the state.

SUMMARY

Formal state regulation of the nursing profession in the United States evolved in the 20th century from the rare occurrence to the commonplace. While state regulation of nursing initially focused on registered nurses, from the 1970s to the present, most states adopted additional statutory and regulatory provisions specific to nursing specialties such as nurse anesthesia.

Institutional and employer policies often have a more immediate effect on nurse anesthesia practice than do state laws or regulations. Nevertheless, because formal state regulation of nurse anesthesia practice is widespread, the possibility always exists of adoption of state laws or regulations that could restrict or undermine nurse anesthesia practice. For this reason, it is imperative that state nurse anesthetist associations, as well as individual nurse anesthetists, closely monitor and be involved with pertinent state statutory and regulatory developments.

REFERENCES

1. Clayton, JE: Licensure of health care professionals. In Macdonald, MG, Meyer, KC, and Essig, B (eds): Health Care Law: A Practical Guide. Matthew Bender, New York, 1991.
2. *Dent v. West Virginia*, 129 US 114 (1889).
3. Bullough, B: The current phase in the development of nurse practice acts. St. Louis University Law Journal 28:365, 1984.
4. Greenlaw, J: Definition and regulation of nursing practice: An historical survey. Law, Medicine, & Health Care 13:117, 1985.
5. Hadley, EH: Nurses and prescriptive authority: A legal and economic analysis. American Journal of Law & Medicine 15:245, 1989.
6. American Nurses' Association: Nursing Practice Act: Suggested State Legislation. American Nurses' Association, Kansas City, MO, 1990.
7. American Nurses' Association: Nursing: A Social Policy Statement. American Nurses' Association, Kansas City, MO, 1980.
8. Gunn, IP: Professional credentialing: Tying hands while protecting the public. CRNA Forum 2:11, 1986.

6

Nongovernmental Regulation of Nurse Anesthesia Practice

Karen L. Zaglaniczny

OUTLINE

OBJECTIVES

On completing this chapter, the reader will be able to:

1. Describe the facilitatory role of the AANA in the advancement of credentialing procedures for CRNAs.
2. Explain the purpose and roles of the Council on Certification, Council on Recertification, and the Continuing Education Program for CRNAs.
3. Review the criteria for certification and development of the National Certification Examination (NCE) for CRNAs.
4. Delineate the recertification process and the categories of recertification for CRNAs.
5. Define the AANA Continuing Education Program.
6. Discuss the credentialing function of clinical privileges in nurse anesthesia practice.

The purpose of this chapter is to describe the nongovernmental regulation of clinical practice for Certified Registered Nurse Anesthetists (CRNAs). For this discussion, nongovernmental regulation of clinical practice will pertain to the credentialing procedures for CRNAs. These procedures include certification, recertification through mandatory continuing education (CE), and clinical privileges. Additional regulatory procedures of CRNA clinical practice are hospital and departmental policies that are congruent with the Joint Commission on Accreditation of Hospitals Organization (JCAHO) and total quality management (TQM) standards. This discussion focuses on describing these credentialing procedures and the facilitatory role of the American Association of Nurse Anesthetists (AANA).

HISTORICAL PERSPECTIVES

The AANA has fostered professional growth and continued competency of CRNAs since its inception. As stated in the AANA philosophy, "The members of this professional association are dedicated to the precept that its members are committed to the advancement of educational standards and practices, which will advance the art and science of anesthesiology and thereby support and enhance quality patient care"[1] (p. 2). Advancement of CRNA practice has been promulgated by the AANA through the certification and recertification processes, implementation of mandatory CE, and the publication of the standards and guidelines related to clinical anesthesia.

One of the objectives of the AANA is to provide CE opportunities for CRNAs. This objective has been met primarily through the use of CE lectures related to nurse anesthesia practice at state and national nurse anesthesia meetings. The historical precedence for CE was established at the first AANA annual meeting held in 1933. Clinical lectures were presented by anesthesia practitioners and included such topics as: "The Induction of an Anesthetic, Intratracheal Anesthesia, Ethylene Anesthesia, and Carbon Dioxide Filtration of Anesthesia."[2] At this meeting, in the first President's Address, Hodgins identified the need for continued growth of the nurse anesthesia profession. She stated, "This present meeting is the first fruit of what might be called an adventure. This spirit of adventure is then the dynamic force that keeps us constantly contrasting what we are and what we may be and supplies the necessary courage to change from static to growing conditions"[2] (p. 80). Nurse anesthesia practice has continued to be in a dynamic state due to the consistent evolution of technologic and scientific advances and the leadership role of the AANA. The promotion of education and practice standards by the AANA has been a paradigm for other professions.

In 1967 and early 1968, the AANA Board of Directors realized that evidence of continued professional excellence was becoming increasingly important to health care and directed the Education Committee to investigate the issue of CE. The committee recommended the awarding of certificates to CRNAs who voluntarily attended CE meetings related to anesthesia practice. At the AANA annual meeting in 1969, this recommendation was implemented through a bylaw change approved by the membership over a 5-year period. This was known as the Continued Professional Excellence Program, a voluntary program in which the member was awarded a Certificate of Professional Excellence after he or she had earned 100 points. The program was discontinued in 1978.

In 1975, the AANA established the Councils on Accreditation, Certification, and Practice. This restructuring occurred partially in awareness of the 1975 US Department of Health, Education, and Welfare (HEW) proposal related to credentialing for health care. In the final report that was published in July 1977, two recommendations, competency measurement and continued competence, were pertinent to nurse anesthesia. The recommendation on competency measurement stated that

> Certification organizations, licensure boards, and professional associations should take steps to recognize and promote the widespread adoption of effective competency measures to determine the qualifications of health personnel. Special attention should be given to the further development of proficiency and equivalency measures for appropriate categories of health manpower[3] (p. 16).

The recommendation on continued competence stated that

> Certification organizations, licensure boards, and professional associations should adopt requirements and procedures that will assure the continued competence of health personnel. Additional studies of the best mechanisms to assure continued competence should be supported on a high-priority basis by professional associations, the proposed national certification commission, state agencies and the federal government[3] (pp. 16–17).

The reorganization of the AANA to include the formation of the Councils was a result of the visionary insights of the board of directors and the membership to further advance the profession of nurse anesthesia. The reasons cited for the restructuring included

1. To overcome the questions of conjugation of membership and recertification by external agencies
2. To allow the AANA to respond more freely to members' requests for increasing political, economic, and government relations activities
3. To provide a mechanism that would separate the evaluation of professional competence from association activities[4]

During the 1960s and 1970s, there was evidence of an increase in public concern not related to the quality and economics of health care but of the competency of health care providers. New challenges regarding the education, competency, practice, and political aspects of nurse anesthesia needed to be addressed by the members and leaders of the AANA.

In 1976, at the AANA annual meeting, the membership voted to approve mandatory CE for recertification. As health care professionals, CRNAs were motivated to support and participate in this credentialing process. Their support was echoed in the introductory statements of the AANA CE program:

> The rapidly changing character and increased complexity of our society demand continued updating of one's knowledge, understanding and skills. It is evident that any improvement in standards and expectations cannot be met without the continuous involvement of knowledgeable and skillful professionals engaged in an ongoing, lifelong growth process.[5]

The program was planned to be implemented on August 1, 1978. To facilitate the implementation, an ad hoc committee on recertification was appointed by the AANA Board of Directors. This committee drafted the initial standards, criteria, and procedures for recertification. At the 1978 AANA annual meeting, the members approved the formation of the Council on Recertification.

CERTIFICATION

Certification has been a requirement for nurse anesthesia practice since 1945. One of the early leaders of the profession, Gertrude Fife, identified the need to establish a national board examination for nurse anesthetists. The national board examination was chosen "to safeguard the surgeon's interest, the interest of the hospitals and the interest of the public."[2] (p. 81). The Credentials Committee of the AANA was organized in 1941. This committee drafted and administered the national certification examination (NCE) to all nurse anesthesia graduates of accredited programs.

Certification is defined as a process by which a nongovernmental agency or association certifies that an individual licensed to practice a profession has met certain standards specified by that profession for specialty practice.[6] The purpose of certification is to assure the public that an individual has mastered a body of knowledge and acquired skills in a particular specialty. *Licensure* refers to a process by which a state government grants permission to individuals to practice their occupation as a way of ensuring that the public health, safety, and welfare will be reasonably protected. Licensure and certification are mechanisms of regulating nurse anesthesia practice. Certification goes beyond licensure by recognizing the acquisition of additional specialized knowledge and establishing certain professional standards.[7]

Council on Certification

The responsibilities for the development and administration of the NCE were transferred to the Council on Certification of Nurse Anesthetists (CCNA) in 1975. The CCNA is an autonomous, certifying agency under the corporate structure of the AANA. The certification program has been approved by the National Commission for Certifying Agencies (NCCA) since 1980. The NCCA approval provides recognition that the CCNA certification program has met the highest national voluntary standards for private certification. A panel of experts from NCCA has reviewed the CCNA certification process and determined that it meets the standards and criteria of the commission.

The CCNA is charged with protecting and serving the public by assuring that individuals who are credentialed have met the predetermined qualifications or standards for providing nurse anesthesia services. The purposes of the CCNA are to

1 Formulate and adopt requirements for eligibility for admission to the certification examination and for the certification of registered nurse anesthetists
2 Formulate, adopt, and administer the certification examination to those registered nurse anesthetists who have met all requirements for examination and have been found eligible by the CCNA
3 Evaluate candidates' performance on the certification examination
4 Grant initial certification to those candidates who pass the certification examination and fulfill all other requirements for certification[8]

The membership of the CCNA includes three CRNA educators, three CRNA practitioners, two anesthesiologists, a nurse anesthesia student, one public member, and one hospital administrator. Members are elected to the CCNA in accordance with the AANA bylaws and can serve for two consecutive 3-year terms.

The eligibility criteria for admission to take the NCE are listed in Table 6–1. To be certified by the CCNA, the applicant must meet all of the eligibility requirements and successfully pass the NCE. If an applicant does not pass the NCE, he or she may retake the examination at the next scheduled date. Currently, the NCE is administered twice a year, in June and December.

TABLE 6–1

ELIGIBILITY REQUIREMENTS FOR THE NATIONAL CERTIFICATION EXAMINATION

- Current registered nurse licensure
- Graduation from an accredited nurse anesthesia educational program
- Completed application form
- Official, notarized transcript that documents the applicant's academic and clinical experiences
- Payment of application fee

Content Validation Procedures for the National Certification Examination

The CCNA has collaborated with national testing agencies to aid in the actual administration of the NCE. Previous testing agencies used by the CCNA include Psychological Corporation (1975–1984) and Assessment Systems, Inc. (ASI) (1984–1991). In the fall of 1991, American College Testing (ACT) was selected to serve as the testing agency.

During the transition to ASI in 1984, representatives from ASI and the CCNA collaborated on the procedures to build a valid, job-related examination to comply with the Uniform Guidelines on Employee Selection Procedures. These guidelines established a uniform federal position prohibiting discrimination in employment practices, particularly in the use of tests.[9] The guidelines addressed the importance of test validation procedures and documentation of a job analysis. Although the guidelines were unclear with respect to voluntary certifying organizations, it is well established in the courts that a validated test is a solid defense against allegations of discrimination.[10] The CCNA recognized that the guidelines could apply to those employers who use the certification credential for employment purposes.

In the Standards for Educational and Psychological Testing, *validity* is described as the appropriateness, meaningfulness, and usefulness of specific inferences made from test scores. Test validation is the process of accumulating evidence to support such inferences.[11] Credentialing examinations are validated through content, criterion, or construct validation strategies. Content validation is the most frequently used strategy for professional certification examinations.

Content validity is defined as the adequacy of the extent to which a test samples the knowledge, skills, and abilities within a selected content domain.[12] Since certification reflects the acquisition of the knowledge, skill, and abilities (KSAs) required for specialty practice, the content validation procedures can link the KSAs to the certification examination.

The process of establishing the content validity of a certification examination begins by examining the job tasks or roles expected of someone who is certified. A standard of performance is established and documented by experts in the profession. A content validity study consists of data showing that the content of the examination is representative of the important aspects of performance expected of an individual who is certified.

Another important link that must be present for an adequate content validity study is the linkage between the aspects of work performance expected of a CRNA and the KSAs required to perform the tasks. Figure 6–1 presents a conceptual overview of the content validation model.

The CCNA delegated the NCE validity process to the members of the CCNA Examination Committee (EC). Membership on this committee includes four CRNA practitioners and one anesthesiologist, who represent a variety of practice and education settings. Three CCNA members also serve as participants. The members of the EC developed 242 task statements that reflected entry-level nurse anesthesia practice. The tasks were organized into a survey and mailed to 1777 graduates of nurse anesthesia programs. The surveys were mailed to CRNAs who had passed the NCE between June 1984 and June 1986. This population was selected to obtain suggestions concerning the essential tasks performed by an entry-level CRNA.[13] Each respondent was asked to make judgments about the extent to which each task was required at job entry, its importance to practice, and the amount of time spent performing each task. Of the 1777 surveys mailed, 669 were returned, a response rate of 37.6 percent. After analysis of the survey data, the CCNA deleted 16 tasks as not being essential for entry into practice.

The EC then detailed the knowledge and skills required to perform each task. The 881 knowledge and skill statements were clustered into content areas that provided the basic structure of the NCE outline. The number of KSAs assigned to each content area determined the relative distribution of questions needed in each area of the NCE outline. The current content outline and percentage of the examination tested in each area are listed in Table 6–2. The first NCE that reflected the content validation procedures was administered in December 1987. The content validation process was repeated by the CCNA in 1992 with support from ACT.

Development of the NCE

The NCE for nurse anesthetists consists of 250 multiple choice questions. Questions are submitted by members of the EC and members of the Academy of Item Writers. The Academy of Item Writers is a group of CRNAs who voluntarily submit examination questions in their area of expertise to

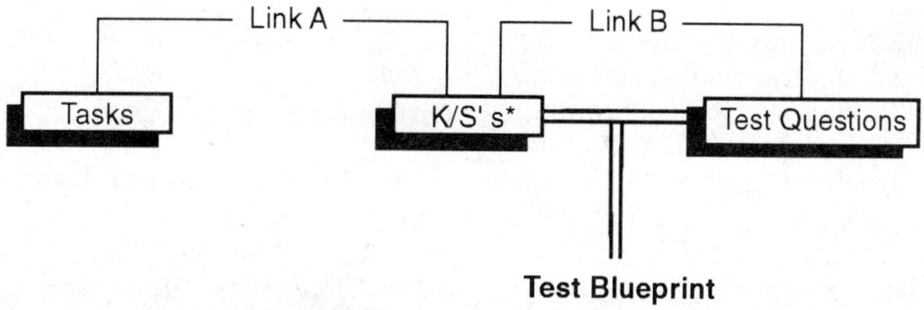

K/S' s* = knowledge and skill statments.

Figure 6–1. Content validation model. (Adapted from Gerbasi, F, Griffis, C, Samph, T, et al: The impact of present testing in the certification process of nurse anesthetists. AANA Journal 55:198–201, 1987.)

TABLE 6–2

COUNCIL ON CERTIFICATION OF NURSE ANESTHETISTS CERTIFICATION EXAMINATION CONTENT OUTLINE

Content	Percent
I. Basic Sciences	30
II. Equipment, Instrumentation, and Technology	5
III. Basic Principles of Anesthesia	31
IV. Advanced Principles of Anesthesia	30
V. Professional Issues	4

the chairperson of the EC. The EC reviews and approves each question for content and format with a representative of the testing agency before it is entered into the approved-item bank. Each examination is computer generated, based on the percentages for each area of the NCE content outline. The CRNA and physician members of the CCNA approve the final draft of the NCE prior to each test administration.

Determination of the Passing Score

Since the December 1987 NCE, the passing score has been determined using the Angoff method. The Angoff method is a criterion-referenced procedure that consists of the following steps:

1. Selection of judges
2. Definition of "acceptable level of performance"
3. Collection of judgments about each test item
4. Combination of judgments to set passing score[14]

The CRNA and physician members of the CCNA and the EC determined the passing score for the December 1987, December 1990, and June 1992 examinations. Following the Angoff procedure, all of the members read each of the 250 test questions and made their best estimate as to the probability that the minimally competent, entry-level CRNA would answer it correctly. The minimum passing score was computed by averaging the probability data generated by each individual for each of the test items for the test as a whole. The actual passing score is confidential information.

The passing score for each NCE administered after December 1987 has varied with the difficulty of the examination. To account for the difference in difficulty levels across examinations, an equating process is used. *Equating* is a statistical procedure that adjusts the number of questions needed to be answered correctly to account for the variations in difficulty levels across test forms.[15] The equating process is accomplished by selecting a group of questions from the June 1992 NCE. These anchor items or equating blocks are representative of the test content and statistical properties. The anchor items or test items with similar performance statistics are then used on subsequent examinations to maintain continuity in difficulty levels. Figure 6–2 graphically depicts the use of anchor or equating items. Equating allows the raw score or passing point to fluctuate and reflect the level of difficulty of the NCE. The equated passing scores are converted to fixed scales to avoid confusion among test candidates and the perception that the passing scores are manipulated for different examinations. The passing scaled score for the NCE is 450.

Following every examination, the testing agency performs an item discrimination analysis on each item. The preliminary item analysis is reviewed by the CRNA and physician members of the CCNA. The CCNA members then discuss the items that are identified to have problem statistics. A decision is made to keep the item as it appears or to give all the test-takers credit for the question on the examination. A final item analysis and calculation of the candidates' scores is performed by the testing agency. The score reports are then mailed to the candidates and program directors.

Future Directions

The CCNA is committed to continually investigating avenues to keep current with new developments related to testing procedures. These include updating the content validation process, investigating testing techniques such as computer adaptive testing and promoting research activities. Representatives from the CCNA participate in

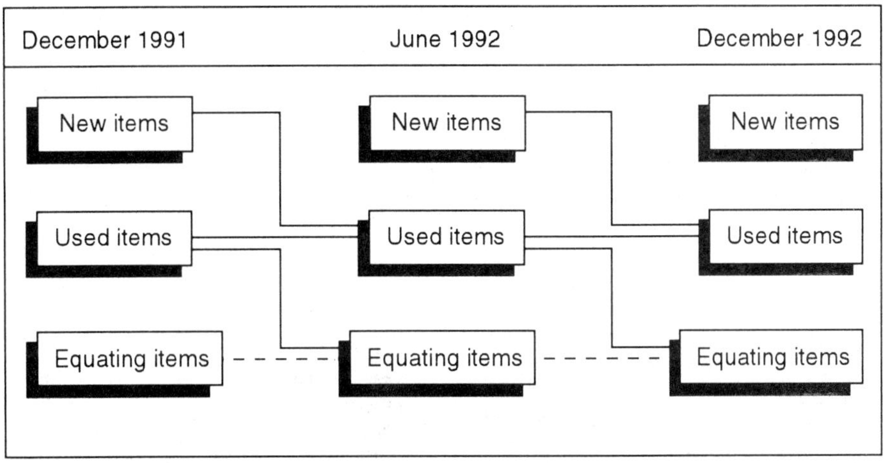

Figure 6–2. Equating process among examinations.

meetings with other agencies associated with professional certification issues. These agencies include the National Organization for Competency Assurance (NOCA), National Commission for Certifying Agencies (NCCA), National Council of State Boards of Nursing (NCSBN), National Specialty Nursing Certifying Organizations (NSNCO), and the American Board of Nursing Specialties (ABNS).

RECERTIFICATION

Following initial certification, a CRNA is eligible to apply for recertification on July 31 and accumulate CE points for 2 years beginning the August 1 following the date of initial certification. Recertification is a voluntary process. CRNAs apply for recertification biennially. Through the recertification process, the Council on Recertification of Nurse Anesthetists (COR) strives to promote the professionalism of CRNAs and the quality of anesthesia care provided to patients by nurse anesthesia practitioners. Recertification is not and cannot be a guarantee of competence to perform all anesthesia procedures. Full recertification is an indication that the CRNA has maintained an unblemished license to practice, has exercised his or her skills, has participated in approved CE activities, and is not known to have developed any impairment that could interfere with the administration of anesthesia.[16] The COR has set forth established guidelines and criteria for recertification with input from the AANA membership.

Council on Recertification

The purposes of the COR are to

1 Recertify qualified CRNAs on a biennial basis.

2 Formulate and adopt criteria for eligibility for recertification of CRNAs based on the maintenance of practice skills, participation in approved CE activities, and other recognized activities conducive to professional proficiency and freedom from known mental or physical impairments that may prevent the professional practice of nurse anesthesia. The practice of anesthesia may include clinical practice and anesthesia-related administrative, educational, and research activities.

3 Formulate and adopt criteria for approval of CE programs and offerings.

4 Formulate and adopt criteria for delegating to recognized CE agencies the authority to approve CE programs and offerings.

5 Develop and maintain mechanisms to provide for a hearing and appellate review for individuals seeking recertification or agencies seeking recognition who have received an adverse decision.

TABLE 6–3

CRITERIA FOR FULL RECERTIFICATION

1. Initial certification by the Council on Certification of Nurse Anesthetists.
2. Current licensure as a registered nurse.
3. Documentation of 40 hours of approved CE within the 2-year period prior to the upcoming August 1 recertification date.
4. Certification of substantial engagement in anesthesia practice during the 2-year period prior to the applicant's upcoming August 1 recertification date.
5. Certification by the applicant that he or she:
   a. Does not suffer from a mental or physical condition that may interfere with the practice of anesthesia;
   b. Does not currently suffer from drug or alcohol addiction or abuse;
   c. Has not been convicted of and is not currently under indictment for any felony;
   d. Has not been the subject of any documented allegations of misconduct, incompetent practice, or unethical behavior;
   e. Has not had his or her registered nurse license revoked, restricted, suspended, or limited by any state, has never surrendered his or her registered nurse license, and is not the subject of a pending action or investigation.

From Criteria for Recertification, with permission.[19]

6 Develop and maintain a mechanism for the investigation and final resolution of charges or other allegations against individuals currently holding recertification by the Council.

7 Make recommendations to the board of directors, councils, and committees in conformity with stated purpose.[17]

The membership of the COR includes four CRNA practitioners, one CRNA educator, the chairman of the CE committee, one anesthesiologist, one surgeon, and one public representative. Members are selected according to the AANA bylaws and are elected to the COR for a term of 3 years with eligibility to be re-elected for one additional term.

Categories of Recertification

Two categories of recertification have been established by the COR, full recertification and interim recertification. The criteria for full recertification are listed in Table 6–3. The process of recertification includes meeting all of the criteria and completing the application procedures.

The CRNA applying for recertification needs to submit the following information to the COR: completed application and fee, documentation of current nursing licensure, completion of 40 hours of approved CE, and documentation of practice by the July 31 deadline. The recertification period is effective for a 2-year period from August 1 through July 31. The recertification status is renewed every 2 years and expires automatically at the end of the recertification period unless renewed.

The category of interim recertification includes provisional recertification and conditional recertification. Provisional recertification may be granted for any of three reasons: pending review of an application, pending fulfillment of the practice requirements, and pending completion of a treatment or rehabilitation program.[16] The COR will grant a CRNA provisional status while reviewing an application if questions arise as to the fulfillment of the established criteria. After completion of the investigation, the COR may grant or deny recertification.

If a CRNA has not been substantially engaged in practice during the 2-year period prior to recertification, provisional recertification may be granted. A CRNA who is participating in a drug, alcohol, or other type of treatment or rehabilitation program may be assigned provisional recertification if all of the other recertification criteria are met. After completion of the rehabilitation or treatment program, the CRNA may receive full recertification.

Conditional recertification is granted to those CRNAs who meet the recertification criteria but have restrictions placed on their professional nursing license. Examples of restricted licensure include professional nursing practice under direct supervision and participation in an alcohol or drug rehabilitation program for a stated period. The status may be changed to full recertification when the restrictions are removed from the license.

The COR has the authority and the ability

to revoke or modify the recertification status of an anesthesia practitioner. Reasons for automatic revocation of recertification include the failure to maintain professional licensure and a judgment by a court of law that the practitioner is mentally incompetent or has committed a felony. Discretionary revocation of recertification is used if the practitioner fails to comply with the established criteria for recertification, intentionally falsifies material fact, or deliberately fails to provide relevant information to the COR. Documented evidence of gross incompetence, unethical conduct, or moral turpitude which, in the opinion of the COR, represents a significant threat to patient well-being, may also influence the decision to enact discretionary revocation of recertification.[18] The recertification status of a CRNA may be modified at any time by the COR to reflect applicable information that is presented.

The COR has established procedures for reconsideration of any modification in the recertification status of a CRNA. These include prompt notification and guidelines for appeal through the Council for Public Interest in Anesthesia. The COR strives to maintain the integrity of the nurse anesthesia profession and to protect the welfare of the public in its decisions about the recertification status of CRNAs.

Future Directions

The COR is dedicated to consistently evaluate and update the criteria and procedures related to recertification. Through the established recertification process, the COR seeks to ensure that nurse anesthesia practitioners maintain the high level of knowledge and skill required for current practice. It also aims to ensure that appropriate limitations are placed on those CRNAs who are known to have developed conditions that might adversely affect their ability to practice. The COR will continue to explore strategies to meet its goals and the needs of the profession.

CONTINUING EDUCATION

CE for CRNAs has been a requirement for recertification since 1978. The AANA CE Committee defines CE as those learning activities intended to build on the educational and experiental bases of the professional nurse anesthetist for the enhancement of clinical, education, administration, research, or theory development to improve public health.[18] The CE program for CRNAs seeks to enhance the professional competence of health care providers in the specialty of nurse anesthesia practice. CE is an organized and evaluative educational process extending beyond basic preparation, promoting the enrichment of knowledge and understanding toward the maintenance of anesthesia expertise. The AANA seeks to assist each member in accepting personal responsibility for safe anesthesia practice. This is achieved by a purposeful CE program that enables all members to contribute effectively to the health care delivery system.[18]

Continuing Education Committee

The CE Committee (CEC) is a standing committee of the AANA. Members are appointed by the president-elect with approval from the board of directors. According to the AANA bylaws, the CEC shall formulate criteria for eligibility for recertification. Such criteria shall be submitted to the COR for evaluation and adoption. The CEC shall also supervise the CE projects conducted by the association, evaluate applications for program approval, and approve refresher courses based on established criteria that are required prior to transference to active recertified membership.[19]

The philosophy of the CEC describes the vital importance of CE to nurse anesthesia practice. The AANA believes that nursing is accountable to the public for promulgating standards of nursing practice that will improve the delivery of nursing services and promote quality patient care. As the national professional association for nurses specializing in anesthesia, the AANA holds itself responsible for providing CE activities that will help maintain excellence in practice. Further, it meets its commitment to society and the profession by upholding standards that promote quality CE activities sponsored by other providers of nurse anesthesia programs.

The CEC is primarily responsible for providing opportunities for continued learning by individual and groups of nurse anesthetists. It believes that lifelong learning is essential for the continued acquisition of the necessary knowledge and skills to maintain competence in practice. The CEC maintains that nurses, by entering the field of anesthesia, hold themselves accountable and responsible for seeking out learning experiences that will improve and advance the practice of anesthesia and the quality of care they provide to their patients.

The CEC believes that CE activities are most effective when the learning needs of participants are taken into consideration and when principles of adult learning are applied. It supports its beliefs by providing standards of CE that include these basic concepts. Furthermore, the committee monitors and appraises the CE activities of other providers to ensure their adherence to the established standards that promote quality CE for nurse anesthetists.[18]

Continuing Education Program

The purpose of the CE program of the AANA is to promote quality educational activities for nurse anesthetists. The program includes standards and criteria for the review, approval, and recognition of CE activities. The CEC, under the guidance of the director of continuing education, oversees the program and continually monitors the system to ensure that the standards and criteria are maintained.

The goals of the CE Program facilitate the promotion of quality CE for nurse anesthetists. They encompass

1 Promoting high-quality CE for nurse anesthetists by implementing a review and recognition process that includes standards and criteria for CE providers

2 Providing a clearly defined application process as well as procedures for the review approval process to guide providers effectively and accurately through it

3 Assisting state associations and other providers of CE in developing skills to offer quality CE in nurse anesthesia

4 Implementing an ongoing process for evaluating the policies, procedures, and criteria of the CE program to appraise the effectiveness of services provided

5 Engaging in strategic long-range planning activities to ensure the continued growth and viability of the AANA's CE program[18]

Each CRNA is required to obtain 40 CE credits every 2 years as part of the recertification criteria. One CE credit is equal to 50 minutes or 1 contact hour. Individual CRNAs must first perform a self-assessment to identify the areas and types of CE activity that correspond to their needs in professional practice. CRNAs elect to participate in the CE activity that provides the most benefit to them in terms of content, location, and cost. The provider of the CE activity is responsible for securing approval for the educational opportunity. The CE program has two types of approval for CE activities, prior approval and nonprior approval. Table 6–4 lists the types of educational activities available for CE credit.

The AANA has established standards and criteria for CE Programs that are used by the CEC to review and approve an application. The standards are listed in Table 6–5. The criteria for each of the standards provide further clarification of their meaning. The CE Committee may withdraw approval status of a CE activity if the provider fails to comply with the established standards and criteria. Educational activities that are not congruent with the AANA CE program phi-

TABLE 6–4

TYPES OF CONTINUING EDUCATIONAL ACTIVITIES

1. Attendance at local, state, and national nurse anesthesia meetings
2. Participation in hospital or anesthesia department in-services
3. Audiovisual media programs such as videos, audiotapes, and computerized instruction
4. Participation in research activities
5. Attendance at college and university courses relevant to anesthesia practice
6. Publication of original papers
7. Clinical anesthesia experiences beyond the requirements of basic preparation

TABLE 6–5

STANDARDS FOR CONTINUING EDUCATION PROGRAMS

I.	Official application for providers
II.	Purpose of continuing education activity
III.	Planning process
IV.	Needs assessment
V.	Learner objectives
VI.	Content of CE activity
VII.	Teaching methods
VIII.	Faculty
IX.	Physical facilities and resources
X.	Recordkeeping
XI.	Verification of attendance
XII.	Evaluation

From Continuing Education Program of the AANA, with permission.[23]

losophy may be denied approval. An appeal mechanism exists for providers or individuals who are not satisfied with a CEC decision.

Prior-Approved CE Activities

Prior approval is the process used to prereview applications and award CE credit based on predetermined criteria. Prior approval by the AANA designates that a CE activity has met specific standards and has been awarded CE credit prior to its actual presentation. In addition, it obliges the provider to assume certain responsibilities for recordkeeping and attendance taking. The program content must be consistent with the overall purpose and goals of the AANA CE program.[18]

The types of activities that are eligible for prior approval include: educational programs sponsored by associations and organizations at the local, state, regional, or national level; in-service programs; provider-directed independent study; self-directed independent study; and research in anesthesia-related fields.

To obtain prior approval, the provider must submit the completed application form to the CEC at least 90 days in advance of the CE activity. Additional materials that are required include the application fee, evaluation form, and certificate of attendance. Notification of approval is furnished in writing within 30 days of receipt of the application. If additional information is required for prior approval, the provider must submit it before the presentation of the CE activity or approval will not be granted. A code number is assigned to the CE activity and must appear on promotional activities, certificates of attendance, attendance records, and correspondence sent to the CE department. The recordkeeping process involves submission of an official AANA attendance record with the names, AANA numbers, and CE credits for each participant within 30 days after completion of the program. Also, the provider must issue a certificate of attendance to all participants.

Nonprior-Approved CE Activities

The nonprior approval process is used to award CE credit to individuals for participation in learning activities that have not been prior-approved by the AANA but which have been approved for CE credit by a recognized professional accreditation or approved organization prior to their presentation. This approval mechanism is initiated by the individual who submits the application. CE activities that may be eligible for nonprior approval are not evaluated until they have been presented and an official AANA application requesting CE approval has been submitted to the CE department. Applications for nonprior approval should be submitted within 60 days after conclusion of the activity.[18]

Examples of activities that are eligible for nonprior approval include educational programs sponsored by other recognized professional associations, in-service programs, provider-directed independent study, college and university courses, acceptance of an original paper for publication, clinical anesthesia experiences, and research in anesthesia-related fields.

The individual or group requesting the CE credit must complete the appropriate application procedures and provide the required documentation. Written notification of approval or denial for CE credit is sent after review of the application. The CEC ensures that the nonprior-approved program meets the standards and criteria for the AANA CE program.

Recordkeeping

The AANA CE department maintains records of CE credits earned by its members and will contract this service for nonmembers. At the end of the recertification period, this documentation is forwarded to the COR. The CE credits are recorded during each year from August 1 through July 31 to coincide with the recertification period. Computer printouts with CE information and the certification/recertification status are mailed to the CE coordinator of each state several times a year. Most states have this printout available at their state meetings. On an annual basis, the AANA CE department sends a transcript of CE credits it has on file to members who are eligible for recertification and to the nonmembers who use its recordkeeping services.

CLINICAL PRIVILEGES

The granting of clinical privileges is one of the methods used by hospitals to credential professional staff members. Each hospital has an established procedure through the Medical Staff Affairs Department for the approval of an individual's clinical privileges to practice his or her specialty. A CRNA can apply for clinical privileges related to anesthesia practice by following their hospital/employer guidelines. It is important to note that the guidelines also depend on the type of setting in which the CRNA is employed. Examples of the guidelines for the granting of clinical privileges at Detroit Receiving Hospital (DRH) and the AANA are described.

Detroit Receiving Hospital Guidelines

As an employee of a hospital, the CRNA usually completes an application (Figure 6–3) and submits it to the Department of Anesthesia Advisory Committee (DAAC). The objectives of the DAAC include

1 Checking the validity of credentials submitted by the applicant, such as academic background, previous clinical experiences, references, and appropriate certification and licensure to practice.

2 Reviewing the application and granting or denying approval of privileges based on the documentation.

3 Forwarding the application to the Medical Staff Credentials Committee for acceptance with final approval granted by the Medical Executive Committee.

4 Reviewing all staff privileges every 2 years based on compliance with acceptable standards of care.[20]

Following the decision to grant, deny, or modify the application for clinical anesthesia privileges, the DAAC conveys its response to the anesthesia provider and forwards the information to Medical Staff Affairs. A flowchart of the application process for DRH is shown in Figure 6–4.

American Association of Nurse Anesthetists Guidelines

The AANA Guidelines for Granting Clinical Privileges to CRNAs describe the qualifications, application process, administrative review, and renewal of clinical privileges for CRNAs. Recommended clinical privileges for the preanesthetic preparation and evaluation, anesthetic induction, maintenance and emergence, postoperative care, and the perianesthetic and clinical support functions are identified (Table 6–6).

The basic qualifications of a CRNA applying for clinical privileges include current licensure as a registered nurse, graduation from an accredited nurse anesthesia educational program, and current professional certification or recertification status.

The CRNA requesting clinical privileges should submit a written and signed application form (Figure 6–5). In the event that the hospital does not have a prescribed form, the CRNA should submit a curriculum vitae. Whether an application form or a curriculum vitae is used, the nurse anesthetist shall

1 Provide detailed information regarding his or her qualifications.

2 Make a specific request for the anesthesia service and anesthesia clinical privileges for which the applicant wishes to be considered.

Text continued on p. 86.

DETROIT RECEIVING HOSPITAL AND UNIVERSITY HEALTH CENTER

APPLICATION FOR CLINICAL PRIVILEGES - ANESTHESIOLOGY

Certified Registered Nurse Anesthetist: ______________________

RN License #: ______________________ Expiration Date: ______

Initial Certification: ______________________ Expiration Date: ______

Recertification #: ______________________ Expiration Date: ______

INSTRUCTIONS TO APPLICANT: Please check ( ) the procedure(s) in which you are proficient and for which you are requesting privileges:

	DEPARTMENTAL RECOMMENDATIONS		
	REQUESTED	**APPROVED**	**DENIED**
1. Selection of administration of anesthesia, including all ancillary methods and all necessary monitoring modalities (noninvasive and invasive) required to provide anesthesia.	1. ❑	❑	❑
2. Administration of anesthesia including all ancillary methods and monitoring modalities (noninvasive and invasive) required to provide anesthesia under the direct supervision of an anesthesiologist or another fully privileged member of the department.	2. ❑	❑	❑
3. Selection and administration of regional anesthesia as described below including all methods required to provide regional anesthesia under the supervision of an anesthesiologist.	3. ❑	❑	❑
A. Topical and infiltration	A. ❑	❑	❑
B. Spinal	B. ❑	❑	❑
C. Epidural	C. ❑	❑	❑
D. Intravenous	D. ❑	❑	❑
E. Upper Extremity Blocks	E. ❑	❑	❑
F. Field Blocks	F. ❑	❑	❑
G. Other (describe) ______________	G. ❑	❑	❑
4. Selection and/or administration of drugs providing analgesia, sedation, and hypnosis.	4. ❑	❑	❑
5. Selection and/or administration of fluids, blood, and blood products.	5. ❑	❑	❑

Figure 6–3. Detroit Receiving Hospital and University Health Center application for clinical privileges—anesthesiology. (From Detroit Receiving Hospital Guidelines for Clinical Privileges, Department of Anesthesia Services Policy Manual, 1992, with permission.)

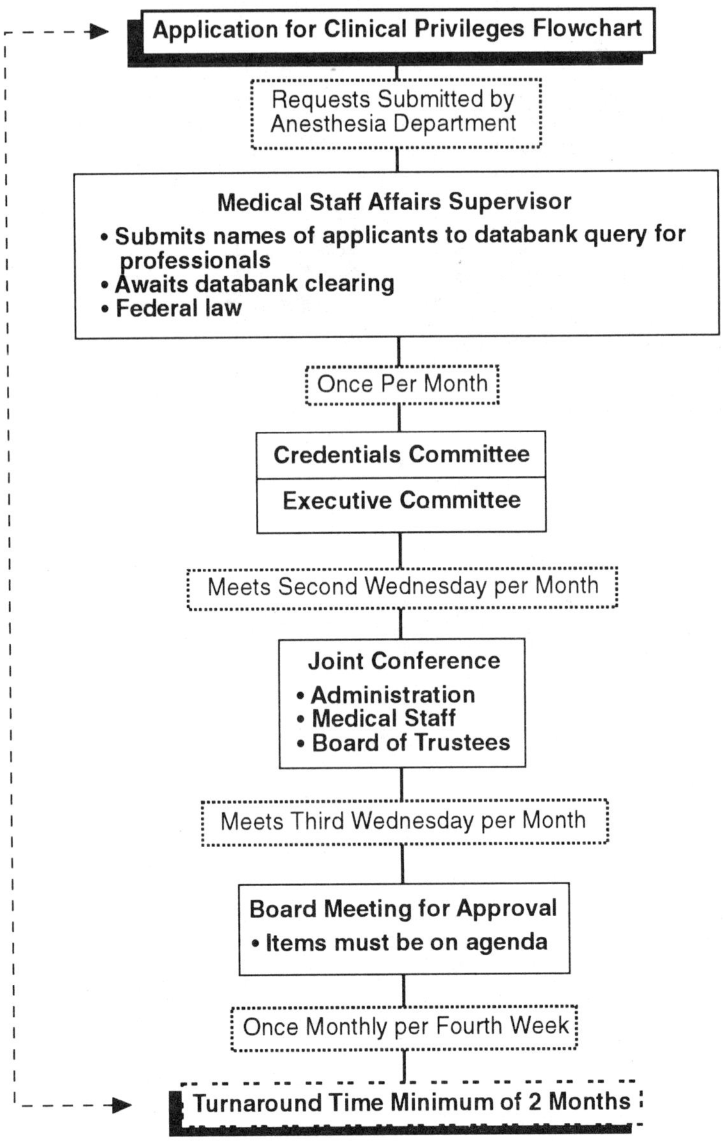

Figure 6–4. Detroit Receiving Hospital Clinical Privileges Flowchart. (From Detroit Receiving Hospital Guidelines for Clinical Privileges, Department of Anesthesia Services Policy Manual, 1992, with permission.)

TABLE 6–6

RECOMMENDED CLINICAL PRIVILEGES

CRNA privileges and responsibilities must be consistent with law and may include, without limitation, the following:

Preanesthetic Preparation and Evaluation

- Obtaining an appropriate health history including biophysical and psychosocial data.
- Conducting an appropriate physical screening assessment.
- Recommending or requesting and evaluating pertinent diagnostic studies.
- Selecting, ordering, and administering preanesthetic medications.
- Documenting the preanesthetic evaluation and obtaining informed consent for anesthesia.

Anesthesia Induction, Maintenance, and Emergence

- Securing, preparing, and providing basic safety checks on all equipment, monitors, supplies, and drugs used for the administration of anesthesia.
- Selecting the anesthetic techniques, agents, and adjunctive drugs and administering an anesthetic consistent with patient needs and procedural requirements.
- Performing tracheal intubation and extubation and providing mechanical ventilation.
- Performing and managing regional anesthetic techniques including, but not limited to, subarachnoid, epidural, and caudal blocks; plexus, major, and peripheral nerve blocks; intravenous regional anesthesia; transtracheal, topical, and local infiltration blocks; intracapsular, peribulbar, intercostal, and retrobulbar blocks.
- Providing appropriate perianesthetic invasive and noninvasive monitoring using current standards and techniques and responding to abnormal findings with corrective action.
- Recognizing and treating cardiac dysrhythmias through the use of perianesthetic electrocardiogram monitoring.
- Recognizing abnormal patient response during anesthesia, selecting and implementing corrective action, and requesting consultation whenever necessary.
- Managing the patient's fluid, blood electrolyte, and acid-base balance.
- Evaluating patient response during emergence from anesthesia and instituting pharmacologic or supportive treatment to ensure the adequacy of patient recovery from anesthesia and adjunctive drugs.
- Providing anesthesia care consistent with infection control and anesthetic safety principles to prevent the spread of disease and prevent harm to the patient, the anesthetist, and others in the anesthetizing environment.
- Documenting, as part of the medical record, all aspects of care in a thorough and timely fashion.

Postanesthesia Care

- Providing a thorough report of the patient's psychological and physical condition, perianesthetic course, and anticipated problems to the postanesthetic health care provider.
- Providing postanesthesia follow-up and evaluation of the patient's response to anesthesia and for potential anesthetic complications, taking appropriate corrective actions and requesting consultation whenever indicated.
- Initiating and administering respiratory support to ensure adequate ventilation and oxygenation in the immediate postanesthesia period.
- Initiating and administering pharmacologic or fluid support of the cardiovascular system during the immediate postanesthesia period to prevent perianesthetic morbidity and mortality.
- Releasing patients from the postanesthesia care unit or discharging patients from the ambulatory surgical setting.

Perianesthetic and Clinical Support Functions

- Inserting peripheral and central intravenous catheters.
- Inserting pulmonary artery catheters.
- Inserting arterial catheters and performing arterial puncture to obtain arterial blood samples.
- Identifying and managing emergency situations, including initiating and/or participating in cardiopulmonary resuscitation that involves airway maintenance, ventilation, tracheal intubation, pharmacologic cardiovascular support, and management of blood, fluid, electrolyte, and acid-base balance.
- Providing consultation and implementation of respiratory and ventilatory care.
- Initiating and modifying pain relief therapy using drugs, regional anesthetic techniques, or other accepted pain relief modalities.
- Selecting and/or prescribing medication and treatment modalities related to theperianesthetic care of the patient, with consultation or collaboration when appropriate.
- Accepting additional responsibilities appropriate to the practice setting that are within the expertise of the individual CRNA.

From Guidelines for Granting Clinical Privileges to the Certified Registered Nurse Anesthetist, with permission.[31]

AANA APPLICATION FOR CLINICAL PRIVILEGES

Date ________________

The undersigned applies for clinical privileges at ______________________________
(Name of Institution)

as delineated in the Addendum to this Application.

Category:

Certified Registered Nurse Anesthetist

PERSONAL DATA

Name ____
(Last) (First) (Middle) Maiden Name If Applicable

Social Security Number ____ - ____ - ____ Telephone ________________

Home Address ____

City ________________ State ____________ Zip __________

Birth Date ______________ Birth Place ____________ Sex __________

Citizenship ______________ Type ________________________

EDUCATION

High School ________________________ Graduation Date __________

City ________________ State ________________________

Nursing School/College

Graduation Date ____________ Degree ________________________

Address ____

City ________________ State ____________ Zip __________

Anesthesia Education Program

Graduation Date ____________ Degree ________________________

Address ____

City ________________ State ____________ Zip __________

Other Education

1. University/College __________________________________
   Address ____
   City ________________ State ____________ Zip __________
   Major ______________ Years Completed ______ Degree ________
2. University/College __________________________________
   Address ____
   City ________________ State ____________ Zip __________
   Major ______________ Years Completed ______ Degree ________
3. University/College __________________________________
   Address ____
   City ________________ State ____________ Zip __________
   Major ______________ Years Completed ______ Degree ________

Figure 6–5. Application form for clinical privileges. (From Guidelines for Granting Privileges to the Certified Registered Nurse Anesthetist. In Professional Practice Manual for the Nurse Anesthetist, 1989, pp 7–9, with permission.)

4. University/College ____________________
Address ____________________
City ____________ State ____________ Zip ____________
Major ____________ Years Completed ________ Degree ________

PROFESSIONAL ORGANIZATION MEMBERSHIPS

1. ____________________
2. ____________________
3. ____________________
4. ____________________

LICENSES: (Submit copies of documents)

State ________ RN License # ____________ Exp. Date ________
Advanced Practice License # (if applicable) ________ Exp. Date ________
State ________ RN License # ____________ Exp. Date ________
Advanced Practice License # (if applicable) ________ Exp. Date ________
State ________ RN License # ____________ Exp. Date ________
Advanced Practice License # (if applicable) ________ Exp. Date ________
CRNA Certification # ____________ Original Date Certified ________
Recertification Expiration Date ______ Basic Cardiac Life Support Expiration Date ____
Other Certification or Licensure Type ________ License # _____ Exp. Date ________

PROFESSIONAL ANESTHESIA EXPERIENCE* (Put present or most recent first)

1. Employed by ____________________
Address ____________ Telephone ____________
City ____________ State ________ Zip ________
Position ____________ Period of Employment ____________
Area of Practice ____________________
2. Employed by ____________________
Address ____________ Telephone ____________
City ____________ State ________ Zip ________
Position ____________ Period of Employment ____________
Area of Practice ____________________

Other Professional Experience*

1. Employed by ____________________
Address ____________ Telephone ____________
City ____________ State ________ Zip ________
Position ____________ Period of Employment ____________
Area of Practice ____________________

CONFIDENTIAL INFORMATION

As part of an application for clinical privileges, hospitals and clinics sometimes ask a variety of questions concerning personal and professional data relating to suitability to administer anesthetics. There are several federal laws relating to discrimination that may affect an institution's ability to inquire as to personal and professional data,

**Attach a list of additional employment experiences or a curriculum vitae.*

Figure 6–5—continued.

Continued

and state laws vary as to questions that may be asked in these applications. It is advised to consult with an attorney in formulating questions to be asked in connection with application for clinical privileges and as to appropriate waivers from applicants permitting background checks.

PROFESSIONAL LIABILITY INSURANCE

❑ Provided by Institution ❑ Provided by Group ❑ Individual Policy

Name of Carrier ____________________

Limits of Liability __________/__________ Policy Number __________

Date of Policy: From ________ To ________

REFERENCES — List three

1. Name ____________________

   Institution ____________________

   Address__________ Business Telephone __________

   City__________ State __________ Zip __________

   How long have you known this person? __________

2. Name ____________________

   Institution ____________________

   Address__________ Business Telephone __________

   City__________ State __________ Zip __________

   How long have you known this person? __________

3. Name ____________________

   Institution ____________________

   Address__________ Business Telephone __________

   City__________ State __________ Zip __________

   How long have you known this person? __________

I consent to release of information necessary for an evaluation of my background, training, professional competence, and ethical character. I affirm that the information included in this document is true to the best of my knowledge.

Signed: ____________________ Date: __________

Addendum to the Application for Clinical Privileges

CLINICAL PRIVILEGES DELINEATION FORM

Type of Request : ❑ Initial ❑ Renewal

Name __________ Category: Certified Registered Nurse Anesthetist

Social Security Number __________

Please check the procedures for which you are making application

❑ Preanesthetic assessment

❑ Requesting laboratory/diagnostic ❑ Cardiopulmonary resuscitation management

❑ Preanesthetic medication ❑ Perianesthetic invasive and noninvasive monitoring

❑ General anesthesia and adjunct drugs ❑ Tracheal intubation/extation

Figure 6–5—continued.

- ❑ Regional techniques
- ❑ Subarachnoid
- ❑ Epidural
- ❑ Caudal
- ❑ Upper extremity
- ❑ Lower extremity
- ❑ Peripheral nerve blocks
- ❑ Infiltration
- ❑ Topical
- ❑ Eye block (peribular, retrobular)
- ❑ Transtracheal
- ❑ Intracapsular
- ❑ Intercostal
- ❑ Other ______________________
- ❑ Emergency/ancillary drugs to maintain physiologic homeostatis and prevent or treat emergencies during the perianesthesia period
- ❑ Mechanical ventilation/oxygen therapy
- ❑ Fluid, electrolyte, acid-base management
- ❑ Blood, blood products, plasma expanders
- ❑ Peripheral intravenous/arterial catheter placement
- ❑ Central venous catheter placement
- ❑ Pulmonary artery catheter placement
- ❑ Chronic pain therapy
- ❑ Postanesthesia care/release
- ❑ Other ______________________

I am mentally and physically capable of performing the privileges I have requested:

Signature: ______________________ Date: ____________

The above nurse anesthetist is granted the full privileges he or she has requested with the following exceptions and/or limitations. (If none, so state).

____

____

Decision: ❑ Approval ❑ Disapproval

Signed, Chief Nurse Anesthetist: ______________________ Date: ________

Signed, Medical Director: ______________________ Date: ________

Signed, Director, Medical/
Professional Staff Office: ______________________ Date: ________

Date Practitioner Notified: ____________

These privileges are granted initially for one coming calender year and must be renewed on a biennial basis. The applicant may request to have privileges changed as required during this period.

For Use by the CRNA Applicant

I have reviewed the approval/disapproval of my application for clinical privileges and staff appointment. If disapproved, adequate explanations of the reasons for disapproval have been explained and provided to me in writing. I have also been provided with a copy of staff rules and regulations including all due process policies and procedures.

______________________________ ____________
Applicant's Signature Date

Figure 6–5—continued.

Continued

INSTRUCTIONS TO APPLICANT: Please check ( ) the procedure(s) in which you are proficient and for which you are requesting privileges:

	DEPARTMENTAL RECOMMENDATIONS		
	REQUESTED	APPROVED	DENIED
6. Full participation in resuscitation measures in any location within the hospital.	6. ❑	❑	❑
7. Participation in recovery room activities.	7. ❑	❑	❑
8. Preoperative and postoperative evaluation of patients.	8. ❑	❑	❑

I am mentally and physically capable of performing the privileges that I have requested.

Signature: ______________________________

It is recommended that the above Certified Registered Nurse Anesthetist be granted the full privileges that he or she has requested above with the exception and/or limitation, if any, as noted above or immediately following: (If none, so state).

____
____
____
____

Signature: ______________________________ ______________
Department Advisory Committee Date

______________________________ ______________
Chief, Department of Anesthesia Date

Figure 6–5—continued.

3 Provide references of persons who have worked with and who can comment on the ability and character of the applicant.

4 Provide information as to whether certification, licensure, or clinical privileges have ever been denied, revoked, suspended or reduced.[21]

The application and any supporting materials is submitted to the Anesthesia Service. Upon receipt, the Anesthesia Service may request a personal interview with the applicant, and after evaluation and review, transmit the application, supporting materials, and its recommendation to the appropriate committee. The Anesthesia Service will recommend privileges to be granted, as well as any conditions that need to be attached to the granting of clinical privileges.

The same committee or body that considers applicants for professional staff membership reviews and evaluates the CRNA's application and supporting materials, the Anesthesia Service's recommendation, and other relevant information. The same committee or body approves or disapproves the Anesthesia Service's recommendation and forwards its decision to the institution's administration. Final privilege granting should be based on preestablished criteria uniformly applied to all applicants.

Requests for renewal of privileges shall be evaluated by the Anesthesia Service, the appropriate professional staff committees, and by institutional administration based on the CRNA's education, training, experience, demonstrated ability, and judgment. The basis for privilege determinations shall include previous quality assessment activities to the extent applicable. Privileges of the CRNA should be reviewed through the above channels at least every 2 years, with appropriate due process available to all anesthesia providers. The CRNA shall assist in the review of the guidelines for nurse anesthesia practice in the institution at least every 2 years.

CRNAs are responsible for seeking clinical privileges that reflect their educational preparation, clinical experience, and level of professional competence. It is incumbent on CRNAs to maintain knowledge of current scientific theories, principles, and techniques related to the field of anesthesia and their current practice situation.

Individual clinical privileges should be delineated regardless of the contractual or employment relationship that exists within the practice setting. This can take a variety of forms, that is, individual clinical privileges approved by medical staff or other bodies or authorized through individualized position descriptions. The privilege-granting process should incorporate results of quality assurance and risk management.

These recommended clinical privileges are not intended to be all-encompassing but should serve only as examples for the preparation of documents required in granting clinical privileges, since all institutions will, of necessity, modify such procedures and documents to meet their individual circumstances. CRNAs should review their clinical privileges on a regular basis. Caution is advised to ascertain that listed privileges are not overly specific or restricted.[21]

SUMMARY

The nongovernmental regulation of credentialing of nurse anesthesia practice comprises the certification and recertification processes through mandatory CE and the approval of clinical privileges. This chapter has described the development and implementation of these major procedures. The AANA, its leadership, and its membership have facilitated the establishment of sound regulatory practices for CRNAs. It is vital that CRNAs continue to actively participate in and support credentialing of their practice and profession. Each individual CRNA, as a member of the specialty profession of nurse anesthesia, is responsible for the commitment to provide quality anesthesia services. This commitment is fostered through continued involvement in professional growth. The AANA is the facilitator of the credentialing procedures; however, it is the responsibility of the individual CRNA to promote the dynamism of the profession.

REFERENCES

1. American Association of Nurse Anesthetists Philosophy. In Bylaws and Standing Rules of the American Association of Nurse Anesthesia. The Association, Park Ridge, IL, 1992.
2. Bankert, M: Watchful Care: A History of America's Nurse Anesthetists. Continuum, New York, 1989.
3. Credentialing Health Manpower. US Department of Health, Education, and Welfare, Washington, DC, 1977.
4. Proposed American Association of Nurse Anesthetists Restructuring Detailed Assembly of States. American Association of Nurse Anesthetists NewsBulletin 1:57, 1978.
5. Continuing Education Program of the American Association of Nurse Anesthetists. The Association, Park Ridge, IL, 1990, p 4.
6. American Nurses' Association: The Study of Credentialing in Nursing: A New Approach, vol I. A Report of the Committee. The Association, Park Ridge, IL, 1979.
7. Scofield, R: Certification: What does it mean? Current Concepts in Nursing 2:6–10, 1988.
8. Council of Certification Bylaws. The Association, Park Ridge, IL, 1989.
9. Civil Service Commission: Uniform guidelines on employee selection procedures. Federal Register 43:166, 1978.
10. Bryant, SK: Voluntary certification and the uniform guidelines on selection procedures: A potential problem for personnel managers. Health Policy and Education 2:135–152, 1981.
11. Standards for Educational and Psychological Testing. American Psychological Association, Washington, DC, 1985.
12. Wohlgemuth, R and Samph, T: A Summary Task Analysis Report for the American Association of State Social Work. 1:1–12, 1983.
13. Zaglaniczny, K: Development of the current certification examination. AANA Journal 58:5–7, 1990.
14. Livingston, S and Zieky, M: Passing Scores: A Manual for Setting Standards of Performance on Educational and Occupational Tests, 19 , pp 1–17.
15. Gerbasi, F, Griffis, C, Samph, T, et al: The impact of present testing in the certification process of nurse anesthetists. AANA Journal 55:198–201, 1987.
16. Council on Recertification of Nurse Anesthetists: Criteria for Recertification, 1990, p 2.
17. Council on Recertification Bylaws. The Association, Park Ridge, IL, 1991.
18. Continuing Education Program of the American Association of Nurse Anesthetists. The Association, Park Ridge, IL, 1990.
19. Appointed committees. In Bylaws and Standing Rules of the American Association of Nurse Anesthetists. The Association, Park Ridge, IL, 1992, p 17.
20. Detroit Receiving Hospital Guidelines for Clinical Privileges. In Department of Anesthesia Services Policy Manual. Detroit, 1992.
21. Guidelines for Granting Clinical Privileges to the Certified Registered Nurse Anesthetist. In Professional Practice Manual for the Nurse Anesthetist, 1989, p 7.

7

Standards of Care in Anesthesia Practice

John G. Aker
Rita M. Rupp

OUTLINE

OBJECTIVES

On completing this chapter, the reader will be able to:

1. Highlight the similarities and differences between practice guidelines, position statements, and promulgated standards of care as published by the AANA, including an understanding of the role each plays in professional practice.
2. Outline the current method of practice guideline development.
3. Define and provide examples for the terms "process" and "outcome" standard.
4. List the sources of professional standards, as well as their respective contributions and influence on clinical practice.
5. Become familiar with current AANA standards for nurse anesthesia practice and selected practice guidelines and position statements, as they relate to clinical practice and other pertinent professional issues.

Perhaps the most definitive means by which a Certified Registered Nurse Anesthetist (CRNA) will be perceived by the public and peers alike is the manner in which he or she maintains a "quality of care" provided to patients. This term, albeit prone to rhetorical abuse, underlies the integrity of nurse anesthesia practice. "Quality of care" is most often defined as that activity involving patient/provider interactions that are solidly based on defined standards of practice. In this chapter, the reader is introduced to new terminologies that relate to anesthesia care, including standards of clinical practice, practice guidelines, and position statements. Although they are distinctly different, for many, these terms are often used interchangeably. Each is a necessary ingredient in determining the quality of care. For purposes of preliminary definition, the reader should refer to Figure 7–1 to conceptualize the relationship of these three terms. Each is discussed in more detail throughout this chapter.

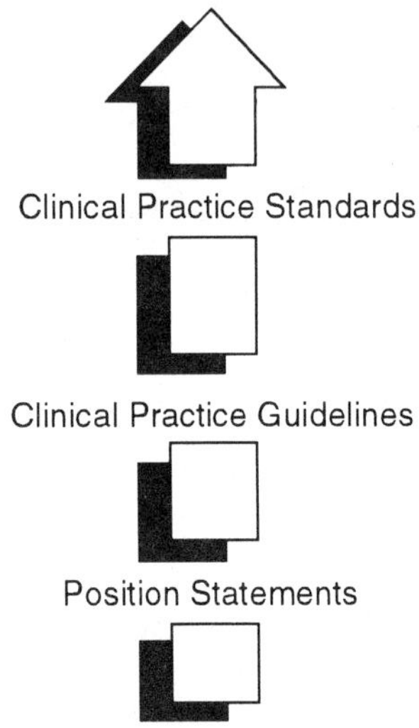

Figure 7–1. *Relationship among clinical practice standards, practice guidelines, and position statements.* Clinical standards represent the highest form of evaluative criteria for clinical practice. They are often originally based on position statements that have been tested and used as practice guidelines before becoming an explicitly stated, mandated standard.

Practice standards remain the ultimate mandate for clinical behavior. A *standard* represents what must be exercised by the prudent nurse anesthetist in similar circumstances. Standards allow for little variation in practice behavior that cannot be justified by a clear and compelling rationale. Practice guidelines are, in fact, guides to decision making or provider behavior that is commonly accepted within the community of anesthesia at large. Practice guidelines are not mandated; rather, they are suggested or advised. Position statements, although legitimate in their intent, have less compelling characteristics than either practice guidelines or standards. They usually represent either a summary of emerging trends on a given topic or popular practice modalities, or they discuss common procedural issues, both clinically and nonclinically related. Either practice guidelines or position statements may eventually evolve into mandated practice standards, given appropriate testing, discussion, and review.

In the last decade, the study of practice standards and associated practice guidelines has received renewed attention by many professional health care groups. This renewal has occurred largely at the behest of public and private pressures brought to bear on the health care community to further define, justify, improve, and document their quality of care. In short, the public, governmental agencies, business, and industry are demanding accountability of health care providers to publicly issue, maintain, and enforce appropriate standards of care.

The establishment and implementation of practice guidelines and standards of practice are an inherent responsibility of a professional organization. In addition, the profession must hold members accountable for using the standards, educate the public relative to the standards, and protect the public from individuals who have not attained or who willfully do not follow the professional standards.[1] The American Association of Nurse Anesthetists (AANA) has maintained this responsibility to the public by promulgating standards (clinical practice and patient monitoring), defining the acceptable level of anesthesia care provided by its members. This activity is largely the responsibility of the AANA Practice Committee, with the advice and consent of AANA membership and the board of directors.

The AANA Board of Directors first adopted standards of practice and published *The Guidelines for Nurse Anesthesia Practice* in

1983, with subsequent revisions in 1989 and 1992.[2] The practice guidelines accomplished three major goals: they clarified the scope of nurse anesthesia practice to the public, delineated the responsibilities for perioperative anesthesia care, and provided a framework for structured support and accountability of the provider to the consumer of anesthesia services. That document included, among other items, "Standards for Nurse Anesthesia Practice," "Patient Monitoring Standards," "Guidelines for Granting Clinical Privileges to Certified Registered Nurse Anesthetists," and a model position description. Today, a larger, more comprehensive compendium entitled "Professional Practice Manual for the Certified Registered Nurse Anesthetist" is available and includes a wide variety of practice-related documents germane to contemporary anesthesia practice, including those mentioned earlier. This manual is divided into eight primary sections, the topics for which are listed in Table 7–1.

STANDARDS OF PRACTICE

Standards are published authoritative statements that describe the professional responsibilities of the membership. Standards promulgated by a profession are representative models that delineate contemporary principles of practice, reflect the philosophic values and clinical priorities of the profession, and provide the foundation by which clinical practice can be evaluated. Furthermore, standards furnish practitioners and the judiciary with confirmation of what constitutes the standard knowledge and skill that the practitioner should apply in the daily care of anesthetized patients. Members of the profession must be accountable to the public for maintaining all published standards.

TABLE 7–1

TOPICS SECTIONS OF THE *PROFESSIONAL PRACTICE MANUAL FOR THE CRNA*

Part I:	Standards and Guidelines Guidelines and Standards for Nurse Anesthesia Practice Guidelines for Obstetric Anesthesia and Conduction Analgesia for the CRNA Postanesthesia Care Standards for the CRNA
Part II:	Qualifications and Capabilities of the CRNA
Part III:	Professional and Legal Issues in Nurse Anesthesia Practice
Part IV:	Synopsis of Anesthesia Outcome Studies
Part V:	Other Considerations in Anesthesia Practice Documenting the Standard of Care: The Anesthesia Record Informed Consent in Anesthesia Infection Control Guidelines for Anesthesia
Part VI:	Quality Assessment and Risk Management AANA Quality Management Initiative Risk Management Guide for the CRNA
Part VII:	AANA Position Statements
Part VIII:	AANA Code of Ethics

Standards can be subdivided into two types: process and outcome. *Process standards* refer to a specific conduct or the method by which a particular task is undertaken. Process standards mandate a particular clinical behavior. Box 7–1 lists the standards for nurse anesthesia practice. Standard 1 (the completion of a preanesthetic visit) and standard VI (documentation of anesthesia care) are examples of process standards (procedural or "how to" standards). The Patient Monitoring Standards, which are an elaboration of standard V of the "Standards for Nurse Anesthesia Practice," are also examples of process standards.

Although current standards include no *outcome standards*, future standards development will likely focus on the requirement of the CRNA to provide data that speaks beyond process to tangible, patient-related results. These standards may, for instance, mandate a particular patient outcome; the incidence of nausea and vomiting in the inpatient postoperatively shall be less than 5 percent, or the occurrence of perioperative myocardial infarction (MI) in patients without previous history of MI shall be less than 0.7 percent. These standards emphasize the importance of maintaining continuous quality improvement data related to anesthesia care.

Outcome standards are not without obvious problems. First, medicine is not an exact science, and for all the best intentions, there will be circumstances affecting patient outcome that are beyond the control of the provider. For instance, if an ASA Class 4E patient presents for surgery, there are likely to be preexisting medical problems that would overwhelm any probability that the

BOX 7–1
STANDARDS FOR NURSE ANESTHESIA PRACTICE
AMERICAN ASSOCIATION OF NURSE ANESTHETISTS

A characteristic of any profession is its responsibility to the public for promulgating standards by which the quality of practice rendered by its members can be assessed. Standards, based on sound philosophy, theory, science, and principles, serve to upgrade clinical practice.

As the representative of the profession, the Board of Directors of the American Association of Nurse Anesthetists adopts and promulgates standards of practice with input from the members of the Association. The primary responsibility for implementing these standards rests with the practitioners, Certified Registered Nurse Anesthetists (CRNAs). As an organization composed of health care providers, the American Association of Nurse Anesthetists recognizes that the principles of anesthesia practice should be clearly described as professional standards that guide the practitioner in maintaining and improving the delivery of quality anesthesia care.

Purpose of Standards

These standards are intended to assist the CRNA practitioner in providing consistent, safe anesthesia care. The standards are descriptive, providing a basis for evaluation of the practice and reflecting the rights of those receiving anesthesia care. The AANA recognizes it may not be possible for the CRNA to comply with each of these standards in certain extraordinary or emergency situations. It is expected that the CRNA should assess each patient situation and utilize professional judgment in selecting a course of action, and that in each case, the CRNA can demonstrate that the decisions made were in the best interest of the patient. In addition, while the standards are intended to encourage high quality patient care, they cannot ensure specific patient outcomes. Their intent is to:

1 Assist the profession in evaluating the quality of care provided by its practitioners.
2 Provide a common base for practitioners to use to coordinate care and unify their efforts in the development of a quality practice.
3 Assist the public in understanding what to expect from the practitioner.
4 Support and preserve the basic rights of the patient.

Standard I

A thorough and complete preanesthetic assessment shall be performed.

Interpretation. The responsibility of the CRNA begins before the actual administration of the anesthesia. Except under unusual or emergency situations, the CRNA has an obligation to determine that relevant tests have been completed and thorough assessment of the patient has been made.

Standard II

Informed consent for the planned anesthetic intervention shall be obtained from the patient or legal guardian.

Interpretation. The CRNA shall obtain or verify that an informed consent has been obtained by another qualified provider. Anesthetic options and risks should be discussed with the patient and/or legal guardian in language the patient and/or legal guardian can understand. The patient's medical record should reflect that informed consent was obtained.

Standard III

A patient-specific plan for anesthesia care shall be formulated.

Interpretation. The plan of care is developed by the CRNA in coordination with appropriate health care providers in a systematic manner based on assessment, analysis, anticipated procedure, patient preference, and current anesthesia principles. It must be coordinated with appropriate health care providers.

BOX 7–1
STANDARDS FOR NURSE ANESTHESIA PRACTICE
AMERICAN ASSOCIATION OF NURSE ANESTHETISTS—*CONTINUED*

Standard IV

The anesthesia care plan shall be skillfully implemented and the plan of care adjusted as needed to adapt to the patient's response to the anesthetic. Vigilance shall be maintained for untoward identifiable reactions and corrective actions initiated as required.

Interpretation. The CRNA shall induce and maintain anesthesia at required levels. The CRNA shall continuously assess the patient's response to the anesthetic and/or surgical intervention and intervene as required to maintain the patient in a homeostatic, physiologic condition.

Standard V

The patient's physiologic condition shall be monitored consistent with both the type of anesthesia care and specific patient needs.

Interpretation. Monitoring modalities shall be instituted in accordance with AANA *Patient Monitoring Standards* (See Box 7–7).

Standard VI

There shall be prompt, complete, and accurate documentation of pertinent information on the patient's record.

Interpretation. Documentation should be criteria-based, reflecting the standards of anesthesia practice. Documentation should include all anesthetic interventions and patient responses. Accurate recording facilitates comprehensive patient care, provides information for retrospective review and research data, and establishes a medical-legal record. The CRNA is responsible for assuring that the care provided by the CRNA is properly documented.

Standard VII

The responsibility for the care of the patient shall be transferred to other qualified providers in a manner that assures continuity of care and patient safety.

Interpretation. The CRNA shall assess the patient's status and determine when it is safe to transfer responsibility for care to other qualified personnel. The CRNA shall accurately report the patient's condition and all essential information to the personnel assuming responsibility for the care of the patient.

Standard VIII

Appropriate safety precautions shall be taken to minimize the risk of fire, explosion, electrical shock, and equipment malfunction.

Interpretation. Safety precautions and controls, as established within the institution, shall be strictly adhered to, so as to minimize the hazards of electricity, fire, and explosion in areas where anesthesia care is provided. The anesthetic machine shall be inspected by the CRNA according to guidelines before use. The CRNA shall check the readiness, availability, cleanliness, and working condition of all equipment to be utilized in the administration of the anesthesia care. Documentation shall be made on the patient's medical record that the anesthesia machine and equipment were checked. Policies for routine safety maintenance checks of anesthesia equipment and monitors shall be developed and adhered to by the appropriate individuals and departments within the institution.

Standard IX

Appropriate safety precautions shall be taken to minimize the risk of infection for the patient, CRNA, and other staff.

Interpretation. Written policies on infection control shall be developed and followed in order to minimize the risk of infectious disease.

Continued

BOX 7–1
STANDARDS FOR NURSE ANESTHESIA PRACTICE
AMERICAN ASSOCIATION OF NURSE ANESTHETISTS—*CONTINUED*

Standard X

Anesthesia care shall be assessed to assure its quality.
Interpretation. The CRNA shall participate in the ongoing review and evaluation of the quality and appropriateness of anesthesia care that he or she provides. Evaluation shall be performed based upon appropriate outcome criteria and reviewed on an ongoing basis.

Standard XI

The CRNA shall participate in a continual process of self-evaluation and strive for excellence in anesthesia practice.
Interpretation. Self-evaluation is accomplished in several ways, including quality assurance, peer review, annual performance appraisal, review of clinical privileges, and ongoing assessment of clinical practice. The CRNA shall incorporate into practice new techniques and knowledge that have been acquired through formal, self-directed study.

Standard XII

The CRNA shall respect and maintain the basic rights of patients, demonstrating concern for personal dignity and human relationships.
Interpretation. The CRNA shall support and preserve the basic rights of patients to privacy, and to independence of expression, decision, and action.

patient might actually improve postoperatively. As such, in some circumstances, provision of a guaranteed outcome is not only impossible but also imprudent. However, this scenario has not prevented outcome data from being applied as a measurement of the quality of hospital services. Several regions of the country now regularly report the outcome data of their patient population in an effort to market their services. Some have claimed that public release of this information has caused irreparable harm to health care facilities that care for much sicker patients. Consequently, it is incumbent on the CRNA to be involved in the acquisition and interpretation of outcome data that accurately reflect the quality of care within the context of its provision.

The reader should carefully note that there is a single standard of care in the practice of anesthesiology. Standards do *not* vary according to the type of practitioner that provides it. Blumenreich[3] states:

> Some people erroneously assume or question whether there is a dual standard of care in the anesthesia field. . . . In fact, because of the nature of anesthesia and the fact that attention and proper monitoring of patients is the overwhelming consideration in the practice of anesthesia, there is, in fact, a single standard of care.

Nurse anesthesia as a separate profession has established its own standard of care. However, this standard of care is not different from that of an anesthesiologist. To quote Blumenreich,[3] "as we know, in the anesthesia field there is, in fact, a rather uniform quality of care between nurse anesthetists and anesthesiologists, and that is further evidence that the 'standard of care' is the same."

PRACTICE GUIDELINE DEVELOPMENT

Practice guidelines can be defined as official policy statements of a professional organization that assist the practitioner in understanding the indications for and performance of clinical procedures (e.g., the administration of anesthesia to obstetric patients) or provide information for the management of a clinical complication or disease process, such as malignant hyperthermia.[4]

Practice guidelines are not only useful in guiding practice, but may also find relevance in education, research, and the development and implementation of continuous quality improvement programs (see Chapter 16).[5] Practice guidelines may assist the instruction of the neophyte anesthetist in the administration of anesthesia for a specific surgical procedure, guide the researcher in the identification and development of methodology for analysis of a specific clinical problem, or serve as the criterion against which one's practice may be examined and improved. Although in concept they do not carry the weight of standards, practice guidelines can and have been used in malpractice litigation when charges of negligence are brought against a CRNA provider.

Woolf[6] describes a process used in the development of practice guidelines and refers to it as "informal consensus development." In this process, a group of "experts" would convene and create a set of guidelines for a particular clinical situation. These guidelines are formulated from the opinions and experiences of the expert panel. Scientific affirmation, or the incorporation of a systematic literature review supporting draft guidelines, is sometimes included. Practice guidelines should ideally be accompanied by interpretive statements that guide the clinician toward understanding and implementing the stated guideline.

Another primary function of practice guidelines is to examine the quality of care provided and to serve as a reminder for providers to practice in a justifiable, prudent, and cost-efficient manner. Many private insurance companies are looking to a future in which they will mandate that the individuals they insure use practice guidelines in an effort to control the cost of health care through the evaluation of use, misuse, or overuse of particular health services.[5] One can also logically conclude that practice guidelines will likely serve in the future as reimbursement tools for the purchasers of health care.

A new and more systematic approach is now emerging in the process for drafting practice guidelines. This approach emphasizes development of specific clinical objectives, an examination of the clinical benefits and harms of the various interventions available, and the acquisition of both expert opinion and scientific evidence to support the guideline's intended objectives.[6] One such government-sponsored body, the Agency for Health Care Policy and Research, has recently published practice guidelines in several areas of general medicine that also have relevance for anesthesiology (e.g., cataracts, pain management). These guidelines were developed to enhance a relative standardization of practice patterns among providers, eliminate excessive waste and cost to patients, and serve as empirically based justification for practice routines.

Effective practice guidelines, such as those referred to above, evolve from the union of scientific evidence, "expert" opinion, and clinical experience. "Expert" opinion must be carefully solicited in a formalized process to assist in the review of scientific data. Individuals must be carefully selected in accordance with the stated practice guideline objectives and must be recognized as experts within the profession. However, input from practitioners must also be solicited to ensure that the guidelines are functional in a variety of practice settings. For example, if a practice guideline mandated the use of transesophageal echocardiography for the detection of air embolism during neurosurgical procedures, it is doubtful that the guidelines would be followed outside a major medical center, as this modality would most likely not be available in smaller hospitals.

For all their apparent advantages, the future of practice guidelines and their eventual importance or influence on standards of care remains in doubt. Today there are many within the medical community who, although they support the concept of practice guidelines, readily admit that many of these guidelines still lack the justification of empirical evidence. In short, much of medical practice today is not based on clear data supporting medical efficacy but rather on established habits and traditional, often dated practice patterns.

PRACTICE GUIDELINE INTERPRETATION

As previously stated, the intent or "spirit" of practice guidelines is to assist the practitioner in deciding which appropriate actions might best apply in specific clinical circumstances.[7] A practice guideline essentially acts as a "proving ground" for what may, in the future, be accepted as a mandated standard. The literal wording of practice guidelines is intentionally tailored to accommodate a range of circumstances, and the interpretation should be flexible enough to allow application to individual patient need. Unlike standards, practice guidelines are not likely to be rigidly applied in all instances, because they are considered "advisory" and viewed as recommended conduct to attain a desirable clinical goal. As previously mentioned, practice guidelines may be so commonly applied by the profession that they constitute a functional standard, characterizing care that a reasonable and prudent practitioner would provide. This fact alone requires all CRNAs to be conversant with the literature pertaining to the transition of a practice guideline to an accepted standard. This is often not an easy distinction and is one that the courts may apply to the detriment of an uninformed nurse anesthetist.

A primary example of practice guidelines for CRNAs is evidenced by *The Guidelines for Obstetrical Anesthesia and Conduction Analgesia for Certified Registered Nurse Anesthetists* (Box 7–2).[8] The guidelines are accompanied by an interpretation that clarifies the intent of the guideline and describes methods to achieve the goal of the guideline. Referring to Box 7–2, the reader will note that guideline III states that a CRNA or other qualified anesthesia provider should be in attendance at all times during regional (conduction) or general anesthesia for an obstetric procedure. The interpretation of this guideline assists the practitioner in decisions related to the simultaneous occurrence of an emergency in another obstetric patient. There are a number of clinical scenarios that may affect the ultimate decision of the practitioner in the care of these patients. The anesthetist who practices in a large medical center will certainly have additional anesthesia personnel available to assist in the concurrent care of an additional obstetric emergency. However, the solo practitioner may be faced with decisions regarding the needs and risks of two simultaneous obstetric emergencies. Therefore, situations do exist in which strict compliance with the guideline may not be possible. This is a distinguishing feature separating practice guidelines and standards.

Guidelines are subject to change over time as additional scientific and clinical information becomes available through research and experience in clinical practice. An example of this was the evolution of the Harvard standards for monitoring patients under anesthesia,[9] which were subsequently modified and adopted by the American Society of Anesthesiologists (ASA) in a document entitled "Guidelines for Patient Care in Anesthesiology". Those guidelines encouraged appropriate intraoperative monitoring of anesthetized patients. However, technologic changes (the availability of pulse oximetry and capnography) and the emerging scientific literature influenced the House of Delegates of the ASA to adopt the Harvard Standards in October 1986. Therefore, what was previously called "Guidelines for Patient Care in Anesthesiology" became "Standards for Basic Intraoperative Monitoring".[10] In December 1986, the AANA Board of Directors endorsed the Harvard Standards and in 1989 developed and published *AANA Patient Monitoring Standards*.

POSITION STATEMENTS

Position statements published by the AANA are documents that serve as suggestions, emerging practice patterns, or recommendations for clinical practice. Position statements may acquaint the practitioner with conduct related to clinical, professional, or generic issues related to anesthesia and nursing. Position statements related to clinical anesthesia practice are not promulgated standards (published as standards by the professional organization) but may refer to practice that is accepted and commonplace within the profession. Accordingly, position statements, like practice guidelines, may form a functional standard although they are not labeled as such. A functional standard would reflect the care that a reasonable and prudent anesthetist would provide his or her patient.

Text cont'd.

BOX 7–2
AMERICAN ASSOCIATION OF NURSE ANESTHETISTS GUIDELINES FOR OBSTETRIC ANESTHESIA AND CONDUCTION ANALGESIA FOR CERTIFIED REGISTERED NURSE ANESTHETISTS

The American Association of Nurse Anesthetists (AANA) advocates high patient safety standards for all anesthesia techniques, including general, regional, local, or monitored anesthesia care. The practice of obstetric anesthesia is by no means an exception. Expectations of the parturient, obstetrician, and the public at large have demanded a reexamination of the quality of anesthesia care offered in the obstetric unit. Quality assessment and improvement activities, legal ramifications of adverse outcomes, and economics have also been instrumental in changing obstetric anesthesia practice. This anesthesia specialty is of dual importance, because the needs of both the mother and the fetus must be assessed and met.

While pregnancy and childbirth are a normal physiologic process, there are many factors that may complicate and play a role in the management of pregnancy, labor, and delivery. The American Academy of Pediatrics and the American College of Obstetricians and Gynecologists (AAP-ACOG) have published *Guidelines for Perinatal Care* which defines levels of perinatal care in terms of facilities, equipment, and personnel to assist hospitals and health care providers in developing policies and procedures for the care of the obstetric patient and the unborn child, including the newborn following birth. (American Academy of Pediatrics, American College of Obstetricians and Gynecologists: Guidelines for Perinatal Care, ed 3. AAP, Elk Grove Village, IL, 1992). Certified Registered Nurse Anesthetists (CRNAs) should make themselves fully aware of these guidelines.

According to Aubry, approximately 20 percent of pregnant women can be identified prenatally to be at risk. They account for approximately 50 to 55 percent of poor pregnancy outcomes. Another 5 to 10 percent of pregnant women can be identified to be at risk for the first time during labor, accounting for another 25 to 30 percent of poor pregnancy outcomes. Another 20 percent of perinatal morbidity and mortality occurs in the approximate 70 percent of pregnant women demonstrating no identifiable risk. (Aubry RH: Identification of the high-risk obstetric patient. In Ryan, GM Jr (ed): Ambulatory Care in Obstetrics and Gynecology. Grune & Stratton, New York, 1980) Furthermore, even if a risk is identified during the antepartum and intrapartum period, transport of such patients to a higher level of obstetric service may be contraindicated or impossible. Therefore, it is imperative that all CRNAs, no matter what their practice setting, work with other health professionals and hospital administration to assure the availability of needed resources, including policies and procedures, to appropriately care for obstetric patients and their newborn infants.

It is further acknowledged that standards and guidelines promulgated by some health care professional groups may not be able to be fully met in certain rural and underserved areas. Nevertheless, it is important that CRNAs who often work in these areas strive to ensure the best conditions possible for obstetric and anesthesia services under the demographic, geographic, and other constraints peculiar to the location. CRNAs must recognize that they are responsible and accountable for their practice, for adherence to generally accepted standards of practice and for compliance with institutional and departmental guidelines.

The tradition of the provision of safe anesthesia care by CRNAs is documented by the positive results of numerous anesthesia outcome studies and decreasing anesthesia malpractice insurance rates. In order to maintain their position as competent providers of anesthesia services in the health care community, CRNAs must continually assess their practice to ensure that it meets or exceeds generally accepted obstetric anesthesia practice.

In recognition of the role of a professional organization in promulgating standards and guidelines, the AANA has developed these Guidelines for Obstetric Anesthesia and Conduction Analgesia to promote the continued safe delivery of obstetric anesthesia care by CRNAs. The AANA, in adopting and publishing these guidelines, is providing a single yardstick for CRNAs to assess their own practice in order to make changes if needed or warranted. Furthermore, these guidelines complement, rather than supplant, the profession's defined standards of care.

Continued

BOX 7–2
AMERICAN ASSOCIATION OF NURSE ANESTHETISTS GUIDELINES FOR OBSTETRIC ANESTHESIA AND CONDUCTION ANALGESIA FOR CERTIFIED REGISTERED NURSE ANESTHETISTS—*CONTINUED*

Qualifications and Availability of Providers

Guideline I

Obstetric anesthesia, whether by conduction techniques (intrathecal, epidural, or caudal epidural block) or general anesthesia techniques should be initiated, monitored, and managed by a CRNA or other qualified anesthesia provider.

Interpretation. A qualified anesthesia provider is a CRNA, an anesthesiologist, or a physician who has been approved by a credentialing body or process to administer or collaborate in the administration of obstetric anesthesia. The anesthesia provider should have the appropriate skills and clinical privileges to administer the types of general or regional anesthesia that may be required for the obstetric patient.

Guideline II

Conduction analgesia (via epidural or intrathecal single dose or via continuous catheter) should be initiated, monitored, and managed by a CRNA or other qualified anesthesia provider.

Interpretation. The course of the conduction analgesia should be monitored and documented by the CRNA or other qualified anesthesia provider. The registered professional nurse providing the patient's obstetric care should monitor the patient and report changes in vital signs, the analgesia level, and other alterations in the laboring patient's condition to the anesthesia provider. Adjustment of analgesia levels should be done by the CRNA or other qualified anesthesia provider.

Guideline III

Conduction or general anesthesia for an obstetric surgical procedure should be administered by a CRNA who is in continuous attendance of the patient unless relieved by another qualified anesthesia provider.

Interpretation. Obstetric surgical procedures may include cesarean section, extraction of retained placenta, uterine manipulation, or other types of procedures. The CRNAs primary obligation is to the patient receiving anesthesia for the obstetric surgical procedures. A simultaneous true emergency with another obstetric patient may dictate that the needs and risks of both patients be weighed and care provided to both patients to minimize the morbidity and mortality of each.

Guideline IV

CRNAs who provide obstetric anesthesia as a component of their practice should make every effort to initiate anesthesia as soon as possible after a decision is made that an obstetric emergency requires an anesthesia service.

Interpretation. Under most circumstances, the response time should be no more than 30 minutes from the time the decision is made until initiation of cesarean section. When this is not possible because of personnel, geographic, or other potential hospital constraints, policies should be in place to provide a plan of action to minimize adverse outcomes resulting from such delays. While transfer of the patient to another hospital is one such option, consideration should be given to the actual time it would take to effect a transfer as opposed to the arrival time of the CRNA as well as other patient considerations.

Guideline V

Prior to the initiation of conduction analgesia, the CRNA should confirm that a physician capable of managing obstetric emergencies is immediately available.

Interpretation. The criteria defining "immediately available" should be documented in institutional policy.

BOX 7–2
AMERICAN ASSOCIATION OF NURSE ANESTHETISTS GUIDELINES FOR OBSTETRIC ANESTHESIA AND CONDUCTION ANALGESIA FOR CERTIFIED REGISTERED NURSE ANESTHETISTS—*CONTINUED*

Guideline VI

The CRNA should be immediately available, as defined by institutional policy, when conduction analgesia is in progress.

Interpretation. The criteria defining "immediately available" should be documented in institutional policy, which must contain a contingency plan for the management of conduction analgesia in the event the CRNA becomes engaged in another anesthetic situation.

Guideline VII

A qualified health care provider, other than the CRNA, should be present during delivery to perform neonatal resuscitation.

Interpretation. Departmental and institutional policies should be developed and approved regarding responsibilities for neonatal resuscitation. Such policies should recognize that in some situations, the CRNA will be the most qualified person available for neonatal resuscitation. While the primary responsibility of the CRNA is to the parturient, any decision to assist in neonatal resuscitation should be made after weighing the risks of diverting attention from the mother's anesthetic or analgesic management and after ensuring that the mother will be continuously monitored.

Preanesthesia Assessment

Guideline VIII

The CRNA should perform a preanesthetic assessment and ensure that informed consent has been obtained prior to initiating obstetric anesthesia or conduction analgesia.

Interpretation. In cases where delays in initiating anesthesia may put the life of the mother or fetus at greater risk, the CRNA must have adequate knowledge of the maternal health history and physical status to tailor an appropriate anesthetic for the patient. Furthermore, the CRNA should weigh the risk of any delay in initiating anesthesia in order to obtain a formal informed consent against the emergency nature of the procedure.

Guideline IX

Prior to initiation of obstetric anesthesia or conduction analgesia, the CRNA must ensure that an evaluation of the parturient, her progress in labor, and the status of the fetus has been performed and documented in the patient's record. An order authorizing this service must be obtained from the attending physician.

Interpretation. The CRNA must ascertain that the attending physician is aware of the patient's status prior to initiation of any analgesia or anesthesia service.

Monitoring and Equipment

Guideline X

In addition to such monitoring as may be indicated from the standpoint of obstetric management, patients receiving conduction analgesia during labor should be monitored as defined in departmental policies. At a minimum, this should include heart rate, blood pressure, and patient comfort level. In addition, oxygen saturation should be monitored and documented if indicated by the condition of the parturient or fetus.

Interpretation. There should be a policy defining monitoring requirements for obstetric patients receiving conduction analgesia during labor which takes into consideration those periods of initiation of analgesia, stabilized levels of analgesia, and reinjection of analgesic drugs. Oxygen saturation should be monitored to document adequacy of oxygenation if significant hypotension or other complications occur or if the fetal heart rate suggests fetal compromise. Compliance with the

Continued

BOX 7–2
AMERICAN ASSOCIATION OF NURSE ANESTHETISTS GUIDELINES FOR OBSTETRIC ANESTHESIA AND CONDUCTION ANALGESIA FOR CERTIFIED REGISTERED NURSE ANESTHETISTS—*CONTINUED*

policy should be demonstrated through appropriate documentation of the monitoring data, including evidence of appropriate intervention as may be indicated by such data.

Guideline XI

Obstetric patients receiving anesthesia for a surgical procedure in a delivery room should be monitored according to the Patient Monitoring Standards of the AANA (See Box 7–7).

Interpretation. It is the responsibility of the CRNA to ensure that appropriate monitoring equipment is available to deliver obstetric anesthesia services or to seek transfer of patients to facilities having such equipment when such a transfer will not further endanger that patient.

Guideline XII

The CRNA should ensure that adequate anesthesia equipment, monitors, and supplies for administering and managing an anesthetic are available in obstetric settings. Such equipment and supplies should be comparable to that found in the operating room for use on surgical patients.

Interpretation. Routine and emergency drugs, supplies, monitoring and resuscitation equipment, including oxygen, intubation equipment, positive pressure breathing devices, and suction, should be available where conduction analgesia or obstetric anesthesia is administered. Appropriate equipment and drugs for resuscitation of the neonate should be available in every delivery room. A defibrillator should be available in the labor and delivery suite.

Protective Measures for Preventing/Managing Potential Complications

Guideline XIII

All obstetric patients who are undergoing an analgesia/anesthesia procedure should be considered to have a full stomach and should be afforded protection from the risks and complications of aspiration pneumonitis.

Interpretation. The patient should take nothing by mouth during labor except small sips of water, ice chips, or a preparation to moisten the mouth and lips. Protection from the morbidity of aspiration may be provided by pharmacologic intervention. If a general anesthetic is to be administered, a rapid sequence induction and intubation with application of cricoid pressure should be performed.

Guideline XIV

All obstetric patients who receive analgesia/anesthesia should have an intravenous catheter inserted and an appropriate type and volume of fluid administered.

Interpretation. Administration of appropriate IV fluids will maintain hydration of the patient. Preloading with fluids is indicated prior to conduction analgesia or obstetric anesthesia. Intravenous cannulation affords direct access for the administration of pharmacologic agents in the event of complications.

Postdelivery Care

Guideline XV

Postanesthesia care should be available, consistent with the analgesia or anesthesia technique administered and the condition and needs of the patient.

Interpretation. Postanesthesia care for the patient receiving major conduction or general anesthesia should be consistent with the AANA *Postanesthesia Care Standards*. This immediate postanesthesia care may be given in the obstetric unit rather than in a postanesthesia care unit. When conduction analgesia is utilized for labor and vaginal delivery, the appropriate monitoring

BOX 7–2
AMERICAN ASSOCIATION OF NURSE ANESTHETISTS GUIDELINES FOR OBSTETRIC ANESTHESIA AND CONDUCTION ANALGESIA FOR CERTIFIED REGISTERED NURSE ANESTHETISTS—*CONTINUED*

modalities to be utilized in the postanesthesia period shall be determined by the patient's condition. The CRNA should remain with the patient until another qualified health care provider accepts responsibility for the patient's care.

Quality Management

Guideline XVI

A quality assessment and improvement program for anesthesia-attended obstetric and neonatal patients should be developed and maintained.

Interpretation. Departmental policies and procedures, in conjunction with the analysis of the annual statistics determined through quality assessment, should be reviewed yearly.

Boxes 7–3 through 7–6 are representative position statements related to clinical anesthesia practice. The position statement titled *Qualified Providers of Conscious Sedation* (Box 7–3) provides guidelines for the registered professional nurse (non-CRNA) who administers conscious sedation. The purpose of these guidelines is to promote the safe care of patients undergoing intravenous (IV) conscious sedation, to address questions raised by nursing organizations and health care facilities relative to the qualifications of non-CRNA providers, and to outline the appropriate care of patients during IV conscious sedation.

Box 7–4 lists specific recommendations for the treatment of malignant hyperthermia with specific reference to the Malignant Hyperthermia Association of the United States (MHAUS). The purpose of this position statement is to increase the provider's awareness of the need to be adequately prepared to treat suspected or unsuspected episodes of malignant hyperthermia. Portions of this position statement are supported by an extensive bibliography. This statement differs from a practice guideline as there are no clinical procedural details for the diagnosis or treatment of malignant hyperthermia.

The position statements, *Administration of Regional Anesthesia* (Box 7–5) and *Utilization of Invasive Monitoring* (Box 7–6), provide information regarding professional consensus for the administration of regional anesthesia and the use of invasive monitoring techniques by the CRNA. These statements may assist the CRNA to develop institutional and departmental policies regarding insertion of central venous, pulmonary artery, and arterial monitoring catheters.

SOURCES OF PROFESSIONAL STANDARDS

In addition to those of the professional organization, standards originate from a number of auxiliary sources.[11] Individual practitioners may develop personal standards. Each practitioner develops warranted clinical habits (e.g., the use of an anesthesia machine checkout list) that are repeated daily. Through repetition, these clinical habits become the personal standards of the practitioner.

Personal standards are acknowledged as an original source of promulgated professional standards and may further evolve into consensus policies and procedures that are subsequently adopted by an anesthesia department and become "departmental standards."[11] As an example, an anesthesia department policy that outlines the care of the patient who has consumed food or beverage within 8 hours of the induction of general anesthesia has evolved from the personal standard of care formulated from clinical experience and scientific affirmation of morbidity that follows aspiration. Departmental policy is formulated from the consensus of the majority of the department

Text continued on p. 108.

BOX 7–3
QUALIFIED PROVIDERS OF CONSCIOUS SEDATION

Position

The AANA believes the safe administration of conscious sedation requires the sole attention of a professional who is educated in the speciality of anesthesia and skilled in the administration of conscious sedation, monitored anesthesia care, and regional and/or general anesthesia.

Purpose

The purpose of this statement is to provide guidance that will improve quality of care when conscious sedation is administered.

Background

Conscious sedation easily may be converted into deep sedation and/or loss of consciousness because of the unique characteristics of the drugs used as well as the physical status and drug sensitivities of the individual patient. The administration of conscious sedation requires constant monitoring of the patient and the ability to respond immediately to any deviation from normal. Conscious sedation should only be provided by an individual who is qualified to select and administer the appropriate drugs and who is capable of managing all anesthetic levels and potential complications including airway management, intubation, and resuscitation. Appropriate monitoring devices, emergency drugs and equipment, and essential support equipment should be immediately available.

Although the AANA believes that optimal care for the patient receiving intravenous conscious sedation is best provided by a qualified anesthesia provider, the association also recognizes the reality of the increased demand for this service, which the current supply of anesthesia providers is unable to fully meet. In recent years, registered professional nurses in selected speciality areas of practice have become increasingly involved in assisting physicians in providing IV conscious sedation. Questions have been raised by nursing organizations and health care institutions concerning the appropriateness, nursing preparation, and patient/procedural requirements for this practice. In an effort to answer some of the concerns and to promote safe care during IV conscious sedation, the AANA has developed suggested guidelines for registered professional nurses who are involved in this patient care activity. (See Addendum: Suggested Guidelines for Registered Professional Nurses who are Engaged in the Administration of IV Conscious Sedation). These suggested guidelines do not supersede or consider the effect of more restrictive relevant laws, regulations, judicial and administrative decisions and interpretations, accepted standards and scopes of practice established by professional nursing organizations and institutional policies applicable to registered professional nurses, which should be reviewed.

Addendum to Position Statement 2.2

Suggested Guidelines for Registered Professional Nurses Engaged in the Administration of IV Conscious Sedation

Preamble. Although optimal care for the patient receiving conscious sedation is best provided by a qualified anesthesia provider, the increased number of surgical and diagnostic procedures being performed and the growth in the number of practice settings in which IV conscious sedation is provided have created a demand that the current supply of anesthesia providers is unable to meet. In recent years, registered professional nurses in selected speciality areas of practice have become increasingly involved in assisting physicians in providing IV conscious sedation. In an effort to promote safe care during IV conscious sedation, to address questions that have been raised by nursing organizations and health care institutions with respect to the qualifications of registered professional nurses involved in this care, and taking into consideration the patient and procedural requirements of this practice, these suggested guidelines have been developed. These suggested guidelines do not supersede or consider the effect of more restrictive relevant laws, regulations, judicial and administrative decisions and interpretations, accepted standards and

BOX 7–3 QUALIFIED PROVIDERS OF CONSCIOUS SEDATION—*CONTINUED*

scopes of practice established by professional nursing organizations, and institutional policies applicable to registered professional nurses which should be reviewed. A registered professional nurse engaged in IV conscious sedation may want to make certain that insurance coverage applies to these activities.

Introduction. Conscious sedation is defined as a minimally depressed level of consciousness that retains the patient's ability to maintain a patent airway independently and continuously and to respond appropriately to physical stimulation and/or verbal command. Conscious sedation easily may be converted into deep sedation and/or loss of consciousness because of the unique characteristics of the drugs as well as the physical status and drug sensitivities of the individual patient. The administration of conscious sedation requires constant monitoring of the patient and the ability to respond immediately to any deviation from normal. Vigilance of the provider and the ability to recognize and intervene in the event complications or undesired outcomes arise are essential requirements for individuals administering conscious sedation.

Suggested Guidelines. The following suggested guidelines require that registered professional nurses administering IV conscious sedation have (1) the requisite knowledge and skills, (2) resuscitation equipment and emergency drugs readily available, and (3) adequate back-up of expert emergency support personnel in the event complications arise.

Management of IV conscious sedation during therapeutic, diagnostic, or surgical procedures by a registered professional nurse must be done in compliance with patient-specific written orders and may be performed by a registered professional nurse provided the following criteria are met:

1 Guidelines for patient monitoring, drug administration, and protocols for dealing with potential complications or emergency situations are available and have been developed in accordance with accepted standards of anesthesia practice.
2 The registered professional nurse managing the care of the patient receiving IV conscious sedation shall have no other responsibilities during the procedure and may not leave the patient unattended or engage in tasks that would compromise continuous monitoring.
3 A qualified professional capable of managing complications that might arise should remain on site until the patient is discharged.
4 A qualified professional authorized to discharge a patient under institutional guidelines remains on site to discharge the patient in accordance with established criteria of the facility.

To be qualified, the registered professional nurse managing the care of patients receiving IV conscious sedation must be able to:

1 Demonstrate the acquired knowledge of anatomy, physiology, pharmacology, cardiac arrhythmia recognition, and complications related to IV conscious sedation and medications.
2 Assess the total patient care requirement during IV conscious sedation. Physiologic measurements should include but not be limited to respiratory rate, saturation, blood pressure, cardiac rate and rhythm, and patient's level of consciousness. Documentation intervals should be dictated by the patient's condition; however, vital signs should be recorded at least every 5 minutes.
3 Understand the principles of oxygen delivery, transport and uptake, and respiratory physiology and understand and be able to use oxygen delivery devices.
4 Anticipate and recognize potential complications of IV conscious sedation in relation to the type of medication being administered.
5 Possess the requisite knowledge and skills to assess, diagnose, and intervene in the event of complications or undesired outcomes and to institute appropriate nursing intervention in compliance with orders (including standing orders) or institutional protocols or guidelines.
6 Demonstrate skill in airway management and resuscitation.
7 Have a thorough understanding and recognition of the legal ramifications of providing this care, especially of their responsibility and liability in the event of an untoward reaction or life-threatening complication.

Each institution or practice setting should have in place an educational/credentialing mechanism that includes a process for evaluating and documenting the individual's demonstration of the

Continued

BOX 7–3
QUALIFIED PROVIDERS OF CONSCIOUS SEDATION—*CONTINUED*

knowledge, skills, and abilities related to the management of patients receiving IV conscious sedation. Evaluation and documentation of competence should occur on a periodic basis.

The following procedural guidelines, which address monitoring modalities, emergency drugs and equipment, and ventilatory support personnel should be incorporated into the institution's/health care facility's policies and procedures for the administration of IV conscious sedation:

1 All patients having local anesthesia with conscious sedation will have a continuous IV in place.
2 All patients receiving IV conscious sedation will be continuously monitored throughout the procedure as well as the recovery phase by electrocardiogram, pulse oximetry, and blood pressure monitors.
3 Supplemental oxygen will be provided to all patients receiving IV conscious sedation per order (including standing orders).
4 An emergency cart must be immediately accessible to every location where IV conscious sedation is administered. This cart must include at least the following: emergency resuscitative drugs, airway and ventilatory adjunct equipment, defibrillator, and a source for administration of 100 percent oxygen. A positive pressure breathing device, oxygen, and appropriate airways must be in each room where IV conscious sedation is administered.
5 Provisions must be in place for back-up personnel who are experts in airway management, emergency intubation, and advanced cardiopulmonary resuscitation if complications arise.
6 Registered professional nurses who are not credentialed anesthesia providers should not administer drugs classified as anesthetics, including but not limited to ketamine, sodium pentothal, methohexital, propofol, etomidate, and nitrous oxide.

Bibliography

Applegeet, CJ: Perioperative nurse must constantly acquire new skills. AORN J 50:950, 1989.

Bell, GD, Bowen, S, Morden, A, et al: Prevention of hypoxaemia during upper gastrointestinal endoscopy by means of oxygen via nasal cannulae. Lancet 1:1022, 1987.

Finnie, G: Conscious sedation and plastic surgery. Speciality Nursing Forum 2:8, 1990.

Fogg, DM: Recommendation for instrument counts: Testing sterilizers with biological indicators: Organizational structure of OR. AORN J 49:1667, 1989.

Guidelines for the elective use of conscious sedation, deep sedation, and general anesthesia in pediatric patients. Pediatrics 76:317, 1985.

Gunn, IP: The many issues regarding IV conscious sedation. Speciality Nursing Forum 2:2, 1990.

Harvard Minimal Monitoring Standards. JAMA 256:8, 1986.

Kallar, SK: Conscious sedation for outpatient surgery. Wellcome Trends in Anesthesiology 9:8, 1991.

Kingsbury, JA: IV conscious sedation: JCAHO and hospital issues. Speciality Nursing Forum 2:7, 1990.

McDonald, JS, et al: A second-time study of the anesthetist's intraoperative period. Br J Anaesth 64:582, 1990.

Murphy, EK: Legal considerations in RN monitoring of intravenous sedation. AORN J 48:1184, 1988.

Needleman, HL: Conscious sedation for pediatric outpatient dental procedures. Int Anesthesiol Clin 27:102, 1989.

Newman, PW: IV conscious sedation: Nursing issues. Speciality Nursing Forum 2:1, 4, 1990.

Petrone, S: Perioperative nurses must prepare themselves to monitor patients receiving local anesthesia. AORN J 50:442, 1989.

Recommended practice: Monitoring the patient receiving local anesthesia. AORN J 50:624, 1989.

Ryder, W and Wright, PA: Dental sedation: A review. Br Dent J 165:207, 1988.

Separation of operator-anesthetist responsibilities. American Association of Nurse Anesthetists Position Statement. Park Ridge, IL, 1988.

Spry, CC: Perioperative nurses should keep monitoring within their speciality. AORN J 51:1071, 1990.

Tucker, MR, Ochs, MW, White, RP Jr: Arterial blood gas levels after midazolam or diazepam administered with or without fentanyl as an intravenous sedative for outpatient surgical procedures. J Oral Maxillofac Surg 44:688, 1986.

US Department of Health and Human Services Office of Medical Applications of Research. Anesthesia and sedation in the dental office. National Institutes of Health (NIH Consensus Development Conference Statement 5:10), Bethesda, MD, 1985.

Watson, DS: Recommended practices for monitoring and administering IV conscious sedation. Speciality Nursing Forum 2:3, 1990.

Watson, DS and James, DS: IV conscious sedation: Implications of monitoring patients receiving local anesthesia. AORN J 51:1512, 1990.

BOX 7–4
PREPAREDNESS FOR TREATMENT OF MALIGNANT HYPERTHERMIA

Position

The American Association of Nurse Anesthetists (AANA) recommends that every anesthetizing location have a well-defined written protocol for the diagnosis and treatment of malignant hyperthermia.

The AANA recognizes the Malignant Hyperthermia Association of the United States (MHAUS) as experts in establishing protocol for the diagnosis and treatment of malignant hyperthermia and advocates that all anesthesia providers and health care facilities adhere to the MHAUS published recommendations.

The AANA believes that the following recommendations of MHAUS are essential practices that should be implemented by anesthesia providers and health care facilities:

1 All anesthesia departments and anesthesia providers should be prepared to treat a malignant hyperthermia episode. (A preoperative and intraoperative treatment protocol is available from MHAUS.)
2 All operating and recovery room personnel should be trained in the recognition and treatment of malignant hyperthermia. (Inservice material can be provided by MHAUS.)
3 A designated cart containing dantrolene (36 vials) and the ancillary medications and equipment as recommended by MHAUS should be immediately available in the anesthetizing and recovery areas. (A list of recommended supplies is available from MHAUS.)
4 A written treatment plan should be posted with the cart in the appropriate area. (A poster is available from MHAUS.)
5 The 24-hour emergency hotline number of the MHAUS/Medical Alert Foundation should be posted on the cart and appropriate areas.

Purpose

To improve patient safety in anesthesia by increasing the awareness of the anesthesia provider of the necessity for thorough preparation to successfully manage a suspected or unsuspected occurrence of malignant hyperthermia.

Background

Malignant hyperthermia is a well-recognized syndrome that can occur in the presence of anesthesia. The morbidity of this syndrome can be quite high if it is not recognized and treated appropriately. The American Association of Nurse Anesthetists believes that thorough preoperative screening and prevention is the first step in protecting the public. Despite the increased awareness among health care professionals and screening for personal and familial history of disease, malignant hyperthermia still occurs. Because of the seriousness of this syndrome and the continued rate of occurrence, the AANA believes that measures should be taken for early detection and treatment of the disease process. With the trend toward more surgical procedures and anesthetics being performed in nontraditional settings, it is imperative that anesthesia practitioners be prepared to handle a malignant hyperthermia crisis in any and all anesthetizing locations.

Bibliography

Allen, GC, Rosenburg, H, and Fletcher, JE: Anesthetic outcome in patients previously tested negative for malignant hyperthermia susceptibility. Anesthesiology 72:619, 1990.

Ashby, D: Malignant hyperthermia: A potential crisis in the postanesthesia care unit. J Post Anesth Nurs 5:279, 1990.

Brownell, AKW and Pauke, TB: Use of local anesthetics in malignant hyperthermia. Can Med Assoc J 134:993, 1986.

DeYoung, R: Malignant Hyperthermia. In: Allan, A, (ed): Post Anesthesia Nursing Review for Certification. American Society for Post Anesthesia Nurses. Richmond, VA, 1986.

Continued

BOX 7–4
PREPAREDNESS FOR TREATMENT OF MALIGNANT HYPERTHERMIA—*CONTINUED*

Drain, C and Christoph, SS: Malignant hyperthermia. In: *The Recovery Room*. Philadelphia: WB Saunders, 1987, pp 516–521.

Gronert, GA, Schulman, SR, and Mott, J: Malignant hyperthermia. In: Miller, RD (ed): Anesthesia, 3rd ed. Churchill Livingstone, New York, 1990, pp 935–956.

Haag, G: Are you prepared for a malignant hyperthermia crisis? AANA Journal 58:250, 1990.

Jordan, LM: Malignant hyperthermia. Today's OR Nurse 9:12, 1987.

Larash, MG, Rosenberg, H, Larach, DR, et al: Prediction of malignant hyperthermia susceptibility by clinical signs. Anesthesiology 66:546, 1987.

Lopez, J, Pablo, M, and Alamo, L: Dantrolene sodium is able to reduce the resting ionic calcium in muscle from humans with malignant hyperthermia. Muscle Nerve 10:77, 1987.

Malignant Hyperthermia: The Role of the CRNA. Malignant Hyperthermia Association of the United States, Westport, CT, 1990.

Managing Malignant Hyperthermia: An Anesthetic Protocol. Malignant Hyperthermia Association of the United States, Westport, CT, 1990.

Mitchell, M: Malignant Hyperthermia: Update 1987. Current Reviews for Post Anesthesia Care Nurses 9:78, 1987.

Muldoon, SM and Karan, S: Testing in malignant hyperthermia: An update. Wellcome Trends in Anesthesiology 8:3, 1990.

Newberry, JE: Malignant hyperthermia in the postanesthesia care unit: A review of current etiology, diagnosis and treatment. J Post Anesth Nurs 5:25, 1990.

Patient Monitoring Standards. Guidelines for Nurse Anesthesia Practice. American Association of Nurse Anesthetists, Park Ridge, IL, 1989.

Pesci, B: Neuromuscular blockade and reversal agents: A primer for postanesthesia nurses. J Post Anesth Nurs 1:42, 1986.

Peter, J: Malignant hyperthermia. In Waugaman, W, Rigor, B, Katz, L, et al (eds): Principles and Practice of Nurse Anesthesia. Appleton & Lange, East Norwalk, CT, 1988, pp 585–599.

Preventing Malignant Hyperthermia: An Anesthetic Protocol. Malignant Hyperthermia Association of the United States, Westport, CT, 1990.

Rosenburg, H: Understanding Malignant Hyperthermia. Malignant Hyperthermia Association of the United States, Darien, CT, 1990.

Sessler, DI: Malignant Hyperthermia. J Pediatr 109:9, 1986.

Stoelting, RK and Miller, RD: Basics of Anesthesia. Churchill Livingstone, New York, 1984, p 400.

Suggested Therapy for Malignant Hyperthermia Emergency. Malignant Hyperthermia Association of the United States, Westport, CT, 1990.

Tomarken, J and Britt, BA: Malignant hyperthermia. Ann Emerg Med 16:1253, 1987.

Waterman, PM: Malignant hyperthermia syndrome. Current Reviews for Recovery Room Nurses 8:131, 1986.

Ward, A, Chaffman, MO, and Sorkin, EM: Dantrolene: A review of its pharmacodynamic and pharmacokinetic properties and therapeutic use in malignant hyperthermia, the neuroleptic syndrome and an update of its use in muscle spasticity. Drugs 32:130, 1986.

BOX 7–5
ADMINISTRATION OF REGIONAL ANESTHESIA BY CERTIFIED REGISTERED NURSE ANESTHETISTS

Position

Regional anesthesia can be administered by a CRNA who has received education and training in the administration of regional anesthetics.

Purpose

To recognize the current professional consensus regarding the administration of regional blocks by CRNAs.

Background

Regional anesthesia requires motor skills and can be performed safely by properly trained professionals. The scope and extent of this training is difficult to define. Didactic and clinical

BOX 7–5
ADMINISTRATION OF REGIONAL ANESTHESIA BY CERTIFIED REGISTERED NURSE ANESTHETISTS—*CONTINUED*

requirements can be set forth in a general way in the curriculum of the school, and these can be reviewed for evidence of fitness by the accrediting and credentialing bodies. Performance of a given number of the more common blocks could be made requisite to completion of the training program.

A point is soon reached, however, beyond which the identification of skill necessary to perform each blocking procedure becomes irrational. No one in anesthesia training, or in practice for that matter, performs all types of regional blocks. Certain fundamental precepts can be stated relative to the safe administration of local anesthetic drugs and to principles of asepsis, nerve localization, and evaluation of the resulting analgesia. Beyond these basic principles, boundaries must be established by fiat and can prove troublesome to defend if exposed to close scrutiny. No statutory or regulatory preclusions for administration of regional anesthesia by CRNAs currently exist in the United States.

Overall, the risks related to regional anesthesia are no greater than those imposed by general anesthesia. To affirm the legitimacy of nurse anesthesia practice and restrict the scope of practice at the same time is to impose restraints that may be inimical to the health of the community.

The nurse anesthetist can function effectively only if all safe and satisfactory procedures are made available and can be utilized on proper indication.

This position reinforces the prevailing positive attitude toward regional anesthesia performed by nurse anesthetists. Since many schools now incorporate this training as part of their programs, there would seem to be no need to belabor this position. Further, it would serve no useful purpose to draw boundaries. As the number of nurse anesthetists who administer blocks increases, the barriers will diminish. This is best developed in an atmosphere of peaceful evolution. The evidence of competent performance of blocks by nurse anesthetists is now overwhelming; the fact that this development is progressing rapidly is undeniable. Let it proceed.

BOX 7–6
POSITION STATEMENT—CERTIFIED REGISTERED NURSE ANESTHETISTS' UTILIZATION OF INVASIVE MONITORING TECHNIQUES

Position

Certified Registered Nurse Anesthetists (CRNAs) are capable of instituting various invasive monitoring techniques as a part of their anesthesia practice in evaluation and treatment of patients. Those CRNAs who have been engaged in anesthesia practice whereby the need for such skills has been limited and who therefore lack the skill or are unable to maintain competence in these procedures must acquire training from a CRNA or other professional skilled in these procedures prior to incorporating such techniques into practice. Competence is defined as including the necessary knowledge and technical skill required to assure patient benefit and safety. The knowledge requirement includes: (1) the normal and abnormal ranges of data that may be derived from the particular monitoring modality and its meaning within the context of the individual patient and the anesthetic and medical procedures being performed; (2) indications and contraindications for such monitoring modalities and any tests that should be performed prior to initiating such procedures; (3) anatomic and physiologic parameters that impact the initiation and maintenance of such monitoring modalities; (4) range of therapeutic actions that may be taken to return abnormal physiologic alterations to normal; and (5) possible complications that can result from such monitoring, including their treatment.

Purpose

This statement is intended to provide guidance to the CRNAs and other individuals involved in the development of institutional, departmental, or nurse anesthesia education program policies

Continued

BOX 7–6
POSITION STATEMENT—CERTIFIED REGISTERED NURSE ANESTHETISTS' UTILIZATION OF INVASIVE MONITORING TECHNIQUES—*CONTINUED*

with regard to the actual insertion of invasive monitoring lines (central venous pressure, arterial, and pulmonary artery catheters) and subsequent monitoring of pertinent physiologic parameters by CRNAs and nurse anesthesia students.

Background

Arterial, central venous, and pulmonary artery monitoring are components of patient assessment within anesthesia and intensive care settings. While every patient may not require such monitoring, many do, and such a need may not always be identified prior to the induction of general anesthesia. Therefore, CRNAs should be prepared to initiate such monitoring modalities and interpret the data derived.

Arterial and/or central venous monitoring may be utilized for patients in whom there is a need for but not limited to (1) continuous assessment of cardiac function—particularly that of the left ventricle—including the impact of anesthesia and/or concurrent medical interventions on such function; (2) maintenance of strict fluid balance or block replacement so that either hypotension or congestive heart failure with pulmonary edema may be prevented; (3) accurate assessment of arterial and venous pressure; (4) assessment of the adequacy of respiratory function to achieve particular therapeutic goals through intermittent sampling to determine arterial blood gas values; and (5) recognition and treatment of air emboli resulting from the positioning of the patient and/or the surgical site.

members that a rapid sequence induction would be the standard of care for the induction of general anesthesia. Future department members are acquainted with this policy and are expected to provide care to patients as outlined by the policy.

Standards may evolve from nonprofessional sources such as insurance companies. Medical malpractice insurance companies may mandate specific clinical behavior such as the use of specific patient monitoring devices for insurability. In 1986, The St. Paul Fire and Marine Company had advised the anesthesia providers it insured to employ pulse oximetry during all anesthetic procedures, and they have encouraged the use of capnography. Today the use of pulse oximetry and capnography is considered standard for all patients under the care of an anesthesia provider. Undoubtedly insurance companies may strongly influence the establishment of standards of care by refusing to insure those who do not use specific monitoring modalities.[12]

Federal agencies (e.g., Health Care Financing Administration) will continue to have an impact on the development of standards. Accrediting agencies such as the Joint Commission on Accreditation of Health Care Organizations (JCAHO) influence the development of practice standards. For instance, JCAHO specifies that all patients presenting for anesthesia receive a comprehensive preoperative and postoperative anesthesia visit (a process standard). The standard was formulated to ensure that all patients in JCAHO-accredited health care facilities would be afforded a preoperative and postoperative visit.

Equipment manufacturers and product standard organizations may publish "voluntary" standards that assist in the operation or purchase of anesthesia-related equipment. Examples include the Z-79 Committee of the American National Standards Institute. The Z-79 Committee has published standards for anesthesia machine construction (the incorporation of a gas-flow ratio protection mechanism to avoid the unintended delivery of hypoxic gas mixtures from the anesthesia machine), as well as the construction and testing of endotracheal tubes, anesthesia ventilators, and oxygen analyzers. The Food and Drug Administration (FDA) is a government organization that has published standards on anesthesia equipment. The FDA *Anesthesia Apparatus Checkout Recommendations*[13] have encouraged the development of anesthesia machine checklists for the preoperative assurance of proper function of the anesthesia machine. This checklist is currently being modified and refined.[14] Although the limits of its usage today are unknown, it is conceivable that this checkout procedure may become the standard for preoperative machine checkout in the future.

A final source of standards is the determination of the standard of care by the judiciary. Anesthesia providers are generally required to meet a national standard of care,[15] which is determined by a judge or jury from testimony of an expert witness. Testimony provided by the expert witness must not be speculative or personal opinion but should convey factual information relative to the case being litigated. Experts who articulate personal opinion and have this opinion accepted by the judge or jury may assist in the establishment of new standards.[16]

INTERPRETATION AND APPLICATION OF PROFESSIONAL PRACTICE STANDARDS

Standards are descriptive of the professional responsibilities for which the practitioner is accountable. Like practice guidelines, standards are constructed from a consensus process involving expert opinion, scientific evidence, and practitioner experience. The literal wording of a standard mandates specific clinical behavior that must be rigidly applied by the professional. In addition, the practitioner must be afforded an environment that is properly equipped to meet the standard. For instance, the *AANA Patient Monitoring Standards* mandate assessment of adequate oxygenation with continuous pulse oximetry. Pulse oximetry must be available to the practitioner for the standard to be met.

How enduring is the intent of the standard following its adoption by a professional organization? Standards reflect the philosophy and the professional responsibilities of the membership, and therefore should be steadfast with time. However, like practice guidelines, standards may require revision to reflect acquired scientific knowledge, changes in technology, and clinical practice. The following discussion highlighting the *Patient Monitoring Standards* illustrates the need for the periodic review and revision of promulgated professional standards.

The *Patient Monitoring Standards,* which appear in Box 7–7, were adopted by the AANA in 1989 and revised in 1992. The standard for monitoring ventilatory adequacy is stated as follows: "Correct placement of an endotracheal tube must be verified by auscultation, chest excursion and end-tidal CO_2 monitoring when available." Since the adoption of the standards, end-tidal CO_2 monitoring has evolved as an accepted monitoring tool for the verification of endotracheal tube placement following endotracheal intubation. Birmingham and colleagues[17] reviewed the detection techniques for esophageal intubation and concluded that end-tidal CO_2 monitoring is the most incontestable monitor for the detection of successful endotracheal intubation. Consequently, end-tidal CO_2 monitoring is now viewed as the standard of care for the detection of correct positioning of the endotracheal tube within the trachea.[18] This standard has evolved because of this technology's availability, nationwide application, and scientific validation. As a result of the advancement in technology and changes in clinical practice since the adoption of the standards, the AANA has recently adopted language mandating the use of end-tidal CO_2 monitoring for verification of proper placement of the endotracheal tube following endotracheal intubation.

Box 7–1 assists the practitioner in outlining the requirements for safe and competent anesthesia care as well as providing the framework for the evaluation of one's professional practice.

The Patient Monitoring Standards elaborate the quantitative and qualitative monitoring that should be used for all patients during anesthesia care. These standards apply to all nurse anesthetists regardless of practice environment. It is the nurse anesthetist's professional responsibility to meet these standards. If the practitioner is unable to comply with these standards, the reasons for noncompliance should be clearly documented on the patient's medical record (the progress note of the medical record, or the anesthesia record itself). While these process standards encourage quality anesthesia care, they do not ensure specific patient outcomes.

BOX 7–7
AMERICAN ASSOCIATION OF NURSE ANESTHETISTS PATIENT MONITORING STANDARDS

Basic to safe anesthesia care is the application of qualitative and quantitative monitoring that enables the anesthetist to administer anesthesia and evaluate its effect in a manner that optimizes desired responses while minimizing the risks of anesthesia. Fundamental to this endeavor is the use of multiple monitoring modalities, which play vital roles in assisting anesthetists to provide conscientious care to patients receiving anesthesia.

These patient monitoring standards are intended to assist the CRNA practitioner in providing consistent, safe anesthesia care. These standards apply to patients undergoing general, regional, or monitored anesthesia care for diagnostic or therapeutic procedures in designated anesthetizing locations. In extenuating circumstances, the CRNA must use clinical judgment in prioritizing and implementing these standards. All of these standards do not normally apply to epidural analgesia for labor or pain management therapy. The standards may be exceeded in any or all respects at any time at the discretion of the anesthetist, as required by individual patient needs.

While the standards are intended to encourage high-quality patient care, they cannot ensure specific patient outcomes. It is recognized that appropriately used monitoring modalities may fail to detect untoward clinical developments. Further, it is recognized by the AANA that under some circumstances certain monitoring standards may not be applicable. While this is a fact of practice, the omission of one or more monitoring standards should be documented and the reason stated on the patient's anesthesia record. Interruptions in monitoring may be unavoidable. Occasionally, the anesthetist must work at some distance from the patient because of an environmental hazard such as, but not limited to, radiation. Under such circumstances, provisions for monitoring the patient must be made and documented on the patient's anesthesia record. Adequate facilities must exist to enable remote patient monitoring. The standards are subject to review and revision from time to time, as indicated by technology and practice.

Anesthesia Providers

Continuous clinical observation and anesthetist vigilance are the basis of safe anesthesia care. The anesthetist, or nurse anesthesia student, shall be in constant attendance of the patient until the responsibility for care has been accepted by another qualified health provider.

Patient Monitors

Ventilation

Purpose. To assess adequate ventilation of the patient. (Standard in effect until October 1, 1992).

Standard. Ventilatory adequacy shall be assessed by continuous auscultation of breath sounds. Correct placement of an endotracheal tube must be verified by auscultation, chest excursion and end-tidal CO_2 monitoring when available. Other quantitative ventilatory devices may be used in conjunction with auscultation, such as spirometry and ventilatory pressure monitors.

Standard. Intubation of the trachea shall be verified by auscultation, chest excursion, and confirmation of carbon dioxide in the expired gas. Controlled or assisted ventilation during the anesthetic shall be monitored continuously with an end-tidal carbon dioxide monitor. Additionally, spirometry and ventilatory pressure monitors may also be used.

Breathing System Disconnect Monitor. When the patient is ventilated by an automatic mechanical ventilator, the integrity of the breathing system shall be monitored by a device that is capable of detecting the disconnection of any component of the breathing system. Such a device shall be equipped with an audible alarm that is activated when its limits are exceeded.

Oxygenation

Purpose. To assess adequate oxygenation of the patient.

Standard. Adequacy of patient oxygenation shall be monitored continuously with pulse oximetry. In addition to pulse oximetry, oxygenation shall also be monitored by observation of skin color, the color of the blood in the surgical field, and arterial blood gas analysis when indicated.

BOX 7–7
AMERICAN ASSOCIATION OF NURSE ANESTHETISTS PATIENT MONITORING STANDARDS—*CONTINUED*

During general anesthesia, the oxygen concentration delivered by the anesthesia machine shall be monitored continuously with an oxygen analyzer with a low-concentration oxygen concentration limit alarm. An oxygen supply failure alarm system shall be operational to warn of low oxygen pressure to the anesthesia machine.

Circulation

Purpose. To assess adequacy of the cardiovascular system.
Standard. Blood pressure and heart rate shall be determined and recorded at least every 5 minutes. The patient's electrocardiogram shall be monitored continuously during the course of the anesthetic.
Circulation shall be assessed by at least one of the following measures: digital palpation of the pulse, auscultation of heart sounds, continuous intra-arterial pressure monitoring, electronic pulse monitoring, or pulse oximetry.

Body Temperature

Purpose. To assess changes in body temperature.
Standard. Body temperature shall be intermittently or continuously monitored and recorded on all patients receiving general anesthesia; the means to monitor temperature shall be immediately available for use on all patients receiving local or regional anesthesia and used when indicated.

Neuromuscular Function

Purpose. To assess neuromuscular function.
Standard. The means to evaluate the patient's neuromuscular function by the use of a nerve stimulator shall be available immediately when neuromuscular blocking agents have been used.

Anesthesia Equipment

A complete equipment safety check shall be performed daily and an abbreviated check of all equipment shall be performed before each anesthetic is administered. All anesthesia machines and monitoring equipment shall conform to the appropriate national and state standards. An ongoing preventative maintenance program shall be established and enforced.

SUMMARY

It is incumbent on all CRNAs to be aware of the practice standards, guidelines, and position statements of their professional association, as all are a measure against which the CRNA can be evaluated. Also, the interpretation of a CRNA's compliance to practice parameters should not be left solely to external agencies, which often lack a clear understanding of the context within which care is provided, resulting in misapplication or unwarranted negative evaluations. The future clearly portends increasing reliance on practice standards and guidelines as the measure of a CRNA's ability to obtain practice rights, reimbursement authority, and statutory and legal recognition.

REFERENCES

1. Metcalf, H and Urwiek, L: Dynamic Administration: The Collected Papers of Mary Follett. Harper & Brothers, New York, 1942.
2. Guidelines and Standards for Nurse Anesthesia Practice. American Association of Nurse Anesthetists, Park Ridge, Il, 1992.
3. Blumenreich, GA: Standard of care. AANA Journal 55(4):312–314, 1987.
4. Woolf, SH: Practice guidelines: A new reality in medicine. Arch Intern Med 150:1812, 1990.
5. Chassin, MR: Practice guidelines: Best hope for quality improvement in the 1990's. J Occup Med 32(12):1199–1206, 1990.

6. Woolf, SH: The process of developing practice guidelines. Decubitus 4(2):28–31, 1991.
7. Field, MJ and Lohr, KN: Clinical Practice Guidelines: Directions for a New Program. National Press Academy, Washington, DC, 1990.
8. Guidelines for Obstetrical Anesthesia and Conduction Analgesia for Certified Registered Nurse Anesthetists. American Association of Nurse Anesthetists, Park Ridge, IL, 1991.
9. Eichhorn, JH, Cooper, JB, Cullen, DJ, et al: Standards for patient monitoring during anesthesia at Harvard Medical School. JAMA 256:1017–1020, 1986.
10. Standards for Basic Intraoperative Monitoring. American Society of Anesthesiologists, Park Ridge, IL, 1986.
11. Eichhorn, JH: Are There Standards for Intraoperative Monitoring? Advances in Anesthesia 5:3, 1988.
12. Gravenstein, JS: Failure to Monitor. In Gravenstein, JS, Newbower, RS, Ream, AK, et al (eds): Essential Invasive Monitoring in Anesthesia. Grune & Stratton, New York, 1980, pp 305–310.
13. Carstensen, P: FDA issues pre-use check out. Anesthesia Patient Safety Foundation Newsletter 1:13, 15, 17, 1986.
14. March, MG and Crowley, JJ: An Evaluation of Anesthesiologists' Present Checkout Methods and the Validity of the FDA Checklist. Anesthesiology 75:724–729, 1991.
15. Blumenreich, GA: The Standard of Care. AANA Journal 59(4):302, 1991.
16. Gild, WM: Expert Witness Sets New Standard for Anesthesia Practice. ASA Newsletter 55:6, 13, 1991.
17. Birmingham, PK, Cheney, FW, and Ward, RJ: Esophageal intubation: A review of detection techniques. Anesth Analg 65:886–891, 1986.
18. Eichhorn, JH: ASA Standards Amended. Anesth Patient Safety Found Newsletter 6:1, 1–6, 1991.

THREE

The Health Care Delivery System and the CRNA

8

The Health Care Delivery System in the United States

Ira P. Gunn

OUTLINE

OBJECTIVES

On completing this chapter, the reader will be able to:

1. Understand, in conceptual terms, the structure of the U.S. health care delivery system.
2. Describe the historical development of the U.S. health care system.
3. Indentify the primary public and private sector roles in the delivery of health care.
4. Indentify major service resources within the health care system.
5. List major problems associated with the current health care delivery system and future perspectives on how a reformed system may address these issues.

The health care system within the United States differs significantly from those in other developed countries. As such, many of its problems are unique; however, all health systems today are overextended, costly, and to some extent present problems relating to patient access. Although the quality and scope of health care resources and technology in the United States are still generally regarded as preeminent, it is clear that the system is in crisis because of its failure to contain costs and serve the basic health care needs of all its citizens.

The configuration of the health care delivery system within the United States is a product of this country's founding economic tenets and the medical profession's influence on its design, as described in Paul Starr's book *The Social Transformation of American Medicine.*[1] Since the late 1800s, state and federal governments legislatively codified much of the structural design of the health care system promulgated by organized medicine. Because of these early and effective attempts at system control, it has taken significant effort to make any statutory or regulatory revision that would enhance system flexibility or accommodate social need.

The current health care crisis has resulted largely from the failure of the health care delivery system and its providers to accommodate change. Some would claim it is the service sector that has abrogated much of its implicit social responsibility. This problem has been manifested in exploding costs, lack of patient access, and inadequate care for some segments of the population. This crisis continues to deepen, affecting every segment of American life, including the U.S. economy.

Health care reform, of which anesthesia payment reform is a small part, has become the predominant political theme of this decade. Exactly what the new look of the health care delivery system will be must await thorough public discussion and legislative imperatives. That system could resemble a modification of our current system, a move to managed care or managed competition, or a single-payer system sponsored by the federal government. Most agree, however, that changes will be sweeping, requiring all providers, including Certified Registered Nurse Anesthetists (CRNAs), to be not only informed consumers but informed policy decision makers. This chapter considers the historical evolution of health care delivery in the United States, its current status, and issues under study.

HISTORICAL OVERVIEW OF THE DEVELOPMENT OF THE HEALTH CARE SYSTEM

While there were a variety of types of physicians in the United States in the late 1800s, the allopathic physicians ultimately won control of the health delivery system. The early design of the system made physicians the gatekeepers to health care and assured that persons seeking care would initially have to be seen by a physician. This was accomplished largely by passage of the Medical Practice Acts that licensed physicians in each of the states, beginning in 1873. While some practice acts were enacted in the late 17th and 18th century, these were all repealed by 1850, due to the chaotic state of medical education and wide variations in the quality of physician providers.

Some of the early practice acts were aimed at setting reimbursement rates for physicians based on their varying levels of competence and education. While some physicians were university educated, others had been trained in apprenticeship programs. It was another quarter-century before the medical educational system was sufficiently stable to allow them to publicly endorse a monopoly over the whole of health care.[2] Bullough,[3] Safreit,[4] and Hadley[5] state that medicine claimed the whole of health care for itself since no other health providers were licensed at the time, including nurses. In the intervening decades, nonphysician health providers have had to work diligently to reclaim their areas of practice through the legislative process (Box 8–1).

Licensing acts not only placed the physician in a position to control the care provided to patients but also essentially extended that control over other health providers. Consequently, their economic control of the health care dollar was assured. Certainly, physicians had more education than other health workers at that time, so it

BOX 8–1
SAMPLE OF MEDICAL PRACTICE DEFINITION IN WHICH MEDICINE CLAIMS THE WHOLE OF HEALTH CARE*

Medical Practice includes any person who shall diagnose, cure, relieve in any degree or profess or attempt to diagnose, cure or relieve any human disease, ailment, defect, abnormality, or complaint, whether of a physical or mental origin, by attendance or advice, by prescribing, using or furnishing any drug, appliance, manipulation, adjustment or [other] method or by any therapeutic agent whatsoever.

*From South Carolina Medical Practice Act, paragraph 40–47–40, Code of Laws of South Carolina, 1976, as amended.

was not difficult for them to achieve dominance. Further, they were organized to achieve that purpose, while organization of other health providers came later. It should be noted that neither the economic stature nor economic rewards for physicians at the turn of the century compare with what they are today. The U.S. population was mostly rural, and the distances patients and their doctors had to travel to see each other took a significant portion of their time, so the number of patients serviced was much smaller than that common today. The pay took the form of a dozen eggs, a couple of chickens, and in some instances money. In addition, there were only a few services that early physicians could provide as medical knowledge was still ill defined or ill understood. Many of those responsibilities today fall within the nature and practice of nursing. Few rural areas had hospitals, and therefore patients were cared for in their homes. Thus, physicians could not rely extensively on nurses or allied health professionals. In fact, except for nurses and pharmacists, many allied health professionals and technicians did not exist.

The physicians' greatest competitors at the turn of the century were the so-called nostrum makers, that is, the makers and sellers of patented medicines. It was not until the passage of the Federal Pure Food and Drug Act in 1906 that the American Medical Association (AMA) began to gain some control over pharmaceuticals and prescription.[1]

While nursing, or nurturing, existed during prehistoric times,[6] as did elements of medicine, formalized nursing in the United States did not appear until physicians were well into the process of seeking licensure. In 1873, there were three schools of nursing.[7] By 1900, there were 432.[7] Many of these schools were established as a cheap source of labor for the developing hospital industry. Florence Nightingale, whose nursing philosophies and traditions influenced early American nursing, did not believe in state or government licensing, but felt that educational programs should be of such quality as to make graduation the sole requisite for professional credibility and recognition.

However, the proliferation of nursing programs in the United States indicated that there was such variation in quality that nursing leaders eventually sought state licensure. Unfortunately, early legislation adopted the practice of registration, wherein the title was protected, but not the practice. That is, the scope of nursing practice was not defined within a registration model as would have been the case under a licensure model. The first state to enact such legislation was North Carolina. Also important and unlike other professional education disciplines in the United States, state boards of nursing were given responsibility for approving nursing educational programs, in addition to registering nurses.[2] In 1938, The National League for Nursing Education began a private sector accreditation program for nursing education. Subsequently its name was changed to the National League for Nursing.[8]

The urbanization of this country also began in earnest with the industrial revolution. In the early 1900s, physicians, church groups, and others began building hospitals for the care of the sick, predominantly in cities. By this time, the germ theory had been enunciated and principles of disinfection and sterilization were being employed that stimulated the growth of hospitals, allowing large numbers of patients to be confined in one institution without the traditional fears of patient-to-patient contamination. Further, because of urbanization and industrialization, few families in cities were well equipped at home to take care of their family members during serious illnesses. Through the efforts of nurses and social workers, the Henry Street Settlement in New York City pioneered the public health movement and the visiting nurse concept for care of the indigent. Congress passed the Sheppard-Towner Act of 1921. This act helped finance public health nurses in training nurse midwives. State laws were passed to register births and license midwives. Soon statistics documented lower maternal and infant mortality at low costs. However, the predictable opposition by organized medicine arose because these programs were not under physician control or direction. This lead to the inevitable discontinuation of the Sheppard-Towner Act.[6,8,9]

Major expansion of community-based hospitals, particularly in rural areas, awaited the passage of the Hill-Burton Act by Congress in 1946. "In its first twenty years 4,678 projects were undertaken, almost half directed to communities with under 10,000 population."[10] Of note, discrimination was a modus operandi of many of the early hospitals in awarding staff membership and clinical privileges. Most often, privileges were restricted to white, male physicians. Early female physicians had to build their own hospitals if they were to benefit from this mode of practice, as did black physicians. Often a qualification for hospital staff privileges was membership in the medical society. At that time, women and blacks were not readily admitted to these societies, and ended in setting up their own societies.[2,8,9] This, of course, was a reflection of the social mores of this nation, until the civil rights legislation of the 1960s.

Health insurance to assist patients in paying for their health care did not get its start until the late 1920s. Interest in health insurance actually had begun in the United States by 1910. The idea put forth at this time was that of universal coverage. Payment for the insurance was to be divided between state government, employers, and employees. Because many physicians believed its emergence was inevitable, many, including the AMA, abandoned their opposition and endorsed these early initiatives. However, World War I intervened, and compulsory insurance began to be cast in the mold of being un-American, and was often termed a "Prussianization of America."

Commercial insurance companies, physicians in New York state, and a labor leader, Samuel Gompers, who preferred higher wages to fringe benefits, began to oppose universal health insurance.[11] In 1925, the New York State Medical Society reported that ". . . health insurance is a dead issue in the United States. . . . It is not conceivable that any serious effort will again be made to subsidize medicine as the handmaiden of the public."[11] A medical historian stated that physicians of the time did not reckon with the great depression that was soon to come, which would threaten the financial security of both physicians and hospitals, and reopen the consideration of health insurance.[11]

In 1929, voluntary health insurance got its start in Dallas, Texas, when 1250 teachers agreed to pay Baylor University Hospital 50 cents a month for hospital insurance. This insurance afforded each teacher 21 days of hospitalization per year. This was the forerunner of Blue Cross, a private, not-for-profit, hospital insurance corporation. Blue Shield, the other part of the "Blues" which covers physician payments, was not formalized until 1946.[12]

The major impetus for the acceptance and spread of private health insurance came from the labor movement shortly after World War II, when the Supreme Court ruled that labor unions could appropriately negotiate or strike over health care benefits for their members. It was at this time that American industry began to offer health benefits to their employees, and today, it is almost unthinkable that major employers would not offer health insurance as an employee benefit.[12] Unfortunately, due to the current health care crisis, this benefit is now perceived by many business leaders as a basis for declining competitiveness and is, consequently, undergoing significant review and change. Retirees are being eliminated from plans promised for life, coverage is being reduced, and beneficiaries are having to pay larger deductibles and copayments.

The most alarming aspect of the current health insurance crisis relates to the potential of losing one's health insurance after being laid off from a job and not being able to qualify for insurance elsewhere because of a prior health problem. Further, the Supreme Court has ruled that companies who self-insure their employees can reduce health coverage for selected health conditions without prior notice or penalty. Many major corporations have become self-insured due to the escalating costs of health insurance, allowed by the Employment Retirement Income Security Act (ERISA). These changes have promoted anxiety in many employees of self-insured companies over their health benefits.

Essentially, as an outgrowth of American medicine's design, the health care delivery system became physician-controlled, acute care–centered, and hospital-based. The payment system was designed to permit physicians to be reimbursed directly by their patients on a fee-for-service basis. Thus medicine had gained through its state licensing acts exclusive privileges and a monopoly as gatekeeper to the delivery of health services in the United States.

Medicine as a state-endorsed monopoly has been traditionally protected from restrictive practices that in the business world would have made individuals, groups, or companies subject to federal and state antitrust laws. It was not until 1976 that the U.S. Supreme Court ruled that the nation's antitrust laws also applied to the professions.[13] Thus, monopolization of markets, conspiring to restrain trade, or price fixing, wherein the profession did not have an exclusive legal prerogative, made them vulnerable to actions under both federal and state antitrust laws. A variety of antitrust allegations have been made against groups of physicians or professional societies with varying results, as they have been against other professionals. However, the cost of such litigation and the length of time required to finalize court decisions have served to reduce the number of actions undertaken under these laws. In some instances either the state or federal governments' antitrust operatives may seek "consent decrees" from persons charged with an antitrust violation to correct situations in which restrictive practices and/or price fixing were alleged.

While many of the arguments the medical profession made for instituting the system as designed were based on quality concerns, there can be little question that the profession was equally concerned about its economic status. Physicians and hospitals have usually been allowed to determine the value of their own services and been given authority to charge what they believed the market would bear. Such practice is usually consistent with our capitalistic system based on the supply and demand theory of a market economy. Unfortunately, the demand for health care services is often significantly influenced by the principal suppliers of that system, the hospital and the physician. Some health policy analysts view the health care system as a traditional market, when it is really an aberration of this model; a view that constitutes a major factor in the current cost crisis in health care.[1,10,12,14]

TODAY'S HEALTH CARE DELIVERY SYSTEM

The basic elements of the health care delivery system resemble, in large measure, the early design created by organized medicine. Today's situation is certainly far more complex and more regulated, but it has yet been largely resistant to change. Consequently, reform measures are well underway.

The major players in the health care delivery system today are health providers (both individuals and institutions or agencies); health payers (health insurers—public and private, industry, individuals); health regulators (public and private); health manufacturers (equipment, pharmaceuticals, etc.); and health clients. In addition to physicians, hospitals have played a major role in influencing today's delivery system.

Hospitals in the United States impact on the delivery of health services in the following ways:

(1) Hospital ownership reflects the pluralism of American society itself. They are owned by the government and by private groups. Those hospitals under private ownership are usually held by various religious, racial, ethnic, and organizational groups. They may be voluntary, nonprofit, or for-profit operations, community-supported at local levels or supported by municipalities, state, or federal governments.

(2) They have also served to define social class and race, including the poor, the wealthy, and a myriad of ethnic groups. While civil rights laws eliminated overt hospital segregation of races, public and private hospitals still often segregate the poor from the wealthy, in more discrete and subtle ways.

(3) Few American hospitals have large endowments and many depend largely on revenues generated from patient services.

(4) Hospitals focus on acute care and high technology, and on surgery in particular due to its revenue potential.

(5) Many consumers perceive a symbiotic relationship between hospitals and physicians; the physician needs hospitals in which to admit patients, and the hospital needs the physician's patients in order to fill beds and pay for its operation. Inherent within this symbiotic relationship, however, are control issues, by medicine as its workhouse, or by administrators as an independent corporate bureaucracy.[10] The doctors are "privileged" to work in hospitals and to admit patients, and have exerted that privileging control, via medical staff policies, to keep other providers out who might afford them competition. Physician influence dominates the hospital environment, especially within the domain of policy making, often to the detriment of other health provider employees, including nurses, therapists, and technicians.

(6) Medical schools, especially university based, have undue influence on the hospital system. They capitalize on virtually all resources causing tensions related to governance and cost.

As these six characteristics are in constant interaction, hospitals are in constant change.[10] "They are affirming and defining mirrors of the culture in which we live, beaming back to us, through the scope and style of the buildings, the organizational personality of the institution and the underlying meaning of the whole enterprise, the values we impute to medicine, technology, wealth, class, and social welfare."[10]

PUBLIC SECTOR ROLES IN HEALTH CARE

Government, at national, state, and local levels, plays substantial roles in health care. Its principal roles relate to financing, delivery, and regulation,[15] although each level of government may approach its role from a different perspective and concept of responsibility. However, secondary roles of government, which directly affect its other roles, include funding of health professions' education and research. Further, each role of government, regardless of jurisdiction, is broader than is immediately apparent. Table 8-1 provides an overview of these roles at varying levels of government.

While the federal government has been a provider of health care services since the Revolutionary War, its role as a major financier of health services came with the enactment of Medicare and Medicaid legislation in 1965.[16] Medicare was conceived as an earned entitlement health insurance program for the elderly paid for by Social Security taxes. The program initially afforded insurance for physician services and hospitalization. Over the years, additional health care providers, including CRNAs, have gained direct reimbursement for services. Many outpatient services are now covered, particularly after the enactment of the Prospective Payment System in 1983, to contain hospital costs. Because patients are now being discharged earlier, as a cost containment measure, coverage for selected home health services was added because many of these patients required continued or rehabilitation care. Medicaid affords health services for the indigent, with the federal government and state governments jointly funding the program and the states operating them. Thus, eligibility for Medicaid is determined by each state, as are any restrictions on health services and reimbursement

TABLE 8–1

MAJOR HEALTH CARE ROLES OF FEDERAL, STATE, AND LOCAL GOVERNMENTS

	Financing	*Delivery*	*Regulation*
Federal	Large role through the Medicare, Medicaid, and other government-sponsored programs; subsidizes selected health professional educational programs; subsidizes much health-related research and other studies.	Operates health care clinics and hospitals for care of military, veterans, Indians, and research subjects at the National Institutes of Health. (Formerly provided services at public health hospitals and clinic for seamen and patients with infectious diseases.)	Regulates health programs it finances through setting conditions for participation, qualification for and conditions and rates for reimbursement, etc.; approves drugs and devices for use in health care; regulates controlled substances distribution; prohibits providers discrimination in care provision; enforces laws having applicability to the nation's health and health care delivery
State	Funds Medicaid with help of federal government, including some long-term care, mental health services, some public health services; subsidizes health professional and occupational education	Operates mental health and mental retardation hospitals, health departments, academic health centers, prison medical facilities	Regulates health and liability insurance; licenses or otherwise credentials health institutions and personnel defining scopes of practice; establishes health codes and standards; enforces standards
Local	Subsidizes public and teaching hospitals; funds local public health departments and clinics; subsidizes some indigent care in the absence of a municipal hospital	Operates clinics and municipal hospitals, operates public health departments.	Establishes and enforces local health codes

rates for providers. Unless reimbursement to selected providers is mandated by federal law, the state determines who will be directly reimbursed for covered services. It should be noted that the federal government today pays approximately 41 percent of all health care costs in this country.[15]

The Health Care Financing Administration (HCFA) is the major payer for the federal government. However, HCFA uses the private insurance industry as its intermediary in reimbursing health services associated with the Medicare Program. HCFA is also responsible for providing the federal portion of funding to the states for their Medicaid programs. Medicaid is usually operated by the State Department of Health, using a private insurer as intermediary.

Workers' compensation programs are state-operated health programs that are designed to pay for health services and disability claims resulting from occupational injury or hazards. While administered through private insurance companies, the state may impose restrictions on services and reimbursement to health care providers and limit disability payments. Like all other health programs, the cost of workers' compensation programs has escalated significantly over the past few years, compounding the overall cost to business and industry for the health services of its workers.

There are multiple other governmental programs aimed at assisting various groups to acquire resources needed to maintain good health. These include maternal and child health programs, which unfortunately have become seriously underfunded in recent years, state rehabilitation programs for children with disabilities, and state mental health programs.

The federal, state, and local governments also bear responsibility for monitoring health care and its delivery, including those national, statewide, or community services essential to the health of all citizens. Monitoring includes assessing the quality and adequacy of health services, the outcomes of care, the adequacy and availability of health personnel and institutional resources, reportable diseases, safety of water and disposal of sewage and other hazardous wastes, environmental conditions having an impact on the public health, food handlers and food service facilities, and so on.

Another significant role of government in health care involves funding much of the basic and applied research associated with disease, injury, treatment modalities, delivery systems, and so on. In addition to establishing and funding the National Institutes of Health, including the Center for Nursing Research, many university and private research groups derive funding from government or private foundations in support of health care and services.

Finally, the government plays a major role in providing educational funding for a variety of health professionals, thus directly affecting the available supply of health manpower. The federal government maintains a Health Manpower Division and a Division of Nursing within the U.S. Department of Health and Human Services (USDHHS) to monitor health human resources and to oversee disbursement of federal funds related to educational funding. Unfortunately, their hands are somewhat tied by congressional appropriations and those for whom these appropriations are destined. These decisions are essentially a function of the political and legislative process rather than in response to bona fide manpower shortages, wherever they exist. In fact, the excess of physicians projected by the end of this century reflects efforts to expand the number of medical schools and the supply of physicians, efforts which date back to the late 1960s.[12] While federal funding for medical education has been reduced, states continue to fund increased numbers of medical schools at the behest of the powerful states' medical education lobbies. At present, federal funding for health education, administered through the USDHHS, amounts to $4.8 billion annually for medical education, while only $400 million is spent for both nursing and allied health education.[17]

The overall spending for medical education has far outstripped that portion of money allotted for nonphysician health care providers, both at the state and federal level. In a study performed in the state of Texas in 1992, it was found that the average cost of preparation of one physician, from the beginning of his or her premed course through medical school and residency, was approximately $650,000 while that of preparing a CRNA was approximately $60,000.[18]

The imbalance in human health resource needs, where there are shortages of nurses (including nurse anesthetists, nurse midwives, and nurse practitioners) and of allied health professionals, is in all probability a function of excess physician production when compared with other health professionals. This also includes the excess money put into medical education compared to that for other health professionals.

Although space limitations prohibit further discussion of government's role in health care delivery, health payers—both government and private—determine directly or indirectly how health care will be delivered, where it will be delivered, what will be delivered, how often, and to whom it will be delivered. Nonphysician health professionals seeking more autonomy in practice and the ability to be reimbursed for their own services ignore at their peril the influence health care funding and reimbursement have on their practice. The skills and capability to influence legislation and regulation are as important in configuring the environment for nurse anesthesia practice as the skills to perform intubations are to the administration of anesthesia.

PRIVATE SECTOR ROLES IN HEALTH CARE

The private sector roles in health care also revolve around education, financing, delivery, research and regulation, although in the latter category this is restricted to credentialing mechanisms such as those involved in accreditation, certification, and recertification. In addition, the private sector is also involved in the research, manufacture, and marketing of health drugs and devices and the education of health professionals who use the drugs and technology. Table 8–2 summarizes the roles of private health care providers, organizations, institutions, and other private sector entities in health care and its delivery.

Additional private sector groups that impact the delivery of health care include a broad variety of health provider associations, consumer health groups, and community activist organizations. While all groups have a general responsibility to their mem-

TABLE 8–2

SUMMARY OF PRIVATE SECTOR ROLES IN HEALTH CARE

	Financing	*Delivery*	*Credentialing/Regulation*
Business/industry	Often provides health insurance for employees; may provide health coverage utilizing HMOs or PPOs. Pays for workers' compensation insurance. Provides coverage for selected addiction rehabilitation.	Operates occupational health clinics; may provide some health maintenance services	May regulate smoking, areas to smoke
Credentialing bodies	Impacts costs of care	Impact delivery of health care services; serve to configure institutional delivery mechanisms, available resources, etc.	Accredit institutional or agency providers; accredit educational programs for preparing health professionals; certify health personnel
Health insurance	For a price, pays for health services; reimburses health professionals and institutions; performs utilization reviews and billing audits	Impacts delivery system based on inherent incentives in insurance policies; providers and services reimbursed; conditions and levels of reimbursement	Determines qualifications for insurance coverage
Health personnel		Provide direct health services. Paid salary or on basis of charge or allowable fees.	
Health institutions*	May have a financing function	Provide health services through organized delivery systems. Reimburse by insurance, health client, for most services rendered as an institution	Often maintain an institutional credentialing for physicians and in some instances for other nonphysician health professionals in independent practice
Professional organizations		Recruitment of new members into the profession to assure adequacy of personnel resources for health care delivery; promote change, innovation in professional practice/health care delivery	Set educational and practice standards for the profession and its members. May participate in or provide quality assurance, risk management programs, or continuing education programs. May publish ethical code for members.
Liability insurers/ product liability insurers	For a price, underwrite costs of malpractice/product-liability claims, defense costs, and/or payments/ judgments		Determine conditions for acquiring liability insurance and liability limits available. Malpractice insurance may be required to obtain institutional clinical privileges.

*Health institutions include hospitals, ambulatory health centers, diagnostic or treatment centers, hospices, long-term care facilities, etc.

bership, professional associations are designed to represent professions and protect the interests of their members as they relate to professional practice. Consumer health groups and community activist groups often provide public watch services concerning health care and identify needs and solutions requiring public and private support to implement solutions. Other groups may be private organizations interested in publicizing the plight of patients with particular disease entities, raising money for research, and educating the public concerning disease. These groups may be national or community in scope; may be defined along racial, age, economic status, or other lines; and may, in some instances, have significant power to influence government and the private sector. The American Association of Retired Persons (AARP), Gray Panthers,

Public Citizen, and diagnosis-specific organizations are but a few of these.

HEALTH RESOURCES IN THE UNITED STATES

Service Providers

While a large number of health professionals engage in private practice, either as individuals or as groups, the health care delivery system today is one of the major employers within the United States. According to the U.S. Bureau of the Census, in 1985 there were approximately 5,715,000 persons employed or otherwise working within the health care delivery system. Of those, approximately 492,000 were physicians, 131,000 dentists, 2.7 million nurses and nurses aides, 172,000 pharmacists, 257,000 therapists (physical, occupational, speech, etc.), and 416,000 laboratory and radiology technicians.[19,20] Approximately 77.0 percent of all health workers were female and about 13.2 percent were black.[19] Ginzberg and Ostow[21] reported that the physician supply in the southern states rose from 94 to 184 per 100,000 population, almost doubling between 1955 and 1988. Considering that the physician supply across the United States was 220 per 100,000 population, the highest in the world in 1985, it is evident that there is a geographic maldistribution of physicians and in other health human resources as well. The fact that there are 615,000 physicians today, projected to reach more than 800,000 by the year 2020, should give pause to policymakers as they consider the eventual impact these numbers will have economically. These numbers do not even take into consideration the additional numbers of allied health support personnel required to support this physician glut.

Hospitals and Institutions

Hospitals, the traditional institutional health provider, are undergoing major financial stresses as government and other payers try to constrain the cost of care. Congressional implementation of the Prospective Payment System as the vehicle for Medicare reimbursement of hospitals has led to shortened hospital stays and lower bed occupancy, prompting closure of many hospitals. These closures were hastened by the advent of freestanding ambulatory health clinics and surgicenters that took many of the profit-making services away from hospitals. Some hospitals have responded by establishing their own hospital-based ambulatory centers, surgicenters, and home health agencies or by entering joint ventures with physicians as a source of patients. The changing reimbursement system for hospital care also prompted entrepreneurs to get into the field, and for-profit hospitals were born. Today, these institutions constitute approximately one third of all hospitals. While many believed that applying market principles to running hospitals would lower the costs of hospitalization, the data are equivocal at best.[22] Further, because of the need to compete for patients, the advertising budgets of hospitals have significantly increased. Again, patients do not normally choose their hospital but rather go where their physician is on staff.

In joint ventures, some hospitals pay physicians on the basis of their admissions or as investors in the hospital. Consequently, the physicians benefit economically from the patient service itself and also from their involvement with the hospital. These arrangements have also spread to freestanding laboratory and radiology services, causing some to question the professional ethics of such practices. The state of Florida has recently passed a law prohibiting physicians from referring patients to professional businesses in which they have an economic interest. That law is now being tested in the courts.

Some hospitals have adopted the principles of Managed Care as a means to effectively compete in the health care market and to cut costs. Managed care, as within health maintenance organizations (HMOs) or associated with preferred provider associations (PPOs), has been touted as an answer to the high cost of health care. In such organizations, payment for health care services may be based on a capitation basis, a fee per person, or in the instance of a preferred provider, a contract for services with a group of providers at a reduced price over that of the market in general. Research is mixed as to the degree of savings and consumer satisfaction with this type of health care delivery.

The American Association of Nurse Anesthetists (AANA) and state nurse anesthetist associations will have to monitor the status and characteristics of managed care groups entering the market place. They must assure that CRNAs, as a group, will not be discriminated against in becoming preferred providers. Again, provider access becomes problematic in the face of the medical profession's traditional control mechanisms exerted at the institutional level.

THE NATIONAL PRACTITIONER DATA BANK

Part of the effort to reform the health care delivery system relates to the need for all professional groups to maintain due diligence in monitoring their own professional performance and to "weed out" those in the profession who are not practicing according to accepted standards of care. Due to general inattention to this professional responsibility by providers, institutional credentialing bodies, and state regulatory agencies, Congress enacted legislation in 1986 that created the National Practitioner Data Bank (NPDB). This law mandated that certain qualified incidents involving substandard care, as well as liability payouts by licensed or certified health professionals or their liability insurer, must be reported to the NPDB for recording on the health professional's profile. The purpose of the legislation is to improve quality of services through identifying health professionals with a significant malpractice history. The law requires agencies and groups responsible for the retention of providers to query the bank before awarding new privileges.[23] In large measure, this law is aimed at eliminating the practice of a health care professional moving from one state to another after being terminated for substandard practices.

FUTURE CONSIDERATIONS

There is little question that the United States is the world leader in high-technology services and tertiary care. However, this nation, which often prides itself as having the best health care system in the world, is not competitive in relation to some of the indices used by the World Health Organization. The most notable measure of these is the U.S. infant mortality rate, which is below 15 other countries. Essentially, the United States and South Africa are the only two developed countries in the world that have not enacted health legislation providing universal access to health care services for all citizens.[24]

Despite spending more than $800 billion on health care this year, approximately 37 to 40 million people in this country are underinsured or uninsured. These people are not below the federal poverty or state poverty levels, so they do not qualify for Medicaid. These people often work, but their employers do not provide health benefits, and their salary is sufficiently low that they cannot purchase health insurance, which today costs approximately $400 to $500 monthly for a family of four. They are also people who, because of their own health problem or that of a family member, cannot obtain health insurance at any cost. The people at greatest risk are single women, children, and low-income minorities. Research evidence clearly demonstrates that many of our children are not being immunized for the preventable diseases. Further, the delay in seeking health care among the underserved groups often makes the care they receive more costly and places them at greater risk for death and/or disability from late detection and treatment. When treated early, many of the complications of diseases can be prevented.

The health delivery system is still, in large measure, acute care–oriented, institutionally based, and physician-controlled. Reform measures are predicted to change at least the degree to which these characteristics will hold sway in the future. The federal government has been slower to respond to health care reform than have the states; currently four states have passed some form of universal health care legislation, and many other state legislatures have them under consideration. However, since many states are in fiscal crisis, their ability to respond to the needs of their citizenry is limited. Some of their efforts include universal health coverage and enactment of taxes, including taxing individual and institutional providers to pay for such care. Other efforts include placing priority for care on underserved populations, including the care of children and pregnant women. The Oregon plan, praised by many health policy analysts for its innovative approach, used a broadly based Health Services Commission to develop a basic, cost-effective package of health services. They planned to greatly expand the Medicaid program and make more than 700 medical services available to beneficiaries.

Because the plan denies certain health services to some beneficiaries, these exclusions have become the center of heated debate regarding the rationing of health services. The USDHHS is soon to rerule on exempting Oregon from the federal Medicaid program, which would allow implementation of this innovative approach to providing health care.

Yanklovich[25] believes that the failure of the American public, legislators, and health policy analysts to achieve consensus with regard to the causes of the health care crisis is at the heart of the inability of the federal government to deal with health care reform. The public lays the blame on the greed of the principle players in health care delivery; legislators and health policy analysts lay the blame on high technology. Many who have studied these problems believe the causes may be far more complex. Most agree, however, that any health care reform must meet criteria that assure broad accessibility of high-quality services to all persons at prices individuals, business, and society can afford. The extent to which we achieve these goals will largely relate to our ability to place people above politics.

In January 1993, a new president of the United States was inaugurated. He campaigned on an agenda for change, one that would include health care reform. A national Health Care Task Force has been charged to propose such a program. The report of the task force is due in May 1993. To what extent it will be successful in achieving sufficient consensus to be enacted into law or will actually be capable of achieving the necessary reforms must await an evaluation and reporting. However, some of the issues that must be debated include the following:

1 *The lack of access to basic health care services based on geographic, social, economic, and other factors.* The solutions to making health care accessible in rural communities are not identical to those of making health care accessible in the inner city or to ethnic communities within large metropolitan areas. Community-centered planning is often essential to resolve some of these problems.

2 *Establishing priorities in health care and assuring cost-effective use of high-technology services.* This will require the identification practice guidelines based on research with regard to the efficacy of high-technology services in treating patients, in addition to performing cost-benefit analyses.

3 *Defining more cost-effective health manpower mixes.* This involves redesigning the health care system and pertinent statutes and regulations to assure its effective function. This will probably entail a reduced reliance on physicians; increased reliance on midlevel providers, such as nurses in advanced practice (CRNAs, certified nurse midwives [CNMs], nurse practitioners [NPs], and some clinical nurse specialists); and empowering the public to take more responsibility for their own health status.

4 *Evaluate privatization.* There is a need to evaluate the impact of privatization of health care in the for-profit mode of the health delivery system and its overall impact on cost-effectiveness.

5 *Tort reform.* Modification of the tort system and alternatives for compensating patients for injuries from health care negligence.

6 *Reimbursement for health service.* Reimbursement methodologies, rates, and identification of payment recipients must be addressed. Fee-for-service medicine creates adverse incentives to cost-effectiveness and is believed by many to be at the heart of escalating health care costs. Historically, there has been an association between the capping of fees and the increase in the number of procedures performed by physicians. While some advocate managed competition or HMOs as a cost-

effective health care delivery system, the savings overall have not been remarkable to date. Many believe that national health insurance with a single-payer system is the only way to eliminate the administrative waste of private insurance and to avoid cost-shifting.

7 *Ethical issues.* Ethical issues such as the prolongation of dying, its impact on the individual, the family, and health resources badly needed by others more likely to benefit within our society need to be reviewed. Intellectual, philosophic, and scientific resources should be used to resolve these issues. Once again, consensus is the culprit in resolving this matter.

8 *Elimination of waste and fraud.* Eliminating waste, fraud, and abuse in the health care delivery system is paramount. Fraud and abuse alone have been estimated at $80 billion annually. The extent to which these could be reduced without excessive expenditures is open to question.[26]

SUMMARY

Because we are all affected by health care issues, it behooves us all, providers and consumers alike, to stay abreast of this rapidly changing arena. We must continually evaluate its impact on us, our families, our patients, and our nation. It is highly possible that the current economic recession in the United States is due, in part, to the impact of the high cost of health care on the ability of U.S. industry to compete in world markets. Keeping abreast, however, is not enough. Each of us must be in a position to make intelligent decisions concerning future proposals for change and involve ourselves in the decision making. To the extent that we can make the welfare of CRNAs and the public congruent and lend our efforts in that direction, we can become winners in any future health care system.

REFERENCES

1. Starr, P: The Social Transformation of American Medicine. Basic Books, New York, 1982.
2. Waddle, F: Licensure: Achievements and limitations. In The Study of Credentialing in Nursing: A New Approach. Vol. 2. Staff Working Papers, American Nurses Association, Kansas City, MO, 1979, pp. 126–132.
3. Bullough, B: Introduction—nursing practice law. In Bullough, B, Bullough, V, and Soukup, M (eds): Nursing Issues and Nursing Strategies of the Eighties. Springer Publishing, New York, 1983, pp. 279–291.
4. Safreit, B: Health care dollars and regulatory sense: The role of advanced practice nursing. Yale J Reg 9:417, 1991.
5. Hadley, EH: Nurses and prescriptive authority: A legal and economic analysis. Am JL Med 15:245, 1989.
6. Donahue, MP: Nursing, The Finest Art. An Illustrated History. CV Mosby, St. Louis, 1985.
7. Nursing organizations: Interrelationships and implications for credentialing. In The Study of Credentialing in Nursing: A New Approach. Staff Working Papers. American Nurses Association, Kansas City, vol. 2. 1979, p. 172.
8. Melosh, B: The Physician's Hand: Work Culture and Conflict in American Nursing. Temple University Press, Philadelphia, 1982, pp. 113–158.
9. Diers, D: Nurse-midwives and nurse anesthetists: The cutting edge in specialist practice. In Aiken, L and Fagin, C (eds): Charting Nursing's Future, Agenda for the 1990's. JB Lippincott, Philadelphia, 1992, pp. 159–180.
10. Stevens, R: In Sickness and in Wealth. Basic Books, New York, 1989.
11. Numbers, RL: The third party: Health insurance in America. In Lee, PR, Estes, DL, and Ramsay, NB (eds): The Nation's Health. Boyd and Fraser Publishing, San Francisco, 1984, pp. 196–204.
12. Califano, JA: America's Health Care Revolution: Who Lives? Who Dies? Who Pays? Random House, New York, 1986.
13. Wing, KR: The Law and the Public's Health, ed 2. Health Administration Press, Ann Arbor, MI, 1985, pp. 177–195.
14. Ribicoff, A and Danaceau, P: The American Medical Machine. Harrow Books, Harper & Row, New York, 1972, pp. 135–167.
15. Brecher, C: The government's role in health care. In Kovner, AR (ed): Health Care Delivery in the United States. Springer Publishing, New York, 1990, pp. 297–323.
16. Brown, ER: Medicare and Medicaid: Bandaids for the old and poor. In Sidel, VW and Sidel, R (eds): Reforming Medicine, Lessons of the Last Quarter Century. Pantheon Books, New York, 1984, pp. 50–76.
17. Health Care Financing Administration, U.S. Department of Health and Human Services. Letter to Michels, KA: American Association of Nurse Anesthetists, from Wynn, BO, Director, Hospital Payment Policy, HCFA, July 27, 1992.
18. Gunn, IP: Promoting a more cost-effective health delivery system through changing the health provider mix. Unpublished paper, 1992.
19. Jonas, S: Health manpower: With an emphasis on physicians. In Kovner, AR (ed): Health Care Delivery in the United States. Springer Publishing, New York, 1990, pp. 50–86.
20. Committee to Study the Role of Allied Health

Personnel, Allied Health Services, Avoiding Crisis. Institute of Medicine, National Academy Press, Washington, DC, 1988.
21. Ginzberg, E and Ostow, M: Grant watch special report: Physician supply strategy: The case of the south. Health Affairs, 11(2):193–197, 1992.
22. Lindorff, D: Marketplace Medicine, The Rise of the For-Profit Hospital Chains. Bantam Books, New York, 1992.
23. Garde, JG: Keeping in balance with the national practitioner data bank. CRNA Forum, 7(1):3, 1990.
24. Schieber, GJ, Poullier, J-P, and Greenwald, LM: Health care systems in twenty-four countries. Health Affairs 10(3):22, 1991.
25. Yankelovich, D and Immerwahr, J: A perception gap. Health Managment Q, 3(3):11, 1991.
26. Wasted health care dollars. Consumer Reports, July 1992, p. 435.

9

Reimbursement for Clinical Services

Daniel C. Simonson
John F. Garde

OUTLINE

OBJECTIVES

On completing this chapter, the reader will be able to:

1. Demonstrate knowledge of the historical context that led to CRNA involvement in securing rights of direct reimbursement.
2. Discuss the theory underlying the prospective payment system and how it affects clinical practice.
3. Describe the Relative Value Scale, and how to establish a unit value for services and determine appropriate fees.
4. Discuss mechanisms involved in anesthesia billing and determining the CRNA's financial worth in the marketplace.

When one person provides a service to another at his or her request, the individual has a right to ask for fair compensation. Nurse anesthetists must not forget that they have made a significant investment both financially and in years of education to acquire their skills. They need not feel embarrassed or demeaned when it comes time to seek fair compensation from patients for the service they have provided.

Traditionally, Certified Registered Nurse Anesthetists (CRNAs) have been employed by physician groups or hospitals who bill for their services; as such, many anesthetists have little understanding of the process, much less the skills to manage the business side of their professional career. If CRNAs seek an employment setting that requires personal management and control of finances, however, they must become fully versed in issues relating to reimbursement and billing. At the very least, each and every CRNA, regardless of practice setting, should be able to determine the exact worth of his or her professional services.

THE HISTORY OF REIMBURSEMENT

In the early years of this century and through the 1950s, CRNAs were usually paid employees of either the surgeon for whom they worked or the hospital. In rural areas, CRNAs often contracted with hospitals to provide services based on fee-for-service structures; that is, a set amount of compensation per case as opposed to straight salary for hours worked.

Private Payers

Blue Cross/Blue Shield was one of the first private payers to emerge during the 1930s. The concept originated in Dallas, Texas, in 1929. Under the leadership of Justine Ford Kimball, PhD, executive vice president of Baylor University, a group of schoolteachers developed an agreement with the university hospital to provide health insurance. For the annual sum of $6.00 per teacher, each participant was assured of receiving 21 days of care in a semiprivate hospital room. Initially, each program involved only an individual hospital, but by 1932, community-wide agreements offered subscribers a choice of hospitals. In 1933, E. A. van Steenwyk, first executive of the Hospital Service Association of St. Paul, Minnesota, conceived the idea of using a blue cross to identify his program on stationery, folders, and other printed material.

Early insurance plans paid only for physician or hospital charges, and they would not directly reimburse other health care providers, such as CRNAs, psychologists, and physical therapists. To obtain payment for their services, these providers would submit charges to the hospital or physician. The hospital or physician would then obtain reimbursement for services as "incident to" their own and pass the money on to the nonreimbursed provider (often after subtracting some type of handling fee). In the case of CRNAs who practiced independently, this usually required contracting with the hospital to gain reimbursement.

The Prospective Payment System

Health care costs continued to escalate under the private payer systems of reimbursement. Reasons cited for this trend were often attributed to the failure of payers to reimburse lower-cost providers (nonphysicians); preferential reimbursement of higher-cost care systems (i.e., hospitals, rather than ambulatory or outpatient services); and the insistence by physicians that inherent harm would come to the physician-patient relationship if the fee-for-service structure were not maintained and strengthened.

In an effort to control escalating medical costs, Medicare instituted a Prospective Payment System (PPS) in 1983. Although initially this legislation affected only Medicare Part A (hospital costs), it would soon have an effect on Medicare Part B (physician and nonphysician costs). Prior to 1983, Medicare reimbursed hospitals for CRNA services on a cost-based system, in which the hospital simply passed along the actual costs of providing the Medicare portion of CRNA services directly to Medicare.

Theory of the Prospective Payment System

It was believed that the cost-plus system provided no real reimbursement incentive for those who provided cost-effective services. Hospitals would provide cost-effective care only when their profits depended on their ability to do so. Moreover, it was believed that if hospital profits also depended on changes in physician behavior relating to hospital resource consumption, hospitals would be more apt to implement strategies for changing physician behavior as opposed to those systems in which hospital profits increased as resource consumption by physicians increased.

Essentially, PPS legislation mandated that a fixed rate for hospital care, covering all Part A services, be paid to hospitals based on a patient's diagnostic-related classification (group) or diagnosis-related group (DRG). This fixed rate was to cover all costs associated with hospital admission, including services provided by nonphysician health providers, whether they were hospital employees or not. The rate of reimbursement for the diagnostic categories was calculated from data derived from the cost-plus system and regionally adjusted. Nearly 400 DRGs were devised and were to be implemented into the existing reimbursement system over a 4-year period.

CRNAs were in great jeopardy under this system, because hospitals, in an effort to cut costs, would have a disincentive to hire CRNAs because their cost would come directly from the hospital DRG payment. The interest of hospitals could best be served by contracting with physicians, since they could still bill under Part B. Not only did hospitals have no incentive to hire CRNAs, physician groups were now in a position of not being able to bill for CRNA services, as their reimbursement was to come from Part A, and the original legislation contained a prohibition against unbundling CRNAs from part A for the purposes of payment. In short, Congress had inadvertently created reimbursement disincentives for the use of CRNAs while bolstering incentives for use of anesthesiologists.

The American Association of Nurse Anesthetists' Response

The plan to correct these potentially devastating measures included several components pursued simultaneously; working with and lobbying both the executive branch, particularly the Health Care Financing Administration (HCFA) and Congress, and undertaking massive effort to educate and motivate CRNAs to become effective lobbyists.

The plan was based on short-term corrections to alleviate reimbursement disincentives. The American Association of Nurse Anesthetists (AANA) requested of Congress an exception to the unbundling provision of PPS for physician-employed CRNAs and a temporary pass-through for costs of hospital-employed CRNAs and private practice contractors. The plan also ensured that future access to reimbursement capability did not create disincentives for use of CRNA services. This would be achieved by paying both CRNAs and anesthesiologists from the same part of Medicare, either Part A or Part B. In this way, competition could be enhanced, and the chance for inadvertent reimbursement disincentives would be minimized.

HCFA eventually rewrote regulations that authorized an exception to the unbundling provision for a 3-year period for physician-employed CRNAs. In 1984, a technical amendment was signed by the President that put a time limit on the pass-through of 3 years and required that a study be forthcoming to determine possible methods of reimbursement that would not discourage the use of CRNAs by hospitals.

The centerpiece of the plan was to seek direct reimbursement for CRNA services from Medicare. The job of the AANA was to convince Congress that CRNAs were concerned about health care costs as well as equitable reimbursement for their services or salaries from employers. Medicare direct reimbursement legislation for CRNAs was introduced in 1983. After massive lobbying efforts by the AANA and CRNAs all over the country, the legislation was passed as part of the Omnibus Budget Reconciliation Act of 1986 with an effective date for direct reimbursement of CRNAs set for January 1, 1989. The unbundling and pass-through provisions achieved earlier were extended to cover the interim period.

As a result of this legislation, all CRNAs, regardless of their practice setting, have the ability to receive reimbursement from Medicare directly or to sign over their billing rights to their employer. All CRNA services are subject to Medicare assignment (no balance billing). A subsequent law also allowed rural hospitals with 500 or fewer surgical cases per year requiring anesthesia and one full-time CRNA to "pass-through" the costs of anesthesia services. In 1992, final regulations were published that detailed procedural definitions of the 1986 legislation. The AANA remains vigilant in its efforts to ensure that these regulations are written and refined in ways that a CRNA's right to gain fair and equitable reimbursement are not infringed.

THE RELATIVE VALUE SCALE

To implement reimbursement law, a system had to be developed to determine appropriate costs and reimbursement rates for each case. To answer this need, a system of "relative value for services" was established that listed all surgical cases requiring anesthesia and assignment of monetary values to each.

Historically, anesthesia charges have been based on direct time involvement, either as a charge for simple time, or as a charge based on a combination of time and the complexity of the anesthetic. The first type, charging for simple time, was prevalent for many years and consisted of determining the number of minutes the anesthetist was involved in rendering anesthesia care and multiplying it by a dollar amount (conversion factor) such as $2 per minute. This method, although attractive in its simplicity, did not allow for the overwhelming differences between types of anesthetics relative to the preparation, skill, or risk involved. Most practitioners agree that the work involved in preparing a parturient for a 1-hour cesarean section is far greater than that required to prepare a healthy 20-year-old for a 1-hour meniscectomy.

To address this inequity, the California Society of Anesthesiologists developed and published the first Relative Value Scale (RVS) in 1966. This publication was the result of a great deal of effort expended to assign a relative base value to all possible surgical procedures for which an anesthetic might be given. The book consisted of a list of surgical procedures by anatomic or functional description, such as head and neck, musculoskeletal, and so on, followed by the number of base units that an anesthetist might charge for the anesthetic. In an additional section, modifier units were listed. These were units to be added to the base for factors such as emergency procedures and extremes of patient risk or age.

After adding together the base and modifier units, the anesthetist would calculate time units at one unit per 15 minutes or portion thereof, and add in that figure. The total number of units was multiplied by the anesthetist's fee per unit (such as $15), and the bill was prepared based on these computations.

Shortly after the initial introduction of this system, a judicial ruling in California determined that the practice was monopolistic, equivalent to "price-fixing." The California Society was enjoined from further publication of the RVS booklet. However, the system worked so well that for many years, until the legal reestablishment of the practice, worn and tattered copies of the initial RVS book were found in the desk drawers of hospitals' professional staff lounge areas and were frequently used by anesthetists to determine their fees.

In the 1970s, insurance companies, seeking to standardize the payments for medical services based on Current Procedural Terminology (CPT) codes, embraced the concept of RVS. Soon many payers had systems in place, and the American Society of Anesthesiologists produced their own relative value guide. Today, most anesthetists bill based on some type of RVS system. The AANA published an RVS for CRNAs, and HCFA has published (in the *Federal Register*) an RVS that Medicare uses in determining payments to CRNAs and anesthesiologists. The greatest variability is in the increment of time for each time unit. Although originally time was calculated based on 15-minute units (and this is the time unit that HCFA uses), it is not unusual for anesthetists to bill using 12- or 10-minute time units. This fact must be considered when comparing the unit charge of competing anesthesia providers.

ESTABLISHING A UNIT VALUE FOR SERVICES

The unit value, also known as the conversion factor, is the basis of a CRNA's fee schedule. From this basic, predetermined charge, the CRNA can convert this figure to a dollar amount by multiplying the conversion factor by the allowable unit value for a particular case. There are a variety of RVSs available for determination of anesthesia fees; they are published by various sources, including Medicare, Medicaid, the American Society of Anesthesiologists, and the local Blue Cross/Blue Shield Insurance carrier.

Before providing examples of this process, it is important to emphasize the difference between what is charged and what is paid. Many third-party payers, such as Medicare and many Blue Cross insurers, ignore the practitioner's charges completely and base payments on their own fee schedule. These payments are often determined by what providers charge "on average" for their services. However, this does not mean that a practitioner must bill using the methodology of these payers. The practitioner's unit value should be based on the particulars of his or her practice, including factors such as personal educational expenses required to provide professional services, overhead expenses, and geographic and market considerations. In non-Medicare cases, CRNAs may balance bill the patient directly to make up the difference between what is charged and what is paid.

Factors that Determine Unit Charge

Many CRNAs are uncomfortable about establishing an appropriate unit charge value. There are several reasons for this. First, practitioners have little experience in formulating an appropriate fee structure based on concrete cost factors. This is complicated by the fact that many CRNAs have little idea of the true value of their services to the patient or the hospital . CRNAs also fear overcharging the patient or the hospital and are reticent about stating clearly and honestly that they are willing to provide services only on the condition that they receive fair and equitable wages. The following factors should be carefully considered when establishing a unit charge.

1. *Cost of living.* This determination should be made on a yearly basis, which yields an approximate cost for securing appropriate housing within a specified geographic area. Consideration should also be given to tax rates, availability of transportation, community services, public services, and so on.
2. *Cost of education.* This cost should be determined from the money invested to secure basic anesthesia education, including direct costs of tuition and fees, future continuing education, licensure, certification, plus indirect costs of missed employment due to moving, and so on.
3. *Availability to secure a client base.* This cost would be measured by one's ability to have sufficient patients available to generate required income. Perhaps very remote, rural areas would not provide sufficient demand for services.
4. *Cost of practice.* This amount would be determined by a yearly analysis of what it costs to secure appropriate equipment, supplies, drugs, liability insurance, billing services, and office overhead.
5. *Quality of life.* This intangible yet important figure would be that amount of money that would convince a CRNA to remain in the community.

Once these dollar amounts have been determined, the CRNA should divide the total amount (costs) by a reasonable estimation of the number of units chargeable per year (based on potential client base). This would yield a reasonable unit charge. The determination of the unit charge should be used in negotiations with the hospital and third-party payers for reimbursement. A word of caution: the CRNA should not be required to subsidize anesthesia care in the community. A CRNA should expect and require reasonable compensation for professional services. If the hospital or other health care facility is not able to meet basic requirements to establish practice, the CRNA should consider other employment.

Determining a Fee

Using the RVS, it is fairly easy to determine the fee to be charged for a particular anesthetic. Base units are determined by referring to a particular anesthetic procedure in the RVS book. Time units are determined by dividing the anesthesia time by 10-, 12-, or typically 15-minute intervals, depending on the policy. The base units are added to the time units to arrive at the total number of units for the procedure. This figure is then multiplied by the CRNA's own conversion factor to arrive at the dollar value of the anesthetic.

Example 1: A 35-Minute Cataract Procedure

Anesthesia for lens surgery
CPT code 00142 .... 4 units
Time: 35 minutes @ 15 minutes/unit . 3 units
Total units .... 7 units
Conversion Factor $30/unit
Charge for anesthetic .... $210 ($30 × 7)

Example 2: A 3-Hour Cholecystectomy

Anesthesia for procedure on upper anterior abdominal wall
CPT code 00700 .... 7 units
Time: 180 minutes @
15 minutes/unit .... 12 units
Total units .... 19 units
Conversion factor $30/unit
Charge for anesthetic ...... $570 ($30 × 19)

Example 3: A 2 ½-Hour Coronary Artery Bypass Graft

Anesthesia for procedure on heart, pericardium, and great vessels of chest, with pump oxygenator
CPT code 00562 .... 25 units
Time: 150 minutes @
15 minutes/unit .... 10 units
Total units .... 35 units
Conversion factor $30/unit
Charge for anesthetic ..... $1050 ($30 × 35)

THE BILLING PROCESS

Obtaining reimbursement for anesthesia services is a systematic process with many possible caveats. The greatest resource for a practicing CRNA to help with problems in billing is the provider relations department of the predominant insurance company in the area. Here, one can obtain information on forms, credentialing, and reimbursement rates. If one is just beginning to bill independently, the first few claims should be hand-carried to the insurer. Asking the provider relations personnel to review the claims for potential errors will smooth the path for subsequent submissions of claims.

Billing for anesthesia services encompasses interactions with three main categories of carriers: commercial carriers (such as Blue Cross/Blue Shield), Medicare, and Medicaid. Initial stages of billing are the same, but variations may occur after payment is received. For instance, payment from a commercial plan often does not cover all of the "allowable" charges (e.g., the fee that the carrier feels is appropriate). This typically results in reimbursement of 80 percent of costs, requiring the provider to balance bill the patient for the remaining 20 percent. For a stepwise billing procedure, refer to Box 9–1.

The Health Care Financing Administration 1500 Form

In the past, it was customary for the patient to pay the provider at the time of service or upon receipt of the bill. The patient was responsible for all charges, and the provider had nothing to do with the insurance company. Patients would fill out their own insurance claim form and send the form with the billing statement to their insurance carrier, which would then reimburse that patient directly.

As of 1991, physicians and CRNAs are required by law to bill Medicare for the patient. Although CRNAs are not required to bill private insurance companies or supplemental policies, it is common for patients, particularly Medicare recipients, to expect that the provider will handle all of the particulars of billing their insurance company. However, given the multitude of insurance carriers, it is impossible to bill all carriers on their own preprinted forms. To standardize the process of billing Medicare directly, HCFA and the American Medical Association developed a comprehensive health insurance claim form. Most private insurance companies have adopted the form as well, so it is now possible to bill insurance companies directly using a single claim form, the HCFA 1500.

Typically, a CRNA completes two forms after administering an anesthetic: a statement of charges for the patient, and an

BOX 9–1
BILLING PROCEDURE

1 a. Obtain insurance information from the patient. This is a vital step in the process that is easily overlooked. For hospital-based anesthetists, this step is usually performed by the admissions office, allowing the anesthetist to receive accurate and timely information. For outpatient or office practices, the surgeon's office may be the appropriate source.
   b. Obtain a photocopy of both sides of the patient's insurance card. If the patient is a Medicare recipient, obtain a copy of any supplemental policy information.
   c. Have patients sign a lifetime authorization signature card and keep it with their records.

2 After performing the anesthetic, prepare a statement of charges (for the patient) and fill out a HCFA 1500 form.

3 Send the HCFA 1500 form to the Medicare carrier or other primary insurance carrier, send the statement to the patient with a notice "your insurance has been billed."

4 An explanation of benefits (EOB) will be returned to the provider from the carrier. Send a copy of the EOB and another HCFA 1500 form to the patient's supplemental insurance company to receive the remaining 20 percent.

5 If the patient has no supplemental carrier, send a bill for the remaining 20 percent to the patient.

HCFA 1500 form, which will go to the insurance company. If the patient has no insurance, they will pay from the statement. If they have insurance, the HCFA 1500 ensures that proper reimbursement is sent to the CRNA. The statement serves only as a reminder to the patient that the insurance company has been billed and to send any payments mistakenly sent to them to the CRNA.

Figure 9–1 provides a composite view of the HCFA 1500 form, completed with hypothetical patient information. This form is the newest version, revised and implemented as of May 1, 1992. The actual claim form is printed in a special red ink to allow carriers the option of using optical scanners to elicit information put on the form by the provider and to aid in automated processing. Box 9–2 provides a stepwise procedure to assist the CRNA in completing the HCFA 1500 form. Note that items 1–12 contain information about the patient and the insured. Items 13–33 address physician or supplier information. It is also helpful to have the claim forms preprinted with the CRNAs name and other consistently used information.

Balance Billing

Balance billing is the practice of billing the patient for the remainder of the fee greater than the allowable charge. It is important to remember that federal law stipulates that CRNAs cannot balance bill Medicare patients. They can, however, legally balance bill patients of private carriers. In most instances, this practice engenders hard feelings between the patients, the insurance companies, and the CRNA, because patients are forced to pay out of pocket for a service they usually believe should be covered by their insurance policy (after deductibles are satisfied). However, the practice may be justified in a case in which an insurance company adheres to an unjustifiably low allowable charge. In this case, billing the patient for the balance may cause the insurer to adjust their allowable charge upward. Unfortunately, this may be the only way to get the attention of the insurer to the problem, if resolution cannot be gained through other means. The following is an example of balance billing using the example of anesthesia provided for cataract and intraocular lens implantation, duration 90 minutes.

Charge for CRNA anesthesia

10 units @ $27/unit	$270.00
Medicare allows	$155.70
Medicare pays 80 percent	$124.56
Patient is responsible for	$31.14
Balance (difference between what medicare allows and you charge)	$114.30

Text continued on p. 140.

BOX 9–2
STEPWISE PROCEDURE TO COMPLETE THE HCFA 1500 FORM

Items 1–8: These items identify the insurance plan, patient demographics, and the relationship of the patient to the insured. Note that the patient and insured can be, and often are, two separate people. A wife can be the insured while her husband is the patient. Or a child can be the patient of a parent with a different surname.

Items 9a–9d: This allows entry of additional policies and covers such situations as Medicare supplemental policies or an insured's policy that covers the patient after the first policy reaches its monetary limits.

Items 10a–10d: These need to be filled out only if appropriate.

Item 11d: This must be filled out. Insurance companies, particularly Medicare, are extremely concerned about instances in which they have paid when another insurer should have paid. The answer here is usually "no," unless the patient states they are covered by another policy. In the case of supplemental insurance, one can still mark "no" and type in the words "secondary only."

Items 12–13: These items require a signature by both the patient and the insured. However, patients and insureds can be asked to sign a "lifetime authorization" card, which authorizes billing in their name and is attached to their chart or account record. If this is the case, it is customary to type "signature on file" in these fields.

Items 14–16: These are usually irrelevant to anesthesia care.

Items 17–17a: This field should contain the name of the surgeon performing the operation. Item 17a is very important for Medicare patients. This is where the anesthetist puts the unique physician identifying number (UPIN) of the surgeon. The number can be obtained from the surgeon's office, or a free printed listing of all physicians UPINs can be obtained from the local Medicare carrier. CRNAs are not currently required to have a UPIN.

Items 18–20: Usually irrelevant to anesthesia care.

Item 21: The field contains the International Classification of Diseases (ICD-9) code for the patient's diagnosis, determined by the surgeon.

Item 22–23: This item is completed if the patient is a subscriber to an insurance plan requiring prior authorization of surgical procedures. The patient is responsible for providing you with this number, and the CRNA will soon become aware of which plans require it.

Item 24:

a. Date of service: As appropriate.
b. Place of service: A code is used to describe the type of setting, such as 22 for outpatient hospital or 24 for ambulatory surgery center.
c. Type of service: The CPT code for the service can be obtained from the CPT code book that lists all surgical anesthesia and medical procedures.
d. Modifiers: These designations are now standardly used by Medicare to describe the type of service. For example, QZ means a nonmedically directed CRNA.
e. Diagnosis code: This refers to the field (1, 2, 3, or 4) in item 21 containing the appropriate diagnosis code relating to the surgery.
f. Charges: Place here the total charge for the anesthetic.
g. Days or units: Charge units for anesthesia are placed here. Although there is no field specified for it, Medicare requires that the minutes of anesthesia time be placed on the HCFA 1500 form. If anesthesia time is not recorded, the claim will be denied.

Item 25: The Federal tax ID number should be the number of the fiscal entity that will be receiving payment. If the CRNA is submitting a bill for himself or herself, this should be the CRNA's number. If the CRNA is employed by someone else or is part of a group, the employer's or group's number should be substituted.

Item 26: The patient account number is for CRNA use. The account number assigned to the patient by the CRNA or billing agent will be placed on the EOB.

Item 27: Accept assignment: By law, CRNAs must accept Medicare assignment. The decision to accept assignment (accept insurance payment as payment in full) with other insurers is at the discretion of the CRNA.

Items 28–30: As appropriate.

Item 31: Although a signature is requested here, a typewritten name and credentials should suffice.

Item 32: As appropriate.

Item 33: The personal identification number (PIN) is assigned to the CRNA by the local carrier.

PLEASE DO NOT STAPLE IN THIS AREA

PICA **HEALTH INSURANCE CLAIM FORM** PICA

CARRIER

1. MEDICARE (Medicare #) X — MEDICAID (Medicaid #) — CHAMPUS (Sponsor's SSN) — CHAMPVA (VA File #) — GROUP HEALTH PLAN (SSN or ID) — FECA BLK LUNG (SSN) — OTHER (ID)

1a. INSURED'S I.D. NUMBER (FOR PROGRAM IN ITEM 1): 000-00-0000 A

2. PATIENT'S NAME (Last Name, First Name, Middle Initial): Doe, Jane E.

3. PATIENT'S BIRTH DATE MM DD YY: 12 09 31 — SEX M ☐ F X

4. INSURED'S NAME (Last Name, First Name, Middle Initial): Doe, John X.

5. PATIENT'S ADDRESS (No., Street): 123 South St.

CITY: Spokane — STATE: WA

ZIP CODE: 99203 — TELEPHONE (Include Area Code): (509) 333-1234

6. PATIENT RELATIONSHIP TO INSURED: Self ☐ Spouse X Child ☐ Other ☐

7. INSURED'S ADDRESS (No., Street): Same

CITY — STATE

ZIP CODE — TELEPHONE (INCLUDE AREA CODE) (   )

8. PATIENT STATUS: Single ☐ Married X Other ☐ — Employed ☐ Full-Time Student ☐ Part-Time Student ☐

9. OTHER INSURED'S NAME (Last Name, First Name, Middle Initial): Same Supplemental Policy

a. OTHER INSURED'S POLICY OR GROUP NUMBER: MS 123-12345

b. OTHER INSURED'S DATE OF BIRTH MM DD YY — SEX M ☐ F ☐

c. EMPLOYER'S NAME OR SCHOOL NAME

d. INSURANCE PLAN NAME OR PROGRAM NAME: Medigap Insurance

10. IS PATIENT'S CONDITION RELATED TO:

a. EMPLOYMENT? (CURRENT OR PREVIOUS) ☐ YES ☐ NO

b. AUTO ACCIDENT? ☐ YES ☐ NO — PLACE (State)

c. OTHER ACCIDENT? ☐ YES ☐ NO

10d. RESERVED FOR LOCAL USE

11. INSURED'S POLICY GROUP OR FECA NUMBER

a. INSURED'S DATE OF BIRTH MM DD YY — SEX M ☐ F ☐

b. EMPLOYER'S NAME OR SCHOOL NAME

c. INSURANCE PLAN NAME OR PROGRAM NAME

d. IS THERE ANOTHER HEALTH BENEFIT PLAN? ☐ YES X NO — *If yes*, return to and complete item 9 a-d. — Secondary Only

READ BACK OF FORM BEFORE COMPLETING & SIGNING THIS FORM.

12. PATIENT'S OR AUTHORIZED PERSON'S SIGNATURE I authorize the release of any medical or other information necessary to process this claim. I also request payment of government benefits either to myself or to the party who accepts assignment below.

SIGNED Signature On File DATE

13. INSURED'S OR AUTHORIZED PERSON'S SIGNATURE I authorize payment of medical benefits to the undersigned physician or supplier for services described below.

SIGNED Signature On File

PATIENT AND INSURED INFORMATION

14. DATE OF CURRENT: MM DD YY — ILLNESS (First symptom) OR INJURY (Accident) OR PREGNANCY (LMP)

15. IF PATIENT HAS HAD SAME OR SIMILAR ILLNESS, GIVE FIRST DATE MM DD YY

16. DATES PATIENT UNABLE TO WORK IN CURRENT OCCUPATION: FROM MM DD YY TO MM DD YY

17. NAME OF REFERRING PHYSICIAN OR OTHER SOURCE: John Q. Surgeon

17a. I.D. NUMBER OF REFERRING PHYSICIAN: A03210

18. HOSPITALIZATION DATES RELATED TO CURRENT SERVICES: FROM MM DD YY TO MM DD YY

19. RESERVED FOR LOCAL USE

20. OUTSIDE LAB? ☐ YES ☐ NO — $ CHARGES

21. DIAGNOSIS OR NATURE OF ILLNESS OR INJURY (RELATE ITEMS 1,2,3 OR 4 TO ITEM 24E BY LINE)

1. 366.10
2. ___ . ___
3. ___ . ___
4. ___ . ___

22. MEDICAID RESUBMISSION CODE — ORIGINAL REF. NO.

23. PRIOR AUTHORIZATION NUMBER

24.

A: DATE(S) OF SERVICE From MM DD YY	To MM DD YY	B: Place of Service	C: Type of Service	D: PROCEDURES, SERVICES, OR SUPPLIES (Explain Unusual Circumstances) CPT/HCPCS	MODIFIER	E: DIAGNOSIS CODE	F: $ CHARGES	G: DAYS OR UNITS	H: EPSDT Family Plan	I: EMG	J: COB	K: RESERVED FOR LOCAL USE
01 01 92	01 01 92	24		00142	QZ	1	324. 00	12				
				Time: 60 minutes								

PHYSICIAN OR SUPPLIER INFORMATION

25. FEDERAL TAX I.D. NUMBER: 12-1234567 — SSN EIN

26. PATIENT'S ACCOUNT NO.: 01234

27. ACCEPT ASSIGNMENT? (For govt. claims, see back) X YES ☐ NO

28. TOTAL CHARGE: $ 324. 00

29. AMOUNT PAID: $

30. BALANCE DUE: $

31. SIGNATURE OF PHYSICIAN OR SUPPLIER INCLUDING DEGREES OR CREDENTIALS (I certify that the statements on the reverse apply to this bill and are made a part thereof.)

Fred Mertz, CRNA

SIGNED DATE

32. NAME AND ADDRESS OF FACILITY WHERE SERVICES WERE RENDERED (If other than home or office)

Spokane Medical Center
S. 26th St.
Spokane, WA 99204

33. PHYSICIAN'S, SUPPLIER'S BILLING NAME, ADDRESS, ZIP CODE & PHONE #

Spokane Anesthesia Services
W. 34th St
Spokane, WA 99204

PIN# 000123456 GRP#

790 0128 (12/90) (OCR) 1 pt.

(APPROVED BY AMA COUNCIL ON MEDICAL SERVICE 8/88) **PLEASE PRINT OR TYPE** FORM HCFA-1500 (12-90) FORM OWCP-1500 FORM RRB-1500

Figure 9–1. HCFA 1500 health insurance claim form. To enhance its readability, the form is reproduced first in its entirety and then in views of its top and bottom halves.

Continued

PLEASE
DO NOT
STAPLE
IN THIS
AREA

PICA

HEALTH INSURANCE CLAIM FORM

PICA

CARRIER

PATIENT AND INSURED INFORMATION

1. MEDICARE [X] (Medicare #) · MEDICAID [ ] (Medicaid #) · CHAMPUS [ ] (Sponsor's SSN) · CHAMPVA [ ] (VA File #) · GROUP HEALTH PLAN [ ] (SSN or ID) · FECA BLK LUNG [ ] (SSN) · OTHER [ ] (ID)	1a. INSURED'S I.D. NUMBER (FOR PROGRAM IN ITEM 1) 000-00-0000 A
2. PATIENT'S NAME (Last Name, First Name, Middle Initial) Doe, Jane E. · 3. PATIENT'S BIRTH DATE MM DD YY 12 09 31 · SEX M [ ] F [X]	4. INSURED'S NAME (Last Name, First Name, Middle Initial) Doe, John X.
5. PATIENT'S ADDRESS (No., Street) 123 South St. · 6. PATIENT RELATIONSHIP TO INSURED Self [ ] Spouse [X] Child [ ] Other [ ]	7. INSURED'S ADDRESS (No., Street) Same
CITY Spokane · STATE WA · 8. PATIENT STATUS Single [ ] Married [X] Other [ ]	CITY · STATE
ZIP CODE 99203 · TELEPHONE (Include Area Code) (509) 333-1234 · Employed [ ] Full-Time Student [ ] Part-Time Student [ ]	ZIP CODE · TELEPHONE (INCLUDE AREA CODE) ( )
9. OTHER INSURED'S NAME (Last Name, First Name, Middle Initial) Same Supplemental Policy · 10. IS PATIENT'S CONDITION RELATED TO:	11. INSURED'S POLICY GROUP OR FECA NUMBER
a. OTHER INSURED'S POLICY OR GROUP NUMBER MS 123-12345 · a. EMPLOYMENT? (CURRENT OR PREVIOUS) [ ] YES [ ] NO	a. INSURED'S DATE OF BIRTH MM DD YY · SEX M [ ] F [ ]
b. OTHER INSURED'S DATE OF BIRTH MM DD YY · SEX M [ ] F [ ] · b. AUTO ACCIDENT? [ ] YES [ ] NO PLACE (State)	b. EMPLOYER'S NAME OR SCHOOL NAME
c. EMPLOYER'S NAME OR SCHOOL NAME · c. OTHER ACCIDENT? [ ] YES [ ] NO	c. INSURANCE PLAN NAME OR PROGRAM NAME
d. INSURANCE PLAN NAME OR PROGRAM NAME Medigap Insurance · 10d. RESERVED FOR LOCAL USE	d. IS THERE ANOTHER HEALTH BENEFIT PLAN? [ ] YES [X] NO Secondary Only *If yes*, return to and complete item 9 a-d
READ BACK OF FORM BEFORE COMPLETING & SIGNING THIS FORM. 12. PATIENT'S OR AUTHORIZED PERSON'S SIGNATURE I authorize the release of any medical or other information necessary to process this claim. I also request payment of government benefits either to myself or to the party who accepts assignment below. SIGNED Signature On File DATE	13. INSURED'S OR AUTHORIZED PERSON'S SIGNATURE I authorize payment of medical benefits to the undersigned physician or supplier for services described below. SIGNED Signature On File

Figure 9–1—continued. Top half.

14. DATE OF CURRENT: MM DD YY — ILLNESS (First symptom) OR INJURY (Accident) OR PREGNANCY(LMP)

15. IF PATIENT HAS HAD SAME OR SIMILAR ILLNESS. GIVE FIRST DATE MM DD YY

16. DATES PATIENT UNABLE TO WORK IN CURRENT OCCUPATION FROM MM DD YY TO MM DD YY

17. NAME OF REFERRING PHYSICIAN OR OTHER SOURCE: John Q. Surgeon

17a. I.D. NUMBER OF REFERRING PHYSICIAN: A03210

18. HOSPITALIZATION DATES RELATED TO CURRENT SERVICES FROM MM DD YY TO MM DD YY

19. RESERVED FOR LOCAL USE

20. OUTSIDE LAB? ☐ YES ☐ NO — $ CHARGES

21. DIAGNOSIS OR NATURE OF ILLNESS OR INJURY. (RELATE ITEMS 1,2,3 OR 4 TO ITEM 24E BY LINE)

1. 366.10
2. ___ . __
3. ___ . __
4. ___ . __

22. MEDICAID RESUBMISSION CODE — ORIGINAL REF. NO.

23. PRIOR AUTHORIZATION NUMBER

24.

	A DATE(S) OF SERVICE From MM DD YY	To MM DD YY	B Place of Service	C Type of Service	D PROCEDURES, SERVICES, OR SUPPLIES (Explain Unusual Circumstances) CPT HCPCS	MODIFIER	E DIAGNOSIS CODE	F $ CHARGES	G DAYS OR UNITS	H EPSDT Family Plan	I EMG	J COB	K RESERVED FOR LOCAL USE
1	01 01 92	01 01 92	24		00142	QZ	1	324. 00	12				
2													
3					Time: 60 minutes								
4													
5													
6													

25. FEDERAL TAX I.D. NUMBER: 12-1234567 — SSN ☐ EIN ☐

26. PATIENT'S ACCOUNT NO: 01234

27. ACCEPT ASSIGNMENT? (For govt. claims, see back): X YES ☐ NO

28. TOTAL CHARGE: $ 324. 00

29. AMOUNT PAID: $

30. BALANCE DUE: $

31. SIGNATURE OF PHYSICIAN OR SUPPLIER INCLUDING DEGREES OR CREDENTIALS (I certify that the statements on the reverse apply to this bill and are made a part thereof.)
Fred Mertz, CRNA
SIGNED — DATE

32. NAME AND ADDRESS OF FACILITY WHERE SERVICES WERE RENDERED (If other than home or office)
Spokane Medical Center
S. 26th St.
Spokane, WA 99204

33. PHYSICIAN'S, SUPPLIER'S BILLING NAME, ADDRESS, ZIP CODE & PHONE #
Spokane Anesthesia Services
W. 34th St
Spokane, WA 99204
PIN# 000123456 — GRP#

PHYSICIAN OR SUPPLIER INFORMATION

790-0128 (12/90) (OCR) 1 pt.

(APPROVED BY AMA COUNCIL ON MEDICAL SERVICE 8/88) — PLEASE PRINT OR TYPE — FORM HCFA-1500 (12-90) FORM OWCP-1500 FORM RRB-1500

Figure 9–1—continued. Bottom half.

TYPES OF INSURANCE PLANS AND HOW THEY REIMBURSE FOR ANESTHESIA

Preferred Provider Organizations (PPOs)

These plans are attempts to control costs by limiting the providers that participants may use for services. Typically, the preferred provider organization (PPO) "prefers" those providers who sign a contract to provide services at a reduced rate to plan members. Historically, these plans have frequently been restrictive to CRNAs, often not allowing them to become preferred providers even if they are willing to sign a contract. Preference is typically given to physician providers.

Health Maintenance Organizations (HMOs)

Health maintenance organizations (HMOs) attempt to limit costs by forcing plan participants to seek all their comprehensive health care needs through the HMO network. Primary care providers refer participants to other primary care providers within the system, such as surgeons, when such services are needed. Large HMOs such as Kaiser Permanente in California and Oregon and Group Health in Washington State own their own hospitals and employ CRNAs directly. However, smaller plans may not be able to justify this expense and will instead contract with certain providers, including CRNAs, for their services.

As opposed to PPOs, which generally allow anyone who will agree to their contract to become a provider, HMOs carefully limit their use of "outside" providers. By contracting with a limited number of providers, HMOs attempt to use the volume of their patients to achieve low contractual rates. Both HMOs and PPOs are often referred to as providers of "managed care," a system which is gaining a wider participant base because of its attempts to control costs through controlled services.

Traditional Plans

These plans represent the bulk of insurance plans today. The traditional plans place no restrictions on participants as to their choice of providers, and usually pay 80 percent of the provider's care, with the participant paying the remaining 20 percent. In the past, participants were expected to pay their bills directly to the provider, then submit copies of their claims to the insurer, who would reimburse 80 percent of the bill. Today, most of those plans accept bills directly from the provider. Variations include paying those providers who sign a contract relinquishing the right to bill the patient over an "allowable" 100% of that amount.

Medicare

Medicare, a federally subsidized health care program, was initially modeled after the "traditional" plan and pays 80 percent of the allowable amount. However, there is often a great disparity between allowable amounts provided by traditional plans and that paid by Medicare. These amounts continue to decline as available health care dollars shrink. Many believe that traditional carriers will eventually more closely ally their allowable charges to those Medicare recognizes.

Supplemental Plans

These plans are meant to supplement Medicare and generally pay the remaining 20 percent of the Medicare allowable amount, plus any deductibles.

Medicaid

Medicaid was devised to provide medical care to the indigent population. These plans are administered by individual states and vary accordingly. Most plans are based on determination of eligibility of the participant and subsequent full payment of the Medicaid allowable fee (generally lower than the Medicare fee) to the provider. Participants may be given "coupons" that they present to the provider at the time of service. These coupons are dated and ensure that the participant receives care only during the eligible period.

Most, if not all, of the aforementioned plans are undergoing rapid and often drastic change in an attempt to control spiraling health care costs. At the very least, CRNAs can expect reimbursement rates will generally decrease in the near future, which will affect anesthetists in *any* practice setting, self-employed or not. Many believe that fee-for-service reimbursement structures are a thing of the past, giving way to the more cost-efficient "managed care" facility where all providers, including physicians, are salaried. Despite this, organized medicine continues to cling to the notion that a fee-for-service system is the only means to maintain the integrity of the physician-client relationship and fights vigorously to sustain the status quo.

Due to the general economic downturn of the early 1990s, (although arguably cyclical) and the fact that about 13 percent of the gross national product (GNP) is given to provide health care, it will not be long until drastic measures are required to restructure a system that is more market sensitive and cost-effective. In fact, since the problems inherent to provision of health care are so great, many state legislatures are debating their own plans, as legislation on the federal level appears interminably mired in indecision and inaction.

It is not the mission of this book to promote or show preference to any particular employment configuration, as CRNAs are employed in virtually every practice setting and should remain free to make those sorts of professional decisions. However, it is incumbent on all CRNAs to become knowledgeable about the issues that will undoubtedly reshape a future health care system that CRNAs will have to practice within. Only with this knowledge can a CRNA be able to retain the right to practice competitively on a level field of play.

DETERMINING YOUR FINANCIAL WORTH

CRNAs, when entering into negotiations with their employers or entertaining the idea of billing for their own services, require a method of determining their productivity in terms of a dollar amount. Since Medicare represents 40 to 50 percent of current surgical patients, examples will be given to determine the payment that would be received for administering an anesthetic to a Medicare participant.

Medicare determines reimbursement based on two major variables, surgical procedure and time. First, a base unit value is determined for the procedure by consulting a list based on the CPT code of the procedure. Second, the time is converted to units by dividing the actual anesthesia time in minutes by 15. Fractional units must now be used, that is, 50 divided by 15 equals 3.3. You can no longer round up to the next unit. In the following examples, several resulting figures are shown to illustrate how payment is made for the procedure. However, the dollar amount in parentheses represents the total payment for the procedure and is the amount that should be used in computing net production.

Example 1: A 76-year-old-man receives a 50-minute anesthetic for cataract surgery. The CRNA is *not medically directed.*

A. Base units are:	4.0
B. Time units: 50 divided by 15 equals:	3.3
C. Total units:	7.3
D. Medicare allowable in locale *x* is $15.75/unit, so allowable charge is:	($114.98)
E. Medicare pays 80 percent of this charge, or:	$91.98
F. Patient or supplemental plan pays remaining 20 percent, or:	$23.00

Example 2: A 67-year-old woman receives a 3-hour and 10-minute anesthetic for abdominal aortic aneurysm. The CRNA is *not medically directed.*

A. Base units are:	8.0
B. Time units: 190 minutes divided by 15:	12.7
C. Total units:	20.7
D. Medicare allowable in locale *x* for non-medically directed CRNA anesthesia is $15.75, so allowable charge is:	($326.03)
E. Medicare pays 80 percent of this charge, or:	$260.82
F. The patient or supplemental plan pays remaining 20 percent, or:	$65.21

Example 3: A 67-year-old woman receives a 3-hour and 10-minute anesthetic for abdominal aortic aneurysm. The CRNA is *medically directed.*

A. Base units are:	8.0
B. Time units: 190 minutes divided by 15:	12.7
C. Total units:	20.7
D. Medicare allowable in locale *x* for medically directed CRNA is $10.50/unit, so allowable charge:	($217.35)
E. Medicare pays 80 percent of this charge, or:	$173.88
F. Patient or supplemental plan pays remaining 20 percent, or:	$43.47

Note: The total amount of income produced by the CRNA in the above three examples is determined by adding the allowable charges (in parentheses) for each procedure, in this case, $658.36.

To determine production, CRNAs should review the cases they have performed for the last month and assign a dollar value to each based on the computations listed earlier. It is important to remember that Medicare has become one of the lowest payers in health care, and allowance should be made for private insurance patients whose payment may be substantially greater. In addition, these figures do not account for balance billing, because it cannot be done by CRNAs under Medicare. Using the Medicare payments will give the CRNA a very conservative estimate of total production.

SUMMARY

The education of every CRNA, whether formally in school or through continuing education, should include attention to the matter of reimbursement and determinations of values for professional services. Because this knowledge has not been universally shared, history has shown that CRNA services have made others within the health care system wealthy, unfortunately at the expense of those entrusted to our care—the patients. Although CRNAs remain unique in nursing in that they have obtained the opportunities of self-employment, reserve, restraint, and responsibility should be the watchwords of any CRNA who chooses to receive direct reimbursement. Without those concerns, such privileges will be short-lived.

GLOSSARY

Allowable charge: The fee that the third party feels is appropriate for a particular service. Third-party payers may pay all or only a portion of that fee.

Carrier: Insurance company; also HCFA's term for the insurance companies with whom it contracts to make payments to Medicare Part B providers (such as CRNAs and anesthesiologists) in a specific area.

Fiscal intermediary: HCFA's term for the insurance companies with whom it contracts to make payments to Part A providers (such as hospitals) in a specific geographic area.

HCFA: Health Care Financing Administration. This is the arm of the federal government that oversees Medicare and Medicaid, which is responsible for establishing reimbursement policy for all Medicare fiscal intermediaries and carriers.

Insured: Person financially responsible for the insurance plan.

Participating provider: A provider who has signed a contract with the carrier to accept a lower payment for services in exchange for some financial incentive. In Medicare, participating providers are given a 5 percent increase in their allowable charge.

Plan: Details of insurance coverage.

Provider: Anesthesia provider.

Subscriber: An enrollee in a health insurance plan.

Third-party payer: A generic term for any system of payment of health care providers other than direct payment by the patient.

10

Asserting Influence in Health Care Policy

Kathleen A. Michels

OUTLINE

OBJECTIVES

On completing this chapter, the reader will be able to:

1. Describe how the AANA is involved in the political and legislative arenas.
2. Discuss how to become politically active.
3. Chart how state and federal governments determine health policy.
4. Give examples of how to influence state and federal legislative processes.

ASSERTING INFLUENCE IN HEALTH CARE POLICY

Democracy means the rule of the people—including you. State and federal legislators can only represent and serve you well if you educate them on health issues through legislative and political involvement. The purpose of this chapter is to provide information on how the American Association of Nurse Anesthetists (AANA) is involved in the political and legislative arenas, how one can become politically active, how state and federal governments determine health policy, and how state and federal legislative processes can be influenced.

AMERICAN ASSOCIATION OF NURSE ANESTHETISTS INVOLVEMENT IN NATIONAL POLITICS AND LEGISLATION

Political Activity

The AANA registered the AANA Separate Segregated Fund, its political action arm, with the Federal Elections Commission in 1983. In addition, the AANA volunteer structure includes an eight-person political action committee (CRNA-PAC). The purpose of the CRNA-PAC is to promote and facilitate the accumulation of voluntary contributions from members of the AANA or others who may legally be solicited into the fund. Distributions from the fund are made by the Committee to support candidates in elections that have national importance. The Committee directs distributions from the fund to support candidates who have taken responsible positions on quality health care.

Legislative and Regulatory Activity

Through membership in the AANA, CRNA interests are represented before federal legislative and regulatory officials. The voice of the AANA is strong because it represents 96 percent of the CRNAs and student nurse anesthetists in the anesthesia profession.

Policy Formation

The legislative positions that AANA lobbyists champion come from the policies adopted by the AANA Board of Directors. Recommendations to the board come from individual CRNAs, state associations, the AANA Government Relations Committee, and resolutions passed at the AANA Annual Meeting. As effective as the association is at representing your views, however, it still requires your personal communication with legislators to enhance the credibility of the association message.

Government Relations Committee

The eight-person AANA Government Relations Committee acts under the belief that CRNAs, as patient advocates and providers of quality anesthesia care, can and do make a difference in influencing legislative changes, both on the state and federal level. The committee monitors, evaluates, and manages legislative and regulatory changes for the profession. The specific functions of the committee are

1. To change and heighten the consciousness of CRNAs and develop their knowledge and understanding of the political process in order to influence legislative and regulatory changes, both on the state and federal level.
2. To develop leadership potential by sharing knowledge, skills, and expertise on behalf of nurse anesthesia and the health needs of the public.
3. To increase visibility and actively influence health policy development.
4. To promote the practice of nurse anesthesia using the legislative and regulatory approach for the advancement of the profession and assuring the public protection and safety in the delivery of anesthesia services.
5. To seek funding for nurse anesthesia students and faculty through the legislative process and other available sources.
6. To seek access to clinical facilities in further developing programs of nurse anesthesia.
7. To monitor and comment on legislative proposals concerning anesthesia practice, education, and human resources.

8 To provide testimony on issues vital to the public interest and the future of the profession.

American Association of Nurse Anesthetists Office of Federal Affairs

The AANA Office of Federal Affairs, in Washington, DC, was opened in July 1990. Its role is to monitor federal government activities and analyze their impact on the nurse anesthesia profession. In addition, it develops draft position papers and statements for approval by the AANA Board of Directors. Information on federal government affairs is shared with the AANA membership in four ways: (1) a weekly "government affairs hotline" of current events that is updated each week by midnight Thursday (the toll-free hotline number is on the back of every AANA membership card); (2) a monthly column in the *AANA NewsBulletin* that describes the political, legislative, and regulatory activities of the association; (3) a bimonthly column in the *AANA Journal* that presents an in-depth analysis of a particular federal health topic; and (4) a written update for the AANA Board of Directors and participants at each AANA Assembly and Annual Meeting.

The AANA Department of Federal Affairs has a professional staff of three people, which includes a director of federal government affairs and two associate directors. The director covers reimbursement and legal issues and is responsible for

- Medicare CRNA fee schedule, conditions of participation, investigations of alleged fraud and abuse, and financing of nurse anesthesia education
- Medicaid reimbursement
- Federal Employees Health Benefits (FEHB) plan reimbursement
- Civilian Health and Medical Program of the Uniformed Services (CHAMPUS) reimbursement
- Senate Finance Committee (reimbursement)
- House Ways and Means Committee (reimbursement)
- House Energy and Commerce Committee (reimbursement)
- Physician Payment Review Commission
- Medical liability/tort reform
- Drug Enforcement Administration
- National practitioner data bank
- General Accounting Office/Office of Management and Budget/Congressional Budget Office
- CRNA-PAC/Federal Elections Commission

One of the associate directors covers education and pay issues and is responsible for

- House and Senate Appropriations Committee
- House and Senate Budget Committees
- Reauthorization of the Nurse Education Act
- Reauthorization of the Higher Education Act
- Reauthorization of the National Health Service Corps
- Division of Nursing nurse anesthesia educational programs
- Office of Rural Health
- Military pay and promotions
- Veterans Administration (VA) pay and promotions
- Indian Health Service pay and promotions

The second associate director covers practice and research issues and is responsible for

- House Energy and Commerce Committee (health programs)
- Senate Labor and Human Resources Committee (health programs)
- Agency for Health Care Policy and Research (AHCPR) Practice Guidelines, including pain management, cataracts, and acquired immunodeficiency syndrome (AIDS)
- AHCPR research
- National Center for Nursing Research
- AIDS, both congressional and Centers for Disease Control

- Access to health care legislation
- Food and Drug Administration
- Trauma Advisory Council

Legislative Contact Network

Many individual CRNAs have a close legislative and political relationship with their members of Congress. The AANA is formalizing that relationship with the development of a Legislative Contact Network. The purpose of the network is to provide CRNA legislative contacts with timely information about legislation of interest to the AANA that we would like their member of Congress to support in some fashion. Examples include introduction of legislation, cosponsorship of legislation, voting for legislation, or amending legislation to include an AANA-endorsed provision. In addition, when appropriate, CRNA legislative contacts may be asked to attend local fundraisers for their member of Congress when the CRNA-PAC has decided to contribute to that member's campaign.

HOW YOU CAN BECOME POLITICALLY ACTIVE

Politics is the use of power for change. Although politics is not always nice or fair, health care professionals must become adept in managing the political process. Otherwise, someone else may exert power on policy decisions that will have a detrimental impact on your professional practice and reimbursement for services.

While political activity takes time and energy, it is the best investment one can make in a career. Politics is an integral part of each of our lives. On a daily basis, our personal relationships involve the art of negotiation and compromise—the essence of politics. In addition, professional relationships revolve around power, teamwork, and creating policies, which are also characteristic of politics. Skills that can be learned by participating in the political process will be useful tools in both your personal and professional lives.

Ways to Get Politically Involved

To be a player in the game of politics, the first thing that one should do is get on the playing field. Do not make the common mistake of thinking that you have to make a major time commitment to some type of political activity to make a difference. Any effort to which you can contribute will make a difference. Start by determining a reasonable time commitment, one that can be realistically followed and completed. The following are suggestions of ways to become politically involved.

- Join your state and/or national associations and participate in their government relations or political action committees.
- Become active in the League of Women Voters, which often is involved in voter registration drives and "get out the vote" campaigns during elections.
- Join your state Democratic or Republican party so that you can pay your "political dues" to the party structure. This is important if you ever want to run for political office.
- Make a generous financial contribution to your state and/or national association's political action committee.
- Approach local talk show hosts about health care issues that you care about or call in to talk to health guests on shows.
- Volunteer to be a speaker on health care issues before local elderly and consumer organizations.
- Build a coalition of individuals like yourself, so that you have the additional power of a collective voice. Then use the coalition as a legislative network for lobbying on issues.
- Participate in professional research, because the database that research provides is key to the shaping of health care policy.
- Run for elective office.
- Campaign to get appointed to a board, commission, or other decision-making body that will influence health policy.
- Invite key decision makers to visit your place of work. There is no more effective way to teach decision makers about the importance of the job you do than by showing them firsthand.

- Write an article on a health care issue for your local newspaper.
- If a legislator or other decision maker does something important on a health care issue of concern to you (such as successfully championing your bill through the legislative process), arrange a media "photo opportunity" at which the decision maker is given an award by your state or national association for his or her efforts.
- Participate in a formal or informal legislative/political internship or fellowship. At the local level, contact your city councilperson's office or mayor's office about any volunteer positions. At the state level, call your state association or the office of your state representative and senator to find out if there are any programs. At the federal level, contact the AANA or the offices of your member of the House of Representatives and your two members of the Senate.
- Host a candidates' night at a meeting of your local or state association to discuss health policy issues.
- Participate in a candidate's election campaign.[1]

Working in a Campaign

When most people think of political action, they usually think of working in an election campaign. Political campaigns can be both exhilarating and frustrating. Part of the reason for the frustration is that most campaigns are chaos. You can imagine how difficult it is to orchestrate every one of the paid staff, as well as hundreds of volunteers. The exhilaration comes from knowing that you have played a part in electing someone to office who cares about the same issues, including health issues, that you do.

If working in a campaign is the political activity that you desire, these are some of the activities to choose from.

Prior to Election Day

- Stuffing envelopes with the candidate's campaign literature
- Putting up yard signs in favor of your candidate
- Distributing campaign literature door-to-door
- Canvassing door-to-door to determine voter opinions
- Staffing phone banks to urge voters to vote for your candidate
- Chauffeuring the candidate to functions (this is an especially good time to talk about health care with candidates because you literally have a captive audience)
- Writing policy papers for the candidate to use
- Participating in mass mailing efforts to registered voters or a targeted audience
- Serving as the candidate's representative at functions
- Building a base of your colleagues so, for example, you can have a "Tuesday CRNA night" at the campaign headquarters during which CRNAs do all the necessary tasks, such as answering the phones, stuffing envelopes, and answering mail
- Hosting a "meet and greet" function for the candidate in your home
- Holding a fundraiser for the candidate in your home
- Making a generous financial contribution to the candidate

On Election Day

- Staffing phone banks to remind voters to vote on election day
- Distributing your candidate's campaign literature at polling places (contingent on election laws)
- Providing transportation and babysitting services to voters
- Watching the polls (to ensure that the voting process is carried out according to the election laws)
- Hosting a victory party for your winning candidate

Networking

It is very rare for a single group alone to promote a piece of legislation, especially a controversial one, through Congress. American society is too complex and diversified for there to be easy consensus on most issues. Therefore, you may need to form coalitions with other groups that have a mutual interest in a given public policy. While alliances may be necessary, approach them with caution because there is usually a price to be paid in terms of needing to compromise or to accommodate the needs of the other groups in the coalition. It is a political call whether or not the benefits of a coalition outweigh the inherent negatives.

There are areas you should consider before formally associating with other groups. You should make sure that there will be an even division of responsibility. You also want to make sure that you can trust the judgment of your partners. There is nothing worse than finding out that you are associated with a campaign that is unethical or irresponsible. By the same token, you do not want to join every coalition. There are limits to how much your organization can do. You should also be concerned about appearing to be active on too many fronts. Being overextended can damage your credibility in the legislative arena as much as being inactive can. Specific parameters should be set when you join a coalition. At a minimum, the coalition ought to be restricted to a specific issue, event, or period. If no such limitations are established, you may find yourself in a situation you cannot easily escape later.[2]

Steps for a Successful Coalition

1. Define and agree on the goal—why is this legislation necessary?
2. Establish guidelines and rules for the coalition. All groups are free to act for themselves, except when they use the name of the coalition.
3. Define tasks.
4. Establish a coordinating committee.
5. Organize resources to complete the necessary elements of the campaign.
6. Keep everyone together and focused on the one area of agreement. Do not let areas of difference or other issues cause infighting.
7. Keep jealous feelings to a minimum. Make sure everyone feels involved and assure them that their individual interests are well represented.
8. Watch legislators' attitudes toward your group to ensure that they are positive.
9. Establish effective communication methods for educating the public. It is important that the coalition speak with one voice.
10. Try to meet at least once a month, if possible, to keep apprised of activities.
11. Keep members informed with a regular update.
12. Investigate any legal requirements that may apply to your coalition, such as lobbying requirements.[3]

Potential Legislative Benefits of Political Activity

Political activity and legislative activity are the flip sides of the same coin. Therefore, always keep in mind that politics may help you achieve your health care policy objectives because the political arena provides access to decision makers. Your relationship with key decision makers may help influence their decisions on vital health policy issues. Your political activity on behalf of a candidate will not always result in the elected candidate voting the way you want, but it does give you the opportunity to eloquently make your case to the candidate. The following are lists of DOs and DON'Ts regarding political activity.

DO

- Build a professional image.
- Work on developing your writing and speaking skills.
- Learn all you can about a candidate's positions before you volunteer to work in his or her campaign.

- Make realistic time commitments about what you can offer a campaign.
- Follow through on your commitments in a responsible manner.
- Have business cards with you at all times for networking.
- Work to expand your network by recruiting other volunteers.
- Vote and encourage others to vote.

DON'T

- Be afraid to volunteer for a low-level task.
- Neglect traditional political organizations.
- Forget to get very clear directions about what the campaign's expectations are of you regarding job responsibilities and time commitments.
- Be discouraged if it takes time to work up to more senior roles in a campaign.
- Put off getting involved until the timing is perfect—it never will be.
- Forget to take fair credit for the work that you have done.

HOW STATE AND FEDERAL GOVERNMENTS DETERMINE HEALTH POLICY

Typical State Legislative Process

As state legislatures take greater initiative in determining health policy, many organizations are taking their first steps into state government affairs. With the exception of Nebraska, state legislatures consist of two houses: the senate (commonly referred to as the upper house) and, depending on the state, either the house or assembly (commonly referred to as the lower house). Bills are identified by state, house of origin, and number; for instance, California Senate Bill 1 (cas1); Nebraska Legislative Bill 3 (ne13); New York Assembly Bill 3695 (nya3695).

State legislatures adopt resolutions and bills. Some resolutions are adopted only by one house; others are adopted by both houses. The substance of resolutions varies; some are used to express legislative concern about a specific issue, and some are simply congratulatory. Most states do not require action by the governor for resolutions to become officially adopted.

Although each legislature has its own unique set of rules and procedures, most bills follow the same general path—introduction, consideration by the first house, consideration by the second house, and consideration by the governor.

Bill Introduction

The state legislative process begins when a bill is introduced. In most states, bills may be introduced only by members or committees of the legislature. In about half the states, bills may not be introduced until the legislature convenes. The remaining states allow the introduction of bills prior to the official convening date for presession study. This practice is called *prefiling.*

Committee Referral and Action

After introduction, bills are referred to a committee for public hearing. The number, structure, and operating procedures of committees are unique to each state. Some states use a joint committee system to review bills, but most states have separate committees in each house dealing with specific subjects, such as health.

Committees usually have the authority to recommend that bills be passed as introduced, passed as amended, substituted by the committee, or killed. Often, bills that would cost money or have some other financial consequence are reviewed by two committees; a policy committee reviews the substance of the bill while the fiscal committee reviews the financial aspects of the bill.

Floor Action

Many bills do not receive committee approval and thus proceed no further. Those bills that are approved by committees (either as introduced, amended, or substituted) proceed to the floor for consideration by the entire chamber. The chamber may pass the bill in the form recommended by the committee(s), amend the bill and pass it, or kill it.

Second Chamber

When a bill is passed by the chamber of origin, it is sent to the second chamber and the procedure is repeated; committee referral, committee action, and floor action in the second chamber. As in the chamber of origin, bills may be approved, amended, substituted, or killed in committee or on the floor.

Concurrence and Conference Actions

Bills that are amended in the second chamber return to the chamber of origin for concurrence. If the chamber of origin concurs with the amended version of the bill passed by the second chamber, the bill is eligible to be sent to the governor for signature. If the chamber of origin does not concur, the second chamber may withdraw the amendments. If the second chamber does not withdraw the amendments, a conference committee is appointed to resolve the differences between the chambers. The report of the conference committee must be approved by both chambers for the bill to move on to the governor.

Governor's Actions

When a bill is approved and passed by the legislature, it is sent to the governor. In most states, the governor may sign a bill into law; veto all or part of the bill (line item veto); or, depending on whether the legislature is in session or adjourned, let the bill die without signature or let it become law without signature. North Carolina is the only state in which the governor does not have veto power.

Vetoed bills are returned to the chamber in which they were introduced. The legislature may pass bills that have been vetoed by the governor if a specified majority of both chambers (usually two thirds) votes to override the veto. Figure 10–1 provides a flowchart of a typical state Legislative process.

Federal Legislative Process

Nowhere are policy and process more intertwined than in the Congress of the United States. Skillful legislators use the legislative process to advance their policy goals. Sponsors often amend the wording of a bill to keep it from being referred to a hostile committee. For instance, an antiabortion amendment may be added to a House appropriations bill and may be germane because it restricts federal funding for abortions. Procedural techniques and policy interact at many stages of the legislative process. "Legislation is like a chess game more than anything else," Representative John D. Dingell (D-MI) has said. "It is a seemingly endless series of moves, until ultimately someone prevails through exhaustion, or brilliance, or because of overwhelming public sentiment for their side."[5]

By the mid-1980s, the federal budget deficit and the complex special budget process that Congress devised for dealing with it resulted in the increased use of omnibus bills. Rather than separate bills going all the way through the normal legislative process, many often unrelated proposals were packaged in a single, large piece of legislation. These so-called omnibus budget reconciliation bills contained literally hundreds of provisions that were supposedly necessary to develop an overall budget plan for the year. The opportunities to debate and amend these bills are often severely limited. Consequently, omnibus bills allow measures that would not normally be approved as separate bills to get adopted. Sometimes this global approach contains provisions that benefit CRNAs, and sometimes it contains provisions that harm CRNAs. A positive example is the authority for CRNAs to receive direct Medicare reimbursement, included in the Omnibus Budget Reconciliation Act of 1986.

Legislative Vehicles

There are four basic forms in which a legislative proposal may be introduced: bills, joint resolutions, concurrent resolutions, and simple resolutions.

Bills are the most common form. They are prefaced by "H.R." in the House and "S." in the Senate, followed by a number assigned based on the order of its introduction during a congressional session.

Joint resolutions may originate in either the House or Senate and are labeled "H. J. Res." or "S. J. Res." followed by a sequential number. The most common usage is to

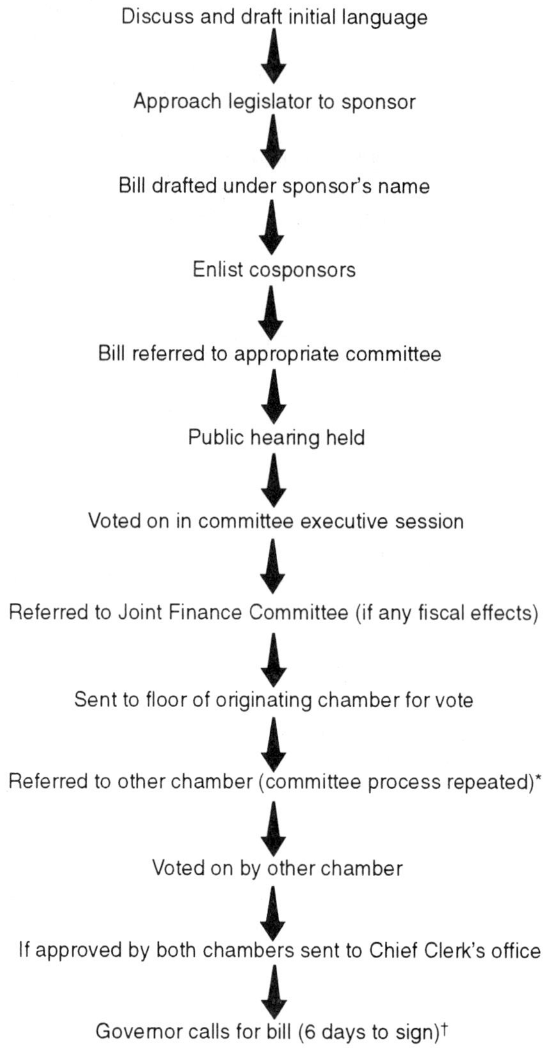

**If bill is revised by other chamber, it returns to the originating chamber. The originating chamber may concur with, disapprove, or modify changes. Bills can go back and forth between chambers several times.*
†If bill is not signed before the end of the session, it is pocket vetoed and sent back to both chambers for override.

Figure 10–1. Typical state legislative process.

continue an existing law. It is subject to the same procedure as bills, unless it is proposing an amendment to the Constitution. If it is the latter, then it must be approved by two-thirds vote of each chamber and be sent directly to the administrator of general services for submission to the states for ratification. Constitutional amendments are not presented to the president for his signature.

Concurrent resolutions are designated by "H. Con. Res." or "S. Con. Res." They must be approved by both the House and Senate before they can become effective. A concurrent resolution does not require the president's signature and does not have the force of law. It expresses the opinion of Congress and is used for matters affecting the operations of both chambers.

Simple resolutions are designated "H. Res." or "S. Res." They are used for a matter concerning the operation of only one chamber and are adopted only by that chamber. They may also be used to create a special investigating committee, change chamber rules, or express the sense of the chamber on specific issues.

Drafting Legislation

Legislation can be drafted by congressional staff or legislative counsels at the request of individual members or committees. Legislation is also drafted by executive branch departments and agencies as well as by interest groups. Much of the legislation dealt with by Congress in any year is comprised of bills reauthorizing expiring laws, bills appropriating money to run the federal government, and bills submitted by the president and the executive branch to implement the administration's programs. Pursuant to the Constitution, revenue legislation originates in the House. By custom, appropriations legislation also originates in the House. All other bills may originate in either chamber.

Introduction and Referral of Bills

Members of the House of Representatives are elected for 2-year terms and senators are elected for 6-year terms. The length of each Congress mirrors the length of a House term—2 years. Each Congress conducts its business in two regular sessions that begin in January of successive years. For example, the first session of the 102nd Congress convened in January 1991; the second session of the 102nd Congress convened in January 1992. Of the 11,824 bills introduced in the House and Senate in the 101st Congress (1989 to 1991), only 1734 were reported by committees and only 484 were enacted into law. Although only a small fraction of all health bills are eventually enacted into law, they stimulate the vigorous debate on the future of health care policy. Any bill that has not received final congressional approval when Congress adjourns automatically dies and must be reintroduced in the next Congress and begin the entire process again.

To become law, proposed legislation must be approved in identical form in both the House and the Senate. The bill is subject to delay, defeat, or substantial modification. "It is very easy to defeat a bill in Congress," President John F. Kennedy once observed. "It is much more difficult to pass one."[6]

Any bill or resolution must be introduced by a representative or senator when Congress is in session. There is no limit to the number of bills a member may introduce. The legislative leader of a proposal is the key to its survival. The fact that a bill has a high-ranking sponsor automatically escalates its importance as a piece of legislation.

A House member may introduce a bill or resolution by handing it to the clerk of the House or placing it in a box at the front of the House chamber, called the "hopper." Senators usually submit their proposals and accompanying statements to clerks in the Senate chamber or may introduce their bills from the Senate floor. If objection to the introduction of the bill is offered by any senator, introduction of the bill is postponed until the next day. It is not uncommon for a representative and a senator to sponsor "companion" (identical) bills, each introducing his or her version simultaneously in their respective chamber. This is done to encourage both chambers to consider the measure simultaneously to dramatize the importance or urgency of the bill and to show broad support for it.

The House or Senate bill is then numbered, referred to the appropriate committee(s), labeled with the sponsor's name, and sent to the Government Printing Office for copies to be made. A representative or senator who is interested in actively promoting legislation often will seek cosponsors. This allows other legislators to jointly introduce the bill and indicate their support for it. Bipartisan sponsorship can be very important, as can endorsement by members of the committee to which the bill will be referred. There is no limit on the number of cosponsors that can be added to a House or Senate bill or resolution. A bill written in the executive branch and proposed as an administration measure usually is introduced by the chairman of the committee that has jurisdiction over the bill's subject matter.

Committees and Subcommittees

STRUCTURE. Committees are the heart of the legislative process. They have existed in the House and the Senate since 1789, and have allowed for a division of work and orderly consideration of legislation. The size of the Senate (100 members) and the House (435 members) makes it extremely difficult for all members to consider each piece of legislation. Consequently, each chamber has established its own committees to study and consider legislation. In turn, committees have established subcommittees to allow even further division of work.

Both the House and Senate have standing (permanent) committees and special (select) committees. There are 22 standing committees in the House and 16 in the Senate. Each standing committee has jurisdiction over certain subject areas of legislation, and all legislation that would affect that particular area of law are referred to that committee of jurisdiction. The number of select committees changes. The select committees are usually investigative in nature, convene for the duration of the matter under investigation, reach a decision or make recommendations, and are then dissolved.

The real nuts and bolts of the legislative process take place in committees and subcommittees, including research, investigation, and public hearings. This is the time to contact your elected legislator and let him or her know what your stand is on the bill. It is at this stage that you have the most ability to influence the movement of a bill. If legislators receive numerous letters in support of a bill, they will relay that to the subcommittee or committee chairman and that often expedites action on the bill. Conversely, if the legislator receives numerous letters opposing the bill, that will be conveyed to the subcommittee or committee chairman and the bill may die in committee without any action being taken.

Membership ratios on committees between the majority and minority parties are determined at the beginning of each Congress and are generally based on the ratio that exists for the entire membership of each chamber plus the political judgment of the majority party. Individuals are assigned to committees by caucus of the respective parties, and these assignments are confirmed by a floor vote. A member usually seeks election to the committee that has jurisdiction over a field in which he or she is most qualified and interested.

Subcommittees and committees are responsible to their parent bodies. However, because of the complexity of their assignments, they have substantial independence and autonomy. The chairman of a committee or subcommittee is a dominant figure in the legislative process because he or she can set the agenda for committee meetings, set up the hearings, and hire the staff. When a bill is referred to a committee, the chairman can either guide it through his or her committee or sit on the bill and effectively kill it.

In Congress, seniority is power. Members rank in seniority on the committee in accordance with their appointment to the committee. The majority member having the most years of service in Congress is usually designated chairman. The most senior member of the minority party is ordinarily designated as "ranking minority member." Better committee assignments and bigger committee staffs usually go hand in hand with tenure on Capitol Hill.

Subcommittee seniority is generally assigned in a similar way, with the full committee determining subcommittee membership and maintaining the same majority/minority ratios. In general, senators may serve on two major legislative committees and one lower-ranking committee. In the House, a representative usually serves on two committees.

COMMITTEE JURISDICTION. Formally, a bill is to be referred to the appropriate committee by the Speaker of the House or the presiding officer of the Senate. Informally, the parliamentarians of the two chambers act on behalf of the Speaker and the Senate presiding officer and actually refer the bills to committees. Bill sponsors may indicate their preferences for referral, although custom, chamber rules, and committee jurisdiction generally govern.

In turn, the chairman of the committee will refer the bill to one of its subcommittees unless the chairman decides to have the full committee act on the proposal. It is important to note that the 1970s witnessed a reform of the seniority system, resulting in restraints on committee chairmen and a diffusion of power from committee chairmen to subcommittees. Each committee has its own method of determining where the predominant policy role and power are exercised, at the full committee or the subcommittee level.

When a bill contains language that cuts across the jurisdiction of two or more committees, it may get a referral to multiple committees. In the Senate, multiple referrals are implemented by unanimous consent agreements. In the House, referral authority remains with the Speaker. There are three types of multiple referrals. First, there is "sequential referral," the most common form, which allows one committee to take action first and then refer the bill on to the second committee. Second is "joint referral," where a bill is referred, within specific time limits, successively to one committee and then to another. An example of joint referral would be bills that deal with Medicare Part B, for which both the House Energy and Commerce Committee and the House Ways and Means Committee share jurisdiction. Third, there is "split referral," where a bill is referred to several committees, each having jurisdiction over specific parts of the bill. Multiple referrals often can kill legislation since several committees are unlikely to agree on a version of the bill or even to report the bill at approximately the same time, if at all. On the other hand, when several committees report a multiply referred bill, the chances of that bill's passage can be greatly enhanced.

Failure of a committee to act on a bill is equivalent to killing it; the measure can be withdrawn from the committee's purview only by a discharge petition signed by a majority of the House membership on House bills, or by adoption of a special resolution in the Senate. Discharge attempts rarely succeed. The full House and Senate seldom question a decision of one of their committees not to report a bill.

REFERRAL TO SUBCOMMITTEE. The first committee action taken on a bill usually is a request for comment by interested agencies of the government, such as the Department of Health and Human Services on health bills. This gives the committee a preliminary indication if they should have the relevant subcommittee hold hearings on a bill. The committee chairperson may then refer the bill to a subcommittee for study and hearings, or it may be considered by the full committee. Subcommittee hearings provide the opportunity for members of Congress, executive branch staff, and representatives of industry, interest groups, and academia to formally present their views and positions on the legislative topic. An increasing trend is to have celebrities testify on particular issues, such as Robert Redford on environmental issues or Elizabeth Taylor on funding for AIDS research. Panels of witnesses are often scheduled together to hear similar perspectives at the same time or to probe the conflicting points of view of the panelists. Witnesses usually give prepared comments and then answer questions from the subcommittee members. The time that each subcommittee member has to ask questions is usually limited by the chairman. Verbatim transcripts of hearings are recorded and generally printed for committee and public use.

Depending on the nature of the bill, hearings may be conducted for a few hours, for several days, or for weeks. The timing and duration of subcommittee hearings depend largely on the discretion of the subcommittee chairman. Most hearings are held in open session. More frequently, the subcommittee chairman will limit the number and type of individuals and organizations that may testify. This is done either to expedite the subcommittee's deliberations or to create a particular attitude at the hearings; for example, only those in favor of a chairman's bill are asked to testify. There has also been an increase, in recent years, in the number of field hearings that are held in the subcommittee chairman's district or state.

On completion of the hearings, the subcommittee "marks up" a bill, which means amending the bill. During this step, a member may offer amendments that he or she supports. As a rule, informal votes are taken on each amendment to obtain a consensus. Because of the political tradeoffs and controversies that occur during markups, they are often closed to the public. The subcommittee has several options regarding actions it may take on the bill. It can

- Fail to take action or complete action on a bill
- Report it favorably without amendments
- Report it favorably with amendments
- Reject the bill
- Report it unfavorably or without recommendation
- Report favorably on a "clean bill." If amendments are adopted that are substantial, the subcommittee may order a "clean bill" introduced, incorporating all amendments in new bill language. The original bill then is put aside and the "clean bill" is then reintroduced,

assigned a new number, and referred to the full committee.

FULL COMMITTEE ACTION. After a subcommittee approves a bill, the full committee can choose from the same options for action that the subcommittee had.

Although the full committee can duplicate the subcommittee's procedures by holding hearings and markup sessions, it seldom does so. Committee discussion is more general, and although amendments may be offered, they are normally fewer than those considered in subcommittee. Committees generally rely on and accept the conclusions of the subcommittee. The full committee then votes on its recommendation to the full House or Senate. This procedure is called "ordering a bill reported." Occasionally a committee may order a bill reported unfavorably, but most of the time a report calls for favorable action because the committee can effectively kill a bill simply by failing to take any action.

When a committee sends a bill to the chamber floor, it explains its reasons in a written statement called a "report," which accompanies the bill. Often, committee members opposing a bill issue dissenting minority statements that are included in the back section of the report. The points made in the dissent section typically signal where the areas of contention are that will arise on the House or Senate floor. The rules of the House and Senate specify some aspects of the contents of reports; for example, they must show changes in existing law. These reports may also include an analysis of the legislative language and a statement of the committee's reasons or intent for passing the bill. In addition, the written statements from government agencies are ordinarily included in the report.

After a bill becomes law, there may be confusion or disagreement about the meaning of the actual legislative language. The committee report is often used to try to determine the "legislative intent" of the bill. For example, when the executive branch writes regulations or the courts rule on legislation, they will often rely on the report background if the law itself is not clear. Each report is given a number; for example, House Report 102-1 designates the first House committee report of the 102nd Congress. Report language is often used by lobbyists to protect their association's interests. For example, the annual health appropriations bill only lists how much money is to be spent for nurse anesthesia educational programs. The accompanying report contains directives to the federal agency that implements the law on how the money is to be spent.

Floor Action

When the full committee has approved a bill, it is reported back to the chamber where it originated. Accounts of floor debate and action taken in each chamber are published daily in the *Congressional Record.* The differences between House and Senate floor procedures are largely the result of the fact that the Senate is of smaller size, which allows greater opportunity for informal arrangements. The larger, more complex House emphasizes rules and precedents. In the House, the completed committee bill is sent to the House Rules Committee to establish the length of time for debate and to determine whether floor amendments will be allowed. Because debate is restricted and the amending process frequently limited, the House is able to dispose of legislation more quickly than the Senate. The Senate, although it has rules and procedures, more often operates by unanimous consent. Each Senate member, even the most junior, is offered a deference rarely seen in the House. The privileges of engaging in unlimited debate, the filibuster, and offering nongermane amendments are highly cherished traditions in the Senate that are not permitted under House rules. Given these conditions, it is not surprising that the Senate may spend days considering a measure that the House has debated and passed in a single afternoon.

Except for the House Rules Committee review, procedures are generally similar in the House and Senate. The bill is placed on a calendar for a vote. When, and sometimes whether, a bill is brought to the floor depends on many factors, including what other legislation is awaiting action, how controversial the measure is, and whether the leadership judges its chances for passage to be improved by immediate action. For example, the leadership may decide to delay taking up a controversial bill until its proponents can gather sufficient support to guarantee its passage. A bill is brought to floor debate by varying procedures. If it is a routine bill, it may await the call of the calendar. If it is urgent or important, it can be taken up in the Senate either by unanimous consent or by a majority vote. The policy committee of the majority party in the Senate schedules the bills that it wants taken up for debate. In the House, debate precedence is granted if a special rule is obtained from the Rules Committee.

House debate is limited by the rule under which the bill is considered. Senate debate is usually unlimited. It can be halted only by unanimous consent or by a "cloture" vote, which requires a three-fifths majority of the entire Senate. Cloture limits senators to 1 hour of debate.

Voting on bills may occur repeatedly before they are finally approved or rejected. The full House or Senate must approve, alter, or reject the committee amendments before the bill itself can be put to a vote. In addition, floor amendments may be offered to further certain objectives. First, members may offer floor amendments to dramatize their stands on issues, even if there is little chance that their amendments may be adopted. Second, some amendments are introduced at the request of the executive branch, a member's constituents, or special interests. Third, some are tactical tools for gauging sentiment for or against a bill. Fourth, others are used to stall action on a bill. Finally, some amendments may be designed to defeat the legislation. One common strategy is to try to load a bill up with so many unattractive amendments that it will eventually collapse under its own weight. Another strategy is to offer a "killer" amendment that if adopted would cause members who initially supported the bill to vote against it on final passage. Conversely, amendments known as "sweeteners" may be offered to attract broader support for the underlying measure.

The Senate has three different methods of voting: voice vote, a standing vote (called a division), and a recorded roll call vote to which members answer "yea" or "nay" when their names are called. The House uses voice and standing votes but has replaced the time-consuming roll calls with an electronic voting device to record the "yeas" and "nays." Another method of voting, used in the House only, is the teller vote. This is where members file up the center aisle past counters; only vote totals are announced. The teller vote is rarely used now, however. The most common method of voting in both the House and Senate is by voice vote.

The House votes on the rule for the bill, various amendments, and then the bill itself. The Senate votes on various amendments and then the bill. Final approval of a bill requires a majority vote of the members present.

Action in the Second Chamber

After a bill is passed in one chamber, it is sent to the other chamber for action. This body may take one of several steps. First, it may pass the bill as is. Second, it may send the bill to its committee of jurisdiction for study or alteration. Third, it may reject the entire bill and advise the other chamber of that fact. Finally, it may simply ignore the bill while it continues work on its own version of the same legislation. Frequently, one chamber may approve a version of a bill that is greatly at variance with the version already passed by the other chamber, and then substitute its amendments for the language of the original bill. This retains, in effect, only the other chamber's bill designation, without the original substance.

Often the second chamber makes only minor changes in the first chamber's bill. If these changes are agreed to by the first chamber, then the bill is sent to the president for signature. However, if the first chamber does not agree to the second chamber's changes, then the bill is sent to a conference committee to reconcile the differences in the two chambers' versions. The chamber that physically possesses the bill requests a conference. If the other chamber does not agree to a conference, then the bill dies.

Conference Committee

Sometimes known as the "third house of Congress," the conference committee usually consists of senior members (conferees) from the committees that have reported the bills. However, designated sponsors of major amendments to the bills also may be appointed to the conference committee. Conferees are appointed by the presiding officer of the Senate and the speaker of the House. The number of conferees may vary, the range usually being from three to nine members from each chamber, depending on the complexity of the bill involved. There does not have to be an equal number of conferees representing each chamber because a majority vote controls the action of each group, so that a large representation on one side does not give that chamber an advantage.

Theoretically, conferees are not allowed to write new legislation when reconciling the two versions before them, but this curb is sometimes bypassed. Many bills have been put into acceptable compromise form only after new language was approved by the conferees. Some of the hardest bargaining in the entire legislative process takes place in the conference committee, and the ironing out of differences may go on for days, weeks, or even months. The real constraining factor for conferees is that the chambers that they represent must accept the compromises. When the conferees have reached agreement, they prepare a conference report embodying their recommendations to each chamber.

The conference report must be approved by each chamber. Consequently, approval of the report is approval of the compromise bill. If no agreement is reached by the conferees, or should either chamber not accept the conference report, the bill dies.

Presidential Action

After a bill has been passed by both the House and the Senate in identical form, it is sent to the White House for action. The president has four options. First, he may sign the bill, date it, and write the word "approved" on the document. The Constitution requires only the president's signature. The president may allow the bill to become law without his signature. This occurs if he takes no action for 10 days (Sundays excepted) when Congress is in session. Third, he may "pocket veto" the bill. This occurs if Congress passes a bill and then adjourns before the president has had the 10-day option to return the bill with a veto. In this instance, the bill will not automatically become law. Fourth, the president may veto the bill within the 10-day option and return it to Congress with a message stating his reasons for the veto. The message is sent to the chamber that originated the bill. If no action is taken there on the veto message, the bill dies. However, Congress can attempt to override the president's veto and enact the bill. The overriding of a veto in each chamber requires a two-thirds vote of those present, who must number a quorum and vote by roll call. If the president's veto is overridden, the bill becomes law, otherwise it dies.

When bills are passed and signed, or passed over a veto, they are given public law numbers in numerical order. They are identified by the Congress that passed them and by the law number, for example, Public Law 101-802 means the 802nd public law passed by the 101st Congress.[7–9] Figure 10–2 designates the flow of legislation through the House and Senate.

Federal Regulatory Process

All rules start with Congress passing, and the president signing, a public law creating a federal program. The law defines the goals of regulatory programs, identifies the agency responsible for achieving them, and contains substantive and procedural guidance as to how the agency is to conduct its work. Rules fill in the details of legislation, with Congress retaining an oversight function. The law usually authorizes the agency to formulate rules to carry out the purposes of the law. For example, within the Department of Health and Human Services, Medicare and Medicaid rules are handled by the Health Care Financing Administration.

The agency of jurisdiction prepares draft rules, which are published in the *Federal Register* each federal working day. The Administrative Procedures Act (APA) establishes a two-step procedure that an agency ordinarily uses for rule making.

First, an agency must publish in the *Federal Register* a notice of proposed rule making, which contains the text of the proposed rules or a description of the subjects and issues involved and an invitation for the

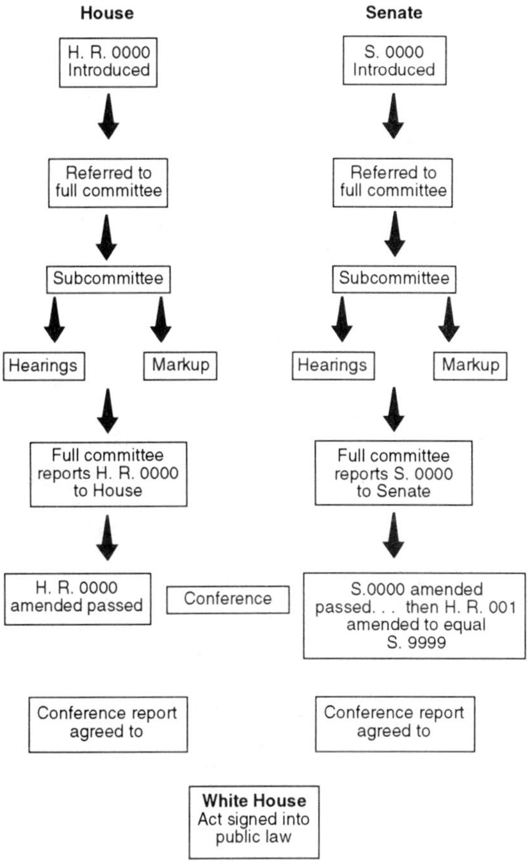

Figure 10–2. Federal legislative process.

public to comment on the rules. Concerned individuals and organizations may submit written comments on the proposed rule, usually within a 30 or 60-day comment period. The comments help bring to the agency's attention information that the agency may not have taken into account in drafting the proposed rule. The content of the final rule may be influenced by the views presented during this period. For example, the Health Care Financing Administration (HCFA) proposed Medicare rule on physician payment reform, which had a major impact on CRNA reimbursement as well, received 95,000 written comments. A significant number of those comments were from CRNAs.

Second, an agency carefully considers the public's comments and, if the agency still believes a rule is necessary, adopts a final rule. Prior to the issuance of a final rule, however, further internal review is done at all levels of the agency and by the White House's Office of Management and Budget. The final rule, with a statement of its basis and purpose, are usually published in the *Federal Register* at least 30 days before its effective date.

Increasingly, rules and rule making play a pivotal role in the policy process by transforming legislative provisions into a blueprint for regulatory program operations. More often than not, the rule-making process is transformed into a battleground of contending interests, where major political and policy issues deferred during the legislative process are resolved, at least until the rules that emerge are themselves challenged. It is not unusual for rule making by an agency to stimulate interest groups to demand new legislation.

HOW YOU CAN INFLUENCE THE LEGISLATIVE PROCESS

The information below references the federal level, but it is usually applicable to the state level as well.

What Is Lobbying?

Lobbying is trying to persuade decision makers to enact measures, such as legislation, favorable to your cause. Alternately, you may want legislation defeated or repealed that is unfavorable to your cause. You are an expert on health care; typically your legislator is not. Your lobbying efforts involve sharing information with a legislator that he or she would not normally have easy access to. Box 10–1 outlines useful information for lobbying.

The normal place to get the answers to the questions cited in Box 10–1 is from your professional organization. Normally, whoever asks you to lobby will provide you with these facts, along with the call for action. You should never be asked to lobby without being armed with the necessary facts. Box 10–2 gives general tips for lobbying.

Methods of Lobbying

The different methods of lobbying include *scheduling a personal visit* with the legislator

BOX 10–1
WHAT DO YOU HAVE TO KNOW TO LOBBY?

To lobby effectively, you have to know your issue and your legislator. You will typically need to know the following things about the bill that deals with your issue:

- What is the number of the bill?
- What is the status of the bill?
- What is the substance of the bill?
- Why is this important to the legislator's constituents?
- What will happen if the bill passes?
- What will happen if it does not pass?
- What is the fiscal estimate on the bill?
- What other groups support the bill?
- What other groups oppose the bill?

Typical questions about your legislator include

- What are his or her past votes on the issue?
- What are his or her positions on health issues generally?
- What political party does he or she belong to?
- What is his or her profession?
- What are his or her legislative interests?
- What are his or her key committee memberships or leadership positions?
- What legislation has he or she introduced?
- What is his or her voting record?
- How long has he or she served in the legislature?
- When is he or she up for reelection?
- Does he or she have an opponent in his or her reelection campaign?

or their health staff person in the district or their state or federal office, *calling* the legislator or their health staff person, *corresponding* with the legislator or their health staff person, or *testifying* at hearings.

How to Make an Appointment for a Personal Visit

Call the legislator's office directly, or else call the U.S. Capitol Switchboard, which can connect you to the legislator's office. The number for the U.S. Capitol Switchboard and other useful federal government information is provided in Table 10–1. When you connect with the office, first ask for the legislative assistant (LA) for health. Tell the LA that you are a CRNA constituent of the legislator and that you want to meet with the legislator for 15 minutes on a specific date to discuss a particular health issue. The health LA may make the appointment for you with the legislator's scheduler or may refer you directly to the scheduler. Make sure you write down the name of the LA and the scheduler, and get a specific time, meeting room number and building, for example, 10:00 AM in Room 205 in the Hart Senate Office Building. Leave your name and phone number where you can be reached if the legislator needs to cancel the meeting. If you request it in advance, the legislator's office can usually arrange for a photographer to be present to take your picture with the legislator. An autographed picture is always a nice memento of your visit, and most offices will be happy to send it to you when developed. If a picture is being taken, request 20 minutes for your visit. Box 10–3 provides many useful tips for personal visits to legislators.

Telephoning

When time is short on an issue, a telephone call may be necessary. Call the legis-

BOX 10–2
GENERAL LOBBYING TIPS

The following basic lobbying tips apply regardless of what type of interaction you have with the legislator.

- Call your state legislative hotline, if they have one, to find out the status of bills; at the federal level the legislative update number is (202) 225-1772.
- Get to know your legislator and his or her staff before you need help on an issue.
- Identify yourself as a voter from a specific congressional district or state. Identify any personal or professional relationships that will add weight and credibility to your position on the issue; for example, "I am the county campaign manager for the legislator" or "I am a member of the (your state) Association of Nurse Anesthetists."
- Clearly identify the bill that concerns you by number and subject matter, for example, S. 1, the reauthorization of the Nurse Education Act. Indicate precisely what action you want the legislator to take (e.g., introduce, cosponsor, support, amend, or oppose the bill).
- State what your position is on this issue and why. Personalize your position by telling the legislator how the issue affects his or her constituency.
- Respect the right of the legislator to disagree with you because of the merits or politics of the situation.
- Ask for a commitment—but do not expect a commitment before all the facts are in.
- Make periodic contact with the legislator. One visit, letter, or phone call will not establish a relationship. Continue to contact the legislator as the issue moves through the process for example, on introduction to cosponsor, to vote in favor at the subcommittee level, to vote in favor at the committee level, to vote in favor on the House or Senate floor, to support your version of the bill in conference committee, to vote for a presidential override.
- Always thank the legislator when he or she has taken positive action on your request.
- Work in conjunction with your state and national association lobbyists on issues, as well as networking with other groups.
- Invite legislators to your nursing meetings and community events; politicians love crowds and cameras.
- Furnish the legislator with your address and telephone number.
- Understand the positions of your association before you lobby.
- Report all contacts to your state or national legislative staff so that appropriate district and national follow-up can occur. This is also valuable for planning future strategy.
- Never leave a legislator out on a political limb by changing your position after the legislator has publicly stated support for a position that you urged him or her to take.
- Do not threaten the legislator with political reprisals.
- Remember that you need the legislator's vote on issues, and he or she needs your vote at election time.
- Invite your legislator to come and see how you practice.

lator at an appropriate time in his or her office. If the legislator is not available, then ask to speak to the health LA. Clearly state your name, that you are a CRNA constituent, the bill number, your position on the bill, and what action you want the legislator to take, for example, "I am Jane Doe, a CRNA constituent of the senator's. I'm calling about S. 1, the reauthorization of the Nurse Education Act, which I support. I would like him to vote in favor of the bill when it comes up for committee action tomorrow. Thank you."

Corresponding with the Legislator

Letter writing techniques are provided in Boxes 10–4 and 10–5, and a sample letter is demonstrated in Figure 10–3.

TABLE 10–1

USEFUL FEDERAL GOVERNMENT PHONE CONTACTS AND INFORMATION*,†

	CONGRESS	
Capitol switchboard	224–3121	Telephone access to House and Senate
Bill Status Office (LEGIS)	225–1772	Update on bills
Library of Congress	287–5000	Research
General Accounting Office	275–6241	Documents
Office of Technology Assessment	228–6590	Reports on technology assessments
Congressional Budget Office	226–2600	Bill cost estimates
Congressional Record Index	275–3121	
	SENATE	
Daily digest	224–2658	Availability of bills
Democratic cloakroom	224–4691	Scheduling information
Republican cloakroom	224–6191	Scheduling information
Democratic cloakroom tape	224–8541	Floor action
Republican cloakroom tape	224–8601	Floor action
Majority leader	224–3135	
Minority leader	224–5556	
Personnel locator	224–3207	
Placement office	224–9167	
	U.S. HOUSE OF REPRESENTATIVES	
Daily digest	225–2868	Availability of bills
Democratic cloakroom	225–7330	Scheduling information
Republican cloakroom	225–7350	Scheduling information
Democratic cloakroom tape	225–7400	Floor action
Republican cloakroom tape	225–7430	Floor action
Speaker	225–8040	
Minority leader	225–0600	
Personnel locator	225–6515	
Placement office	226–6731	
	EXECUTIVE BRANCH AND OTHER SELECTED WASHINGTON NUMBERS	
White House switchboard	456–1414	
Office of the Vice-President	224–2424	
Department of Health and Human Services	245–6296	
Government Printing Office (GPO)	275–2051	
GPO publications and order desk	783–3238	
Supreme Court	479–3000	
Federal Register status unit	523–5230	
Presidential bill signatures	456–2226	
Public law no. assigned to act	523–5230	
Centrex for U.S. government	655–4000	Agency locator

*All have 202 area codes.
†LEGIS.

BOX 10–3
DOS AND DON'TS REGARDING PERSONAL VISITS WITH LEGISLATORS

DO:

- Give as much notice in scheduling your appointment as possible, at least 2 weeks.
- Make an appointment rather than dropping by, because it will greatly increase your chances of seeing the legislator; schedule the specific amount of time that you need—15 minutes is normally sufficient. Tell the appointments person what you want to talk about so the legislator may ask his or her staff person that handles that topic to sit in on the meeting.
- If the legislator is unavailable when you want to meet, it is definitely worthwhile to meet with the health LA. He or she can become your best friend in the office. Rest assured that if you try to circumvent or ignore staff, you will find it difficult to get staff cooperation in the future.
- Before making your appointment, find out if other nurses have already made appointments. Team lobbying is more effective. If you are in a group, select a spokesperson to lead the discussion.
- Be punctual.
- Be professional in your appearance and approach. Carry business cards with you so that you can network at all times.
- Address legislators by "Representative" or "Senator" until they tell you to call them something different.
- Identify yourself immediately as a constituent and a CRNA when you meet with the legislator; public officials meet too many people to remember everyone.
- Assume that legislators do not understand your issue; if they do they will tell you, if they do not you have saved them from looking foolish.
- Have an outline of the points that you want to make.
- If you cannot answer a question knowledgeably, tell the legislator that you or your association will send him or her the information as soon as possible and then do so.
- Do not take up the entire 15 minutes with your presentation; allow at least 5 minutes for the legislator to ask questions.
- Listen carefully to the legislator's view on your issue.
- Ask the legislator to help promote support with his or her colleagues on your issue.
- Ask for your legislator's advice on ways to lobby your issue.
- Ask the legislator what the opposition says about your issue and rebut the arguments if you can.
- Ask your legislator to keep an open mind on your issue even if he or she states that he or she currently opposes your position. Remember that controversial legislation and regulation usually result in compromise. Be ready with alternatives or solutions as well as with criticisms.
- Leave your legislator with a one-page fact sheet on the issue, your position, and exactly what you want him or her to do. Provide articles or data that backs up your view, if possible.
- Keep the door open for further discussion even if the legislator's attitude appears to be negative. Leave on a positive note.
- Follow up with a thank-you letter for the visit and again include a summary of the points that you made.

DON'T:

- Be angry if the legislator cannot meet with you when it is convenient for you; make another appointment or meet with the health LA.
- Visit your legislator at home without an invitation.
- Call your legislator off the floor of his or her respective chamber unless it is truly an emergency.
- Visit the legislator more than once on an issue unless you have something new to say.
- Expect an on-the-spot endorsement of your bill or issue.
- Portray your personal opinion on an issue as that of the association; if your personal position differs from the association, make that clear to the legislator.

Continued

BOX 10–3
DOS AND DON'TS REGARDING PERSONAL VISITS WITH LEGISLATORS—*CONTINUED*

- Let a legislator sidetrack you on another issue for the entire meeting so he or she does not have to address your issue.
- "Cry wolf" on every issue; overreacting diminishes credibility.
- Forget that the impression that you leave is as important as the substance of your discussion.
- Repeat off-the-record comments of one legislator to another—keep them confidential.
- Criticize your legislator for introducing a bill that you dislike, without finding out if the legislator is serious about pushing the bill.

BOX 10–4
ADDRESS THE LETTER PROPERLY

House member:	The Honorable ____________ U.S. House of Representatives Washington, DC 20515
Senate member:	The Honorable ____________ U.S. Senate Washington, DC 20510
President:	The Honorable ____________ President of the United States Washington, DC 20500

WESTERN UNION

1 *Public opinion message:* It may be addressed to any elected official and must be a message of a political nature. You can send a message of 20 words for a fixed price. This message will be telexed to the U.S. Capitol within an hour.

2 *Mailgram:* This option provides next morning delivery of the message. You can send a message of 1 to 50 words, which includes the names and addresses of you and the recipient.

3 *Message to multiple members:* The options include sending a message of up to 40 words to either all representatives, all senators, or all members of Congress.

OVERNIGHT/SECOND DAY DELIVERY

United Parcel Service (UPS), Federal Express, and the U.S. Postal Service all provide overnight and 2-day delivery service.

Testifying at Public Hearings

An effective presentation by a CRNA at a health hearing could have a great impact on the ultimate fate of a bill. During hearings on legislation, representatives from professional associations, special interest groups, the executive branch, academia, and interested members of Congress are invited to speak. Your audience can be expected to be members of Congress, members of the press, congressional staff members, and lobbyists for organizations interested in the bill. The number of people in the audience will depend on the controversial nature of the legislation. At the federal level, hearings are usually scheduled in the morning because the House and Senate normally go into session around noon. Once Congress is in session, there is always a chance that a floor vote will require committee members to leave to go vote, which has a disruptive effect on the hearing.

BOX 10–5
DOS AND DON'TS OF LETTER WRITING

DO:

- Contact your own representative and two senators. As a constituent, you have a better chance of influencing their actions than you would by writing to the entire Senate and House of Representatives.
- Consider the factor of timing. Try to write when the bill is still in committee and awaiting action.
- Address the letter properly.
- Write legibly or type your letter for easiest reading.
- Use your personal stationery unless you have been asked to write on your association's or employer's letterhead.
- Sign your full name and address to the letter—so you can be contacted back. Envelopes are sometimes lost. Be sure the address that you give is within the legislator's district.
- Write to your legislator at his or her office rather than at home, so that your correspondence is filed to receive a response and for future reference.
- Mention the fact that you have a personal connection with the legislator (if indeed you do) because the staffer reading the letter will be more inclined to forward it directly to the legislator.
- Stick to one subject per letter and limit the letter to one page, if possible. If you need to include copies of articles or research data, attach them to the letter.
- Identify the bill number and popular name, if possible, for example, S. 1, the reauthorization of the Nurse Education Act.
- Clearly state your position and why you have taken that position in the first paragraph.
- Personalize the effect of the bill on you, your family, your practice, your community, your state. Form letters and petitions are not considered as valuable as personal letters.
- Request the legislator to communicate his or her position on the bill to you.
- Write to say "thank you" for a favorable vote to let your legislator know that you appreciate a job well done. Make sure to mention helpful staff in your thank-you letter.
- Send copies of your correspondence with legislators and their responses to the AANA Washington, DC office.

DON'T:

- Become a "pen pal" and write on every issue being considered.
- Apologize for taking up the legislator's time—it is what they are elected for.
- Send a copy to a senator when you have written to a representative or vice versa.
- Be insulted if you receive a form letter in reply—legislators receive thousands of letters. After a few letters have been received regarding a particular issue, a standard form letter is written by a staff member and approved by the legislator. This form letter is then sent as a reply to all those people writing about that issue.
- Send form letters or petitions, unless it is the only way a contact will be made.
- Forget to write and say thank you when legislators do something you approve of.
- Postpone writing; there is never a truly convenient time.

The twofold objective of association testimony is to inform and persuade. What you have to say is important, but how well you say it is just as important. Your presentation can be very effective because you will be speaking as one directly affected by the proposal being considered, because you have special knowledge of the subject, or because you represent the viewpoint of many CRNAs. Your appearance increases the likelihood that your association will be consulted on other issues. A hearing can be instrumental in establishing permanent lines of communication with legislators.

SCOPE OF TESTIMONY. Every piece of testimony should include the following:

The Honorable (name of Senator)
Address
Washington, D.C. 20510

Dear Senator ______________:

I am writing to express my strong support for S. 1, the bill to reauthorize the Nurse Education Act. I would like you to cosponsor this important bill because it provides funds for nurse anesthesia educational programs, student traineeships, and faculty development.

The education of certified registered nurse anesthetists (CRNAs) is especially important now because of the severe shortage of anesthesia providers in this country. The CRNA shortage has affected your district as evidenced by _________.

I appreciate your consideration of this critical piece of legislation and hope you will cosponsor it. I would appreciate hearing from you regarding your position on this issue.

Sincerely,

Figure 10–3. Sample letter to senators.

1. Identification of individuals appearing
   a. Name, title, and place of work.
   b. Background to establish credibility as a witness.
   c. Identity of organization and constituency you are representing.
2. Identification of legislation or issue
   a. Specify bill by number, issue by title.
   b. State your position briefly and early.
   c. Paraphrase your understanding of the intent or purpose of the legislation or issue.
3. Areas under consideration
   a. Define them.
   b. If supportive, explain why.
   c. If opposed, state why and give alternatives if any exist.
4. Lengthier explanation of your position and your rationale
5. Summation including what you would like to see accomplished
6. Thanks for being allowed to present your views

Boxes 10–6 and 10–7 provide more useful information for testifying.

The importance of individual congressional committees to health issues varies with changing circumstances, such as committee jurisdiction, the personality and political strength of individual committee chairmen, and the current prominence of an individual health issue during a session of Congress. For the most part, however, the most influential committees are those that deal with the funding of discretionary health programs like the Nurse Education Act (appropriation and budget committees) and those that deal with the financing of entitlement programs like Medicare and Medicaid (authorization committees). Following are descriptions of the health-related committees of the Senate and the House of Representatives that have jurisdiction over the issues that are of greatest concern to CRNAs. Their jurisdictions and important subcommittees are detailed, as well as how to contact these committees.

HEALTH-RELATED COMMITTEES OF THE U.S. SENATE

Appropriations

S-128 Capitol Building, Washington, DC 20510-6025; phone (202) 224-3471. **Jurisdiction:** All discretionary funding for federal

BOX 10–6
PRELIMINARY INFORMATION NECESSARY BEFORE TESTIFYING

Before you testify on a bill, you should have been provided with the following information by your staff person:

- What are the key provisions in the legislation?
- What are the arguments on both sides of the issue?
- Who are its supporters and opponents?
- What is the bill's impact on your practice?
- Has there been any prior hearing on this topic before the panel? Can you get copies of those earlier testimonies?
- What other interest groups and associations are testifying and what are their concerns with the legislation?
- What are the concerns of the individual committee members?
- Will the legislation have a significant impact on any of the constituents of the committee members?
- Does the chairman have a special interest in the bill?
- What amendments are expected to be offered during the markup process? Will the amendments alter your association's position? Do you need to propose any amendments?
- What arguments will be used to oppose your association's position? Your testimony should counter those arguments.
- What are the committee's rules of procedure?
- What districts are represented by the committee members?
- Has your staff suggested "friendly questions" to the committee members that they may ask you to help you expand on your testimony?

BOX 10–7
DOS AND DON'TS OF TESTIFYING

DO:

- Arrive promptly. Witnesses will usually be allowed to enter a hearing room first, before the public. When you arrive, inform committee staff that you are there.
- At the state level, you may need to fill out a witness registration slip, where you indicate whether you are for or against the bill. Persons who wish to speak indicate so on the registration slip. At the state level, if you have traveled some distance to appear and will be returning home that day, note that fact on the registration slip. The committee chairperson will often call such witnesses early in the hearing to allow for their travel time.
- Be prepared to wait. There may be other bills heard before yours. It is also difficult to judge how long each speaker will take. Do not be surprised if you have to wait for some time before being called on.
- If possible, bring a copy of the bill with you. This will allow you to refer to specific sections in your presentation or when answering questions.
- Providing copies of written testimony to the committee is advised even for those who present oral testimony. At the federal level the committee staff will inform you of how many copies of testimony are necessary for the committee.
- A longer written testimony will usually be submitted for the record. You will usually be presenting 5- or 10-minute remarks that are a brief summary of the lengthier text. Rehearse your presentation thoroughly and time it. Do not exceed your time limit under any circumstances. In fact, some committee rooms have green, yellow, and red lights to let you know how you are managing your time. Regardless of where you are in your prepared remarks, when the red light goes on you should finish your sentence, and say thank you.

Continued

BOX 10–7
DOS AND DON'TS OF TESTIFYING—*CONTINUED*

- Usually the message in a piece of testimony is so vital that a script is essential for complete accuracy; however, do not use the script as a crutch, burying your eyes in it.
- Tailor the text delivery and style of your testimony to fit your own personality. It should be simple, focused, and natural. The end result should be like a conversation between you and someone that you like.
- Work with the staff person who is drafting your testimony so that you are comfortable with the way the ideas are expressed. A good use of your familiar expressions and real-life examples in the testimony will make you feel better and make the testimony seem more genuine.
- Be prepared to answer questions. The association staff should go over anticipated questions that you may receive from the committee and provide you with possible answers. Hearing tough questions in advance is much better than encountering them for the first time at a hearing.
- If you are testifying on a controversial topic, be prepared for media at the hearing. Work with your staff person on how to handle a media interview if requested.
- Your staff will not sit at the witness table with you, but they can sit right behind you in case you need some help.
- If neither you nor your staff person know an answer to a question, admit it and offer to supply the information later for the record.

DON'T:

- Assume that all committee members are familiar with all aspects of the bill: That is the purpose of the hearing. Review the specific provisions of the bill that are of concern.
- Repeat at length the points made by a previous speaker. If you have something to add to what was said, by all means do so. If not, simply note your agreement with the earlier speaker and move on to the rest of your presentation. To be effective, your presentation must be somewhat flexible. Pay attention to what other speakers are saying.
- Attempt to answer questions for which you do not have answers or facts. If you are requested to appear by a staff member of a trade association, ask the committee chairperson if that staff member can respond with better facts or experience than you might have. You may also offer to provide additional information after the hearing.
- Be disappointed if only one or two legislators show up for the hearing. That does not diminish your testimony—often legislators have two or more hearings scheduled for the same time. Be comforted that everything you say is going into the hearing record and will be closely studied by the committee staff.[10,11]

programs. **Key Subcommittee:** Labor, Health and Human Services, Education, and Related Agencies, SD-186 Dirksen Senate Office Building, Washington, DC 20510; phone (202) 224-7283. **Jurisdiction:** Nurse anesthesia education funding, National Center for Nursing Research, AIDS funding.

Armed Services

SR-228 Russell Senate Office Building, Washington, DC 20510-6050; phone (202) 224-3871. **Jurisdiction:** Military funding, including CHAMPUS. **Key Subcommittee:** Manpower and Personnel, same address as full committee. **Jurisdiction:** CRNA pay and education funding; CRNA bonus pay for Desert Storm activity.

Budget

SD-621 Dirksen Senate Office Building, Washington, DC 20510-6100; phone (202) 224-0642. **Jurisdiction:** Total health funding and financing ceiling.

Governmental Affairs

SD-340 Dirksen senate Office Building, Washington, DC 20510-6250; phone (202)

224-4751. **Jurisdiction:** Federal worker issues. **Key Subcommittee:** Federal Services, Post Office, and Civil Service, SH-601 Hart Senate Office Building, Washington, DC 20510; phone (202) 224-2245. **Jurisdiction:** The Federal Employees Health Benefits (FEHB) Program reimbursement for CRNAs.

Finance

SD-205 Dirksen Senate Office Building, Washington, DC 20510-6200; phone (202) 224-4515. **Jurisdiction:** Taxes, Medicare, and Medicaid. **Key Subcommittee:** Health for Families and the Uninsured, full committee address. **Key Subcommittee:** Medicare and Long-term Care, full committee address.

Labor and Human Resources

SD-428 Dirksen Senate Office Building, Washington, DC 20510-6300; phone (202) 224-5375. **Jurisdiction:** Health authorizations and reauthorizations, including nurse anesthesia education funding.

HEALTH-RELATED COMMITTEES OF THE U.S. HOUSE OF REPRESENTATIVES

Appropriations

H-218 Capitol Building, Washington DC 20515-6015; phone (202) 225-2771. **Jurisdiction:** All discretionary funding for federal programs. **Key Subcommittee:** Labor, Health and Human Services, Education, and Related Agencies, 2358 Rayburn House Office Building, Washington, DC 20515; phone (202) 225-3508. **Jurisdiction:** Nurse anesthesia education funding, National Center for Nursing Research, AIDS funding.

Armed Services

2120 Rayburn House Office Building, Washington, DC 20515-6035; phone (202) 225-4151. **Jurisdiction:** Military funding, including CHAMPUS. **Key Subcommittee:** Military Personnel and Compensation, 2343 Rayburn House Office Building, Washington, DC 20515; phone (202) 225-7560. **Jurisdiction:** CRNA pay and education funding; CRNA bonus pay for Desert Storm activity.

Budget

214 O'Neill House Office Building, Washington, DC 20515-6065; phone (202) 226-7200. **Jurisdiction:** Total health funding and financing ceiling.

Energy and Commerce

2125 Rayburn House Office Building, Washington, DC 20515-6115; phone (202) 225-2927. **Jurisdiction:** Public Health and health facilities. **Key Subcommittee:** Health and the Environment, 2415 Rayburn House Office Building, Washington, DC 20515; phone (202) 225-4952. **Jurisdiction:** Health authorizations and reauthorizations, including nurse anesthesia education funding, Medicaid and shared jurisdiction with Ways and Means Committee over Medicare Part B.

Post Office and Civil Service

309 Cannon House Office Building, Washington, DC 20515-6243; phone (202) 225-4054. **Jurisdiction:** Federal worker issues. **Key Subcommittee:** Compensation and Employee Benefits, 515 O'Neill House Office Building, Washington, DC 20515; phone (202) 226-7546. **Jurisdiction:** FEHB Program reimbursement for CRNAs.

Ways and Means

1102 Longworth House Office Building, Washington, DC 20515-6348; phone (202) 225-3625. **Jurisdiction:** Taxes and Medicare. **Key Subcommittee:** Health, 1114 Longworth House Office Building, Washington, DC 20515; phone (202) 225-7785. **Jurisdiction:** Medicare Part A and shared jurisdiction with Energy and Commerce Committee over Medicare Part B.

HOW TO OBTAIN CONGRESSIONAL DOCUMENTS

Bills, Reports, and Public Laws

One copy of six different items (bills, reports, public laws) may be requested in writing daily from the Senate Document Room; phone orders are not accepted. One copy of 12 different items may be requested in writing daily from the House Document Room; phone orders of up to 6 items are accepted. Multiple copies of one item are not available. Please enclose a self-addressed gummed label to facilitate the return mailing.

Senate Document Room
B-04 Hart Building
Washington, DC 20510
(202) 224-7860

Hearing Documents

A free copy of a House or Senate committee print or hearing record can be requested by sending a self-addressed label to the publications clerk of the committee from which the document was issued. Mail requests for prints and records may also be sent to: Superintendent of Documents, Government Printing Office, Congressional Sales Office, Washington, DC 20402-9315; phone (202) 275-3030. The GPO documents are not free as are the committee documents. Hearing records are generally available 2 months after the close of hearings.

OTHER FEDERAL GOVERNMENT INFORMATION

Other sources of information, for both the legislative and executive branches of the federal government, are provided in Table 10–1.

SUMMARY

It is hoped that the information provided in this chapter, on how the AANA is involved in the political and legislative arenas, will provide you with the impetus to assert your own influence in health care policy. Educating yourself on the political process will give you the power to have input on those issues that will ultimately be affecting you. This input will allow you to educate legislators on health issues and put the democratic process in motion.

GLOSSARY

Act: Term for legislation that has passed both chambers of Congress and has been signed by the president or passed by a two-thirds majority in a presidential veto override, thus becoming law.

Amendment: A proposal of a legislator to change the language or content in a bill.

Bill: Legislative proposal originating in either chamber of Congress and designated "HR" in the House and "S" in the Senate. The bill number is usually assigned in the order in which legislation is introduced from the beginning of each 2-year congressional term.

Calendar: The agenda or list of pending business before either chamber of Congress or before a committee.

Chamber: Meeting place for the total membership of the House or Senate, as opposed to committee rooms.

Cloture: Process by which debate (or filibuster) can be limited in the Senate, other than by unanimous consent. Requires the vote of 60 senators present and voting. Under cloture, each senator is limited to 1 hour of debate.

Conference Committee: The more controversial a bill may be the more likely it will pass the Senate and House in different forms. Unless either body is willing to accept the changes of the other, the two versions must go to a conference committee. This means that a committee (the number is not fixed), chosen from the originating Senate and House committees, is appointed to work out a compromise. An agreement, if reached, is known as a "conference report." It must then be approved by both the Senate and the House.

Congressional Record: Daily printed account of the proceedings of both the House and Senate chambers, with debate, statements, and so on reported verbatim.

Executive session: Meeting of a committee at which only the committee's members, and no public or press, are allowed to attend.

Federal Register: Daily printed account of

the activities of federal agencies, including rule making.

Filibuster: A device, used only in the Senate, to delay or prevent a vote by time-consuming talk. This tactic is often used by a minority in an effort to prevent a vote on a bill that would probably pass if brought to a vote. Can be stopped only by a 60-member vote of the senators present and voting.

Law: An act of Congress that has been signed by the president or passed over his veto by the Congress.

Markup: After public hearings, a subcommittee will go into executive (either closed or open) session to start the "markup" of a bill, that is, to write amendments into it, delete sections, or revise the language. Views of both sides are stated in detail and at the conclusion of deliberation, a vote is taken to determine subcommittee action. It may decide to report the bill favorably to the full committee, with or without amendments, or suggest that the bill be tabled. Each member of the subcommittee has one vote.

Omnibus bill: A legislative proposal concerning several separate but related items.

Quorum: Number of members whose presence is needed to conduct business. This would be a majority of the members, or 51 in the Senate and 218 in the House. Any member may object to the conduct of business without a quorum and thus force a roll call to bring in absentees. Roll calls are frequently used as a delaying tactic. Much legislation is passed without a quorum because it is noncontroversial. If a point of order is made that a quorum is not present, the only business that can be done is either a motion to adjourn or a motion to direct the sergeant-at-arms to request the attendance of absentees.

Roll call vote: Members vote as their names are called by the clerk of the chamber.

Rule of germaneness: Used to knock out language that does not pertain to the purpose of the bill. Also used to kill an appropriation where the expenditure has not been previously authorized by a separate bill. The Senate may impose the rule on itself under a unanimous consent agreement to limit debate on a pending matter. A two-thirds vote is necessary to retain the language.

Standing vote: An unrecorded vote taken when all members in favor of a proposal stand and are counted and then all members opposed stand and are counted.

Veto: Action taken by the President rejecting a bill presented to him by Congress for his signature. When Congress is in session, the President has 10 days, excluding Sundays, to veto a bill or it automatically becomes law.

Voice vote: The presiding officer of either chamber calls for "yeas" and "nays" to determine the results.

REFERENCES

1. Mason, DJ and Talbott, SW: Political Action Handbook for Nurses. Addison-Wesley, Menlo Park, CA, 1985.
2. Lederer, JC: Legislate success: Learn to lobby. ASAE Association Management, 29–32, December 1987.
3. When you need a coalition. ASAE Association Management: 1, 1990.
4. From Idea to Law: The State Legislative Process, State Net, Sacramento, CA, 1989.
5. Pressures in Congress. The Washington Post, A14, June 26, 1983.
6. Oleszek, WJ: Congressional Procedures and the Policy Process, ed 3., CQ Press, Washington, DC, 1989.
7. Davies J: Legislative Law and Process, ed 2., West Publishing, St. Paul, MN, 1986.
8. Congress and Health. National Health Council, New York, 1989.
9. How Congress Works, ed 2., Congressional Quarterly, Washington, DC, 1991.
10. Gwyn, KH: Presenting testimony before a congressional committee. ASAE Government Relations 2:1–10, 1992.
11. Testifying with Impact, rev ed., Chamber of Commerce of the United States, Washington, DC, 1983.

BIBLIOGRAPHY

Bacchus, WI: Inside the Legislative Process. Westview Press, Boulder, CO., 1983.

Bryner, G: Bureaucratic Discretion: Laws and Policy in Federal Regulatory Agencies. Pergamon Press, New York, 1987.

Congress A to Z: CQ's Ready Reference Encyclopedia. Congressional Quarterly, Washington, DC, 1988.

Davidson, RH and Olezsek, WJ: Congress and Its Members, ed 3. CQ Press, Washington, DC, 1990.

Dodd, LC and Oppenheimer, BI(eds): Congress Reconsidered, ed 4. CQ Press, Washington, DC, 1990.

Froman, LA Jr: The Congressional Process: Strategies, Rules, and Procedures. Little, Brown, Boston, 1967.

Meier, K: Regulation: Politics, Bureaucracy and Economics. St. Martin's Press, New York, 1985.

Smith, S: Call to Order: Floor Politics in the House and Senate. Brookings Institution, Washington DC, 1989.

FOUR

Practice Patterns of the CRNA

11

Assessing and Selecting Practice Settings and Employment Options

Mark C. Hamelink
Tom L. McKibban
Peter Staver
Kimberley Walker

OUTLINE

PRACTICE SETTINGS
Hospital Employment
Outpatient Surgery Centers
Health Maintenance Organizations
Physician Offices
Academic Practices
Veterans Administration Hospitals
Armed Forces
Nonclinical Positions
Locum Tenums
Volunteer Organizations
FACTORS TO CONSIDER IN SELECTING EMPLOYMENT
Personal Considerations
Professional Considerations
Scope of Practice
Professional relationships and autonomy
Credentialing
Business Considerations
Practice Configurations
Solo practice
Group practice
Institution-based practice
EMPLOYMENT CONTRACTS
Contract Law
Four Corners Doctrine
Construed against the drafting party
Parole Evidence Rule
Contract Negotiation
BENEFIT PACKAGES
Health and Medical Insurance
Life Insurance
Disability Benefits
Pension and/or Profit Sharing Plans
Professional Liability Insurance
RESUMES AND INTERVIEW TECHNIQUES
Getting Organized
Drafting Your Resume
Writing a Cover Letter
Preparing for the Interview
Interviewing
Miscellaneous Tips for Interviewing

OBJECTIVES

On completing this chapter, the reader will to able to:

1. Understand functional concepts and relationships of the health care team.
2. Identify and evaluate key factors in assessing employment options.
3. Contrast the advantages and disadvantages of employment settings.
4. Establish personal guidelines for evaluating and selecting employment.
5. Describe the importance of employment contracts, their essential elements, and basic components of contract law.
6. Provide direction for negotiating an employment agreement.
7. Assist the CRNA in preparing a professional resume and interviewing.

PRACTICE SETTINGS

When assessing and selecting practice settings, one must consider a myriad of factors, all of which will culminate to determine the probability of a successful and satisfying professional career. These factors relate both to the clinical role of the Certified Registered Nurse Anesthetist (CRNA) and the role as a member of the health care community and society at large. Among the more critical issues with which the CRNA must be concerned are state statutory requirements affecting practice, liability considerations, and individual and personal practice or lifestyle preferences. This chapter deals with the more pragmatic issues of selecting and moving into new practice settings from the perspective of either the graduating student or the CRNA already in practice.

CRNAs can choose from many different employment settings, including hospitals, ambulatory care centers, health maintenance organizations (HMOs), Veterans Administration Hospitals, the armed forces, academic institutions, or associated industries, such as anesthesia pharmaceutical and equipment companies. New positions are becoming increasingly available outside of the operating room setting where CRNAs have been traditionally employed by either the hospital or an anesthesia group. Each setting has unique advantages and disadvantages.

Hospital Employment

The hospital setting offers many advantages, one of which is readily available support services such as laboratory and radiology services. Quick access to a competently staffed laboratory and radiology department greatly benefits the anesthetist in taking care of a difficult patient or a patient who encounters anesthesia or surgical complications. Medical staff support services, from a variety of disciplines, are also important to the anesthetist and are usually readily available in the hospital setting. Consultations from medical internists, cardiologists, pulmonologists, and primary care physicians are beneficial when making difficult decisions regarding preoperative clearance or when handling an unstable patient during the perioperative period.

There are many different types of employment options available within the hospital setting. The CRNA may work as an independent contractor or as an employee of a group of anesthesiologists, a CRNA group, physician group, or the hospital itself. Each option offers a different set of benefits and drawbacks. Most CRNAs practicing in hospitals are employed by either a physician, CRNA group, or hospital. When entering any of these employment settings, it is important to have a solid, concise, written contractual agreement signed by both parties. Reimbursement may be based on salary, hourly wage, anesthesia productivity, or a combination of these mechanisms; expected reimbursement should be included in the contractual agreement with the employer.

Employees, in contrast to independent contractors, enjoy several advantages, the most valuable of which is a satisfactory and usually extensive benefit package. Benefits included in this package may include health, disability, life and liability insurance; educational leave and expenses; retirement; and paid vacation, holidays, sick leave, and bereavement. The employer is usually responsible for providing relief coverage when the anesthetist is off-duty. Time off, both in terms of regular call coverage and extended vacation time, is a very valuable commodity.

As an employee, the CRNA will not have to worry about the business aspects of anesthesia services. Billing and collections are the responsibility of the employer. Thus, the hospital setting offers several advantages, primarily the benefit package and freedom from business responsibilities. However, there are several disadvantages to the hospital setting. Hospitals are highly regulated health care facilities, controlled in part by federal and state agencies. These agency requirements increase the amount of paperwork required of the anesthesia department. The CRNA is often directly involved in assisting the anesthesia department in meeting these agencies' requirements. These requirements are intended to improve the quality of care delivered to the patient, but completing the paperwork and documentation can prove to be stressful, time-consuming, and expensive.

Acute care hospitals provide services 24 hours a day, requiring the anesthesia department to have anesthetists available at all times. In the hospital setting, CRNAs are likely required to take call or work overtime to meet these human resources needs. On-call duties, although in some circumstances lucrative, can prove to be restrictive even when taken from home; this is especially true in the small hospital setting. CRNAs should consider the potential impact of call responsibilities on their life-style and on their rate of compensation. Too often, CRNAs are not adequately compensated by the employer for call duties, as call is considered a normal part of the overall compensation package. The CRNA should carefully determine whether there is any significant drop in wage for call duties in comparison to what they would make during regular operating room hours and adjust their contract or work agreement accordingly.

With all the benefits of hospital employment, it is paramount that CRNAs employed by an MD group or hospital determine if there are any restrictions to clinical practice imposed by hospital or departmental policy. In some facilities, CRNAs are not allowed to do certain cases such as open heart, neuroanesthesia, or other high-risk cases. In addition, some hospitals restrict CRNAs from administering regional anesthesia or inserting invasive monitoring lines. If these restrictions exist, CRNAs should consider carefully whether or not they can work within these limitations.

Outpatient Surgery Centers

An outpatient surgery center offers many advantages as an employment setting. Surgery centers operate primarily during daytime hours, typically from 7:00 AM to 5:00 PM, and there is often little or no on-call requirement. Outpatient surgery centers usually create a relaxed atmosphere, resulting in pleasant working conditions. Surgeries may be less complicated than inpatient procedures, and the patients often are healthier than those cared for in the hospital setting. However, outpatient surgical centers often lack the extensive support services and personnel that an inpatient setting may provide.

CRNAs may work in an outpatient center as an independent contractor or as an employee. If self-employed, they may realize an above-average income due to the volume of cases. However, as a self-employed anesthetist, CRNAs will be required to pay for their own benefits and probably will have to provide anesthesia coverage on those days they wish to take off. Currently there is a great shortage of anesthesia providers, and relief is both hard to find and expensive. CRNAs employed by these centers, or by anesthesia groups within the centers, tend to be paid less than those employed in the hospital setting. This appears to be a tradeoff for the better hours, lack of call, and a less stressful atmosphere.

Health Maintenance Organizations

HMOs are alternative health care delivery systems. In the original "staff model" HMOs, the anesthesia provider was a salaried employee. The HMO, although popular in certain areas of the country, is experiencing increased competition with preferred provider organizations and independent practice associations (IPAs). Both of these organizations have resulted from attempts to hold down the cost of health care by providing comprehensive services, under contract, by a mix of providers. Health care providers working with PPOs and IPAs are paid on a fee-for-service basis, whereas those with HMOs will likely be salaried employees.

The advantages of working for an HMO are good benefit packages, separation from the business side of the practice, and a noncompetitive atmosphere with colleagues. The benefit package may include health, dental, disability, liability and life insurance, continuing education stipends, paid days off, retirement, and stock options.

HMO employment also has disadvantages; some HMOs are not financially healthy, so ascertain the organization's fiscal status prior to entering an employment agreement. This can be accomplished in a number of ways: obtain and review a recent financial statement from the HMO, or check with the state insurance department, local medical society, and local physicians and CRNAs. Information regarding the stability of an HMO can be obtained by visiting the hospital with which the HMO is associated.

If CRNAs work as an independent contractor with the HMO rather than as an employee, they will probably be required to provide services at a discounted rate under a contractual agreement with the HMO. As with any employment contract, check it closely and have it reviewed by an attorney.

Physician Offices

Physician and dentist offices have become popular employment settings for CRNAs. Opthamologists, plastic surgeons, oral surgeons, ear, nose, and throat (ENT) surgeons, and dentists are among those who have found CRNAs to be valuable and cost-effective providers of anesthesia.

There are many benefits to practicing in the office setting. The working conditions are often pleasant and relaxed, and the hours are reasonable, with on-call rarely involved. Moreover, the office setting can be financially lucrative, especially for CRNAs who work on a fee-for-service basis. Since income is generated largely on the basis of the volume of cases, CRNAs usually do well in a busy office. If working on a fee-for-service basis, the CRNA is probably considered self-employed and is responsible for personal benefits and vacation coverage. If it is a large office, there may be more than one anesthetist, potentially simplifying any coverage problems.

There are also negatives to working in the office setting, one of which is variable or lack of time off. If working for one physician, the CRNA may have to plan time off around the surgeon's schedule. If working with several physicians, the CRNA may have to arrange for anesthesia coverage while away; coverage is often difficult to find, particularly when the coverage must also be acceptable to the physician(s).

A self-employed CRNA may be responsible for billing or be required to rely on the physician to provide billing services. If the physician's office does the billing, they will probably do it for a percentage of the amount collected. This arrangement should be part of the contract. The CRNA can check with local anesthesia providers to predict what the collection rate would be and determine a reasonable or customary charge for doing billing and collections. If the physician's office will be performing these services, make sure that their billing and collection practices are satisfactory.

Depending on a single physician's case load for income can be a disadvantage. If the physician becomes ill, decides to slow down, or changes practice style, income will decrease. In the working agreement with the physician, plan on including the option to supplement income by working elsewhere.

The CRNA should look at the type and number of surgeries the physician or dentist plans on doing with anesthesia assistance. This will give a general idea of income potential. It is also important to look at the patient population served. Medicare, Medicaid, commercial insurance, and private individual payers may have different reimbursement and collection rates. For example, Medicare may pay only 40 percent of a charge, whereas a commercial insurer may pay 100 percent of the same charge.

Above all, the CRNA should understand clearly that office practice settings, although often quite satisfying, require an appreciation that the ultimate responsibility for the patient often rests with the CRNA exclusively, in terms of anesthesia-related complications. This requires that the CRNA be well experienced, educated in the full range of anesthetic techniques, and maintain certification in advanced resuscitation skills. The benefits of entrepreneurial practice require constant vigilance, concentration, and attention to every aspect of patient perioperative care.

Academic Practices

Many opportunities exist for CRNAs in nurse anesthesia education, encompassing clinical, didactic, and research areas. The academic setting offers several advantages. The benefit package at many universities is exceptional, offering free tuition to continue personal education. Some universities also forgo family members' tuition. Academic careers also allow a greater balance between clinical practice, classroom teaching, scientific writing, professional service, and a variety of research opportunities. Considerable flexibility in personal scheduling usually exists. On-call duties and overtime are less often required, and this can be an important life-style consideration. Historically, universities have not compensated CRNAs in terms of salary as well as those in other settings. However, they usually do offer good benefits and academic advancement incentives.

An academic career today is often predicated on the requirement that CRNAs achieve some advanced academic degree. Most faculty members hold at least a masters degree; however, many colleges and universities will require a doctoral degree in an appropriate field before the CRNA has access to tenure, promotable professorial lines, or membership in academic senates or other governing bodies. The number of doctorally prepared CRNAs is increasing at a rapid rate, which is vital in stabilizing nurse anesthesia programs within academic institutions. Currently, there is a great demand for CRNA faculty at both the masters and doctoral level.

Veterans Administration Hospitals

Veterans Administration (VA) hospitals are another viable option of employment for CRNAs. The VA offers an above-average benefits package, including health and life insurance, vacation, paid holidays, sick leave, a good retirement plan, continuing education opportunities, and a thrift savings plan. As a federal employee, there is no need for the CRNA to secure malpractice liability insurance. Since the Nurse Locality Pay Act of 1990 was enacted, salary is based on a local community salary survey. It is set to be competitive with the local CRNA labor market. There are 172 VA sites in the United States and one may transfer (if there is a vacancy) without losing accrued benefits. The disadvantages are similar to those of the hospital setting; on-call and overtime may be required. It should be noted that there is an active professional organization of VA-employed CRNAs that deals with the major issues confronting a VA-employed CRNA.

Armed Forces

The different branches of the United States Armed Forces are another avenue of employment available to nurse anesthetists. The salary and very competitive benefit packages in the different branches are basically the same. Historically, the salary scale has been much lower than that of the private sector, but the exceptional benefit package helps offset that deficiency. If CRNAs retire after 20 years of service, they receive 20 percent of their base pay as retirement pay. They also will have the opportunity to travel and work in many different geographic locations around the world. CRNAs in the armed forces have traditionally enjoyed significant autonomy in their practice settings and have contributed much to the expansion of nurse anesthesia practice over the years.

Nonclinical Positions

There are many opportunities outside of patient care available to the CRNA. Pharmaceutical and anesthesia equipment companies use CRNAs as employees or consultants for their expertise in a variety of areas including sales, education, research and product development, and evaluation. The salary and benefits vary greatly throughout the industry. In addition, an increasing number of CRNAs work primarily as researchers in private industry or government. Usually these CRNAs are prepared at the doctoral level.

Some CRNAs have formed their own consulting businesses in the areas of respiratory care, home health care services, payer billing, or in executive positions of health care-related businesses and professional organizations.

Locum Tenums

An increasingly popular employment option is temporary or "locum tenums" employment. A CRNA may arrange for and contract work independently or use one of the many employment/placement agencies. Temporary employment offers the ability to dictate when and where one will work, which is a clear advantage for some CRNAs. The abilities to work and adapt to new and varied settings are key to making this employment option successful. Temporary employment offers the opportunity to travel and experience a variety of settings. Financial compensation is often very good but generally does not include benefits. Unless there are many anesthesia sites local to the CRNA, most temporary employment arrangements include extensive travel. For the unencumbered CRNA, the opportunity to travel and explore employment options through short-term contracting may be ideal. Drawbacks of locum tenums employment include lack of benefits, long-term security, and a consistent work environment.

Volunteer Organizations

In addition to the previously mentioned employment settings, opportunities with religious orders, missionary societies, and humanitarian world aid organizations exist. These positions offer a chance to contribute to humanitarian causes and promote health in disadvantaged populations and Third World countries. They often present unique challenges related to their diverse practice settings and may contrast considerably with familiar practice settings and routines. Many CRNAs and other health professionals volunteer for short- or long-term service without compensation (often paying their own expenses) as a public service. The rewards of volunteering often surpass any sacrifices made. The Council on Public Interest maintains a directory of religious and humanitarian organizations with opportunities for CRNAs. Time commitments range from a few days to a year or more.

FACTORS TO CONSIDER IN SELECTING EMPLOYMENT

Personal Considerations

An evaluation of one's personal goals, desires, and needs is an important first step in evaluating a practice setting. If the CRNA is married and has children, they need to be involved in the decision process. If the spouse is also a professional, he or she needs to evaluate opportunities available in the area. A look at the schools available will be necessary to evaluate whether or not they meet the needs and expectations of the family.

Consider the religious and ethnic background of the community; visit churches if that is an important factor in decision making. Religious and ethnic backgrounds can greatly influence the social attitude of the community. These attitudes should be assessed to determine if they are in conflict with personal philosophies or will allow the family to fit in comfortably. If the CRNA wants to be involved with the various organizations within the community, find out what organizations are active in the area. Determine if employers expect employee involvement in civic or service organizations in the community.

Evaluate housing opportunities carefully in an area prior to committing to employment. Whether buying or renting, CRNAs should consult a realtor to see what is available. Realtors are one of the best sources of community information and often serve as willing tour guides for perspective residents. Consider future needs as well as current desires.

If moving to a small community, make sure it can meet anticipated medical needs. If specialists such as obstetricians or pediatricians are important, make sure they are available. CRNAs should also make sure they are comfortable with the quality of health care available in the community. It is also an important consideration that when living in a community, it is wise to use the local hospital and/or physicians. Ignoring this aspect may influence your credibility within the medical community.

Explore area shopping, industry, and community resources. Furthermore, try to get an idea about the financial stability of the local business community. Cultural and recreational opportunities are important factors to consider. If CRNAs have special interests, hobbies, or activities, it is important to examine the relevant opportunities the community offers.

Consideration should be given to geographic location. Study the climate of the area to ensure it is acceptable. The CRNA may have to trade off different options for geographic concerns; desirable areas may offer less attractive financial packages due to an overabundant supply of providers and a lessened demand for services.

Remember that relocating is an expensive and sometimes traumatic endeavor for all family members, so consider their needs when making a relocation decision. In any relocation, compromises and tradeoffs will be necessary. List important nonprofessional considerations for the job search. It may be helpful to describe the "ideal or perfect" setting to live and work. Prioritize the list to help evaluate what compromises to make and how to weigh various pieces of information discovered in the search.

Because the demand for CRNAs is high, there are hundreds of professional placement agencies around the country that routinely seek graduating CRNAs or those considering a change in practice settings. These agencies are easy to locate via professional journals or bulletins. Most often, there is no cost to the CRNA for these services. However, a substantial finder's fee will be assessed to the potential employer, often in an amount equal to 5 to 20 percent of the annual compensation of the position to be filled. If the CRNA chooses to use such an agency, he or she should be prepared for an aggressive search that requires a prepared resume and clear guidelines about the type of career position sought.

Professional Considerations

Scope of Practice

When deciding on an employment setting, it is important for CRNAs to determine what types of anesthesia they would like to practice and to what extent they wish to use their full scope of abilities. If this is not agreed on with the employer ahead of time, the CRNA may be required to perform anesthesia that he or she finds undesirable or is unprepared to do, or he or she may be limited in practicing anesthesia in the manner anticipated. Key areas to examine are the elements of anesthesia practice one is expected to perform, those elements one may have the opportunity to perform, and any areas in which one may be excluded from practicing.

Most settings expect the CRNA to provide general anesthesia for a variety of patients. However, CRNAs may not want to do cardiovascular or intracranial procedures or others such as pregnancy terminations. This should be expressed, discussed, and resolved prior to employment. If the CRNA is employed to do a specific type of case, make sure this is included in the employment arrangement.

The right to administer regional anesthesia is an important consideration when outlining a scope of practice. Some facilities and groups do not allow CRNAs to provide regional anesthesia, and this can become not only a professional but a political issue. The CRNA should never accept employment in a setting in which there are practice restrictions based on the argument that quality of care would be sacrificed if CRNAs are allowed to administer regional anesthesia. This argument is specious at best, and is rarely, if ever, justified on the basis of quality improvement data. CRNAs practicing in a particular setting may be the best source of information regarding the involvement of CRNAs in regional anesthesia.

Anesthesia providers are becoming increasingly involved in areas outside the traditional operating room setting, which offer expanded practice options for CRNAs. Prior to employment, practice opportunities in anesthesia-related services should be discussed. CRNA input into preoperative evaluations, recovery room management, postoperative follow-up, invasive monitoring, pain management, ventilator management, resuscitation, department decision making, and quality assurance activities varies greatly among practice settings. Desired involvement in a particular area, such as pain management, should be expressed to determine institutional and staff response prior to employment.

Always review CRNA privilege forms and requirements, job descriptions, and department policies to help delineate the available scope of practice. Although many potential employers offer promises for the future, current employees may offer insight into actual practice.

The caseload of a prospective facility should be appraised to determine a comfort level with the caseload. Practice settings may offer greater (or fewer) opportunities in a special interest area such as cardiovascular, pediatric, obstetric, or trauma anesthesia. Give extra consideration to practice settings that offer the most desirable anesthesia caseload and distribution.

When evaluating a facility, particularly a small facility, inspect the type of equipment available. If practice includes invasive monitoring or continuous regional anesthesia, make sure there is proper equipment. Determine who is responsible for obtaining, servicing, and maintaining anesthesia and related equipment. CRNAs should be comfortable with the anesthesia and monitoring equipment the facility has available, avoiding situations that compromise standards of anesthesia care or entail undue patient risk.

Many facilities require participation of CRNAs in inservice education activities. This is an excellent opportunity for CRNAs to expose their practice style, professional responsibilities, and general clinical acumen to a wide variety of other health care professionals. Success in any practice setting will necessarily include CRNA participation within the team of health care providers, whether in independent practice or group-employed practice. CRNA-conducted inservice education is an excellent venue to start this "networking" responsibility. Assess the facilities' expectations of provider responsibilities in this area.

Professional Relationships and Autonomy

The ability to relate with co-workers is essential for long-term job satisfaction. The philosophy, goals, and work ethic of the anesthesia department should be considered. Homogeneity within a department or institution is not always possible or desirable; nevertheless, a reasonable understanding and acceptance of anesthesia providers and staff is necessary for long-term satisfaction. For instance, it may be difficult for a new graduate to assimilate into a department comprised of older, established providers. Likewise, someone who aggressively likes to try new and varied techniques may feel limited in a department with an established conservative approach to anesthetic management.

The degree of professional autonomy in nurse anesthesia varies greatly among practice settings. Ensure that the employment setting allows the desired level of autonomy. Determine who works with the CRNA and the nature of the working relationships. Specifically identify the working relationships among CRNAs, anesthesiologists, surgeons, supervisors, and administrators.

If you are working for a small group of surgeons, discuss with them in advance the issue of autonomy. Find out their expectations including the conduct of preoperative and postoperative rounds (as is required by the AANA clinical standards). Determine if CRNAs have the authority to order preoperative medications and tests when they believe they are necessary. Evaluate hospital policies and regulations that govern nurse anesthesia practice rights. Other CRNAs in the facility may provide valuable information regarding how much autonomy they have in their practice. If only one CRNA works in the practice, contact the CRNA who vacated the position.

The level of autonomy accorded to CRNAs working in the anesthesia care team varies from group to group. Some anesthesia groups may use the nurse anesthetist as an extra set of hands, whereas others will expect the nurse anesthetist to practice independently with physicians serving as consultants when needed. CRNAs may be expected to make preoperative and postoperative rounds, order appropriate preoperative medications and tests, and manage immediate postanesthesia care. Other practices may require the CRNA to seek consultation before making any change or adjustment in anesthesia administration or exclude CRNAs from preoperative and postoperative management. Before signing an employment contract, the CRNA should be comfortable with the practice arrangements. During the interview, ask the anesthesiologists what their expectations are and express views on work preferences and the anesthesia care team concept. Visit with the other CRNAs. Ask how they practice and how much autonomy they are allowed.

Credentialing

An important aspect of employment is how CRNAs are credentialed. CRNAs may be credentialed under several different headings, including allied health professionals, advanced registered nurse practitioner staff, associate staff, or possibly some other manner external to the medical staff. The most popular appears to be allied health professional.

The area of credentialing and staff membership is evolving and expanding for anesthetists. When interviewing, ask the hospital or group how hospital privileges are governed. In many facilities, CRNAs are regulated by the medical staff. Determine the right to attend medical staff meetings. Additional concerns include the right to due process, peer review, committee membership, and voting privileges. Attendance and input into medical staff and committee meetings enhance the ability to influence decision making. Attendance at medical staff and business meetings is a valuable way to remain informed and influence decision making. Medical staff membership may be regulated by state statutes and medical and hospital bylaws. The Joint Commission for Accreditation of Health Care Organizations (JCAHO) currently allows for full medical staff membership for CRNAs provided they are considered "licensed independent practitioners" by their respective states and hospitals. CRNAs may or may not have medical staff voting privileges, depending on the state and facility where they practice. Determine which committees are open for CRNA membership in the place of employment. Committees may have an important influence on how the CRNA practices, therefore it is important to be active on them.

Business Considerations

Business has been defined as any endeavor for the purpose of earning a profit or making a living. The overall concept can be viewed as encompassing the basis for entering, structuring, and managing available practice settings. Independent or group contractual businesses, related to the practice of anesthesia services, usually provide great flexibility to the entrepreneur in selecting practice environments. This opportunity is unequalled by other health care professions because of the great demand for providers. Frequently, the business of anesthesia is limited only by the preferences of the anesthesia practitioner or geographic location. It is now becoming more common for CRNAs to become part of or responsible for securing personal or group contractual arrangements. There are several CRNA educational groups that provide cogent and timely instruction on how to start and manage private business arrangements.

Even for those CRNAs who are employed by institutions or groups, there is a great need for each to become conversant with basic principles of economics, business dealings, and reimbursement trends. Whether personally responsible for a business or a "part" of a larger business consortium, the CRNA can no longer be ignorant of the economics of practice. It is a requisite of practice that all CRNAs be able to calculate their financial worth to a practice setting in order to ensure that they are compensated accordingly (see Chapter 9).

Practice Configurations

All practice settings involve a form of employment. Individuals may, for example, employ themselves, as in the case of a sole practitioner, where they are solely responsible for the terms of their employment; selection of salary and fringe benefits is limited only by the economic constraints of the practice. Alternatively, one may be employed by a group of anesthesia practitioners, either CRNA or anesthetists (MDA) or a combination of both. Employment in this setting may include the option to own a portion of the practice either as a shareholder or partner. In this environment, salary and fringe benefits will be largely controlled by the economic constraints of the group as well as certain regulations regarding fringe benefits. If the CRNA is a partner or shareholder, he or she may have a voice in the delegation of responsibilities as well as the benefits of employment by the group. Finally, employment by a large corporation such as a hospital is a frequently encountered option. In this environment, CRNAs are likely to have little say in the salary and fringe benefits available or in the particular responsibilities associated with their position. However, just as in the case of the sole practitioner, the same business considerations play on the practice setting of a large corporation. A number of available practice settings are possible, recognizing that individual practitioners may combine practice settings to comply with their preferences or with the preferences of communities or administrators.

Economics is not the only factor affecting the business of anesthesia. Other equally important factors include the social and political environment, professional liability, and regulatory or professional control issues. Any given practice setting is necessarily a combination of all of these factors. Frequently the decision to select a given practice setting is as much a matter of the practitioner's willingness to address each of these factors as it is a matter of opportunity. Generally, the larger the employer, the more distanced the employee is from each of these factors. Simply stated, the employee can become a cog in the wheel simply by performing his or her professional function.

No one practice setting is necessarily better than the others. Several practice settings will be reviewed in this section, with an emphasis on the advantages and disadvantages of each. The results will better prepare the anesthesia practitioner to evaluate each practice setting and to select the single or combination of settings that affords the most rewarding and comfortable environment.

Solo Practice

Autonomy is the cornerstone of the solo practice setting. Autonomy will always include the economic factors related to the business of anesthesia but, depending on the location of the practice, may not involve autonomy in the practice of anesthesia. It is entirely possible to be a sole practitioner working for a group of anesthesia practitioners or a large hospital. Looking first to the economic factors, the sole practitioner's motivation for this practice setting may be the absolute control the practitioner has over economic factors. The salary, benefits, work hours, and security of the practice are a function of the personal preferences of the sole practitioner. There is no "vote." There are no considerations in decision making other than the goals and preferences of the practitioner.

The truly independent-minded sole practitioner may elect to practice in an area where there are no other anesthesia providers, thereby extending his or her autonomy of practice. Frequently, practitioners who pursue this practice setting are active in the governance of the facility where they practice. They serve on various committees, seek out and use the benefits of staff privileges, and participate as active members in the overall "community" of the hospital where they practice. Keep in mind, however, that this level of professional autonomy is not required of the sole practitioner. It is merely available.

The primary disadvantage of solo practice also lies in its autonomy. Sole practitioners rely on themselves for job security, income, benefits, and retirement considerations. The sole practitioner bears a heavy burden of responsibility and availability, often 24 hours a day. The sole practitioner's political awareness is as important, if not more important, than professional abilities, as these skills are required to make the practice secure. Finally, the sole practitioner is more immediately impacted by the economic realities of anesthesia practice. Third-party insurance decisions can have an immediate and occasionally detrimental effect on the business of anesthesia.

If the CRNA is considering a sole practice setting, there are three essential people to consult prior to establishing practice. The first is another CRNA who is experienced in a similar practice environment. This resource can be invaluable not only in assisting to locate and set up practice, but also as a confidant and resource when dealing with problems. The next person to develop a working relationship with is a certified public accountant (CPA). Few people are as intimately familiar with tax and accounting considerations, either individually or for business. The CPA can provide valuable advice in this arena. Finally the advice of an attorney experienced in the business of anesthesia is required. This advice and council is better sought while setting up a practice than after an unexpected problem is encountered.

Group Practice

Employment with a group of anesthesia providers usually offers less autonomy than does solo practice; however, with the decrease in autonomy also comes a decrease in responsibility and required availability. Group practices are as varied as the imagination. Group practices involving CRNA and MDA shareholders or partners are becoming increasingly popular, but are still less common than groups involving only one or the other as shareholders or partners. The autonomy of group practice is primarily a factor of the practitioner's involvement in the group. A shareholder or partner enjoys much more control of the group than does an employee of the group who routinely has no control of the group's practice. Perhaps the most immediate difference a practitioner encounters in the group practice versus the sole practice is the employment contract. The employment contract will detail the financial rewards and the professional duties and obligations of the anesthesia practitioner. As such, it deserves careful consideration and will be discussed in more detail later. One can, however, make generalizations about employment with, or participation in, a group practice.

Group practices offer varying degrees of autonomy depending on the size and makeup of the group and the geographic area in which the practice is located. In smaller groups, the level of autonomy can approach that of the sole practitioner, with the most significant difference being the vote of the other practitioners. In any group practice, participants sacrifice some individual goals for the good of the group. If practitioners enjoy similar family circumstances, obligations, and financial responsibilities, these sacrifices are negligible, but if practitioners differ significantly in age, their goals in practice likely vary. The younger practitioner may be interested in maximizing salary in the hope of purchasing a home or establishing a family while the older practitioner may be interested in acquiring deferred compensation benefits and retirement packages. These are not insurmountable differences and are easily balanced when the group is established and when new members join the group. Professional advice from a CPA and a qualified attorney should be considered essential items in the formation of a professional group practice.

If losing some of the economic autonomy of the sole practitioner can be considered a disadvantage of group practice, then sharing the responsibility of the professional practice can be considered one of its advantages. There is an additional level of security and confidence associated with a fellow professional. This perception is not limited to the practitioner but also extends to other health care professionals who rely on anesthesia services. In addition, the availability of several anesthesia providers traditionally permits the group to be more active in the politics of the practice environment without unduly taxing any single provider. Finally, in group practice, the structure of the group frequently provides rotating call schedules, continuing education, and vacation time for members.

Keep in mind that it is entirely possible to be employed by a group practice without any involvement in the group itself. Generally, the anesthesia provider who is considering employment with a group is also interested in either forming a group, joining a group, or obtaining an option to join the group as a shareholder or partner in the future. This participation in the group offers financial rewards and an opportunity to control the practice setting. It also offers the novice practitioner exposure to the disadvantages of group practice.

One of the primary hazards of a group practice lies in joining or establishing the group without professional assistance. A partnership or small corporation (close-held corporation) is frequently compared to a marriage. Potential members must first meet, consider their respective desires and goals for professional practice, and form a basis of trust with one another. Participation in group practice is always a major step in a career. The results of that participation will form the basis for professional practice, determine financial rewards and job security, and impact the family. These considerations are not actually a disadvantage to group practice unless they are not fully addressed when the group forms or accepts additional members. An attorney experienced in corporate law and structure can address these considerations in the form of voting, buy/sell agreements, compensation options, and employment contracts. Properly addressed, these considerations can result in significant advantages to a group practice. Ignored, they form the basis for the majority of disputes, legal actions, and breakups of professional groups.

Group practices generally take the form of partnerships or professional corporations. Partnerships are generally disfavored because of professional liability considerations. Simply stated, if one partner is sued in the performance of his duties for the partnership, all the general partners may be equally liable. Contrast the corporate setting, where if a shareholder is sued in the performance of his duties for the corporation, the shareholder and corporation may be liable, but the remaining shareholders are not liable. This is an oversimplification of the liability consideration a practitioner should consider in electing the form of group practice. There are also tax considerations, control considerations, and expansion of the group practice at issue.

For our purposes, we will look at partnerships and corporations without defining their actual structures. With few legal differences, the same considerations apply for the practitioner in either setting with only two major exceptions. First, if you are joining a partnership group practice, seek competent legal advice regarding individual liability for alleged malpractice claims and for tax considerations. An attorney should ask for several documents which include copies of the buy/sell agreement, the employment contract, and the professional liability insurance policy.

The second major exception is actually a misconception. Buy/sell agreements (sometimes called stock redemption agreements) are routinely thought of as a corporate document. A buy/sell agreement is as much a part of a partnership practice as it is a corporate practice. Any time individuals join together for the purpose of an enterprise they should consider a buy/sell agreement. The form of their relationship does not lessen the importance of legal planning; the buy/sell agreement is one of the most important documents to consider in establishing or joining a professional practice, addressing those concerns every practitioner hopes will never arise. The buy/sell agreement provides a method by which the members value the group practice. Occasionally this is an actual dollar amount, but more commonly it is an agreed method of valuing the practice, such as by net book value. The buy/sell agreement sets forth the terms and conditions on which a member voluntarily leaves the group or, alternatively, may be forced out of the group. These terms include the amount of money the member is entitled to receive and the method of payment when the member leaves the group. The buy/sell agreement should also address disability and retirement of a member. It should contain a requirement that all members of the group are required to actively practice on behalf of the group and should define the results if a member cannot or does not actively practice. The buy/sell agreement should define the method of termination if the group ceases to practice as a group. Finally, buy/sell agreements frequently provide insurance for each member. If a practitioner is a group member, disability and life insurance provisions will generally be in the buy/sell agreement and not in the employment contract. The buy/sell agreement frequently forms the basis for a member's job security and willingness to contribute to the success of the group.

If the CRNA is contemplating joining a group practice already in existence, the buy/sell agreement is one of the first documents that should be reviewed. It can offer enormous insight into the group members and their expectations in running the practice. Practitioners who are going to work for a group with an expectation of eventual partnership should ask to review the buy/sell agreement before signing an employment contract. While the group has no obligation to show the document at that time, an opportunity to review the buy/sell agreement will be invaluable in determining whether to join this group in the future. A buy/sell agreement is a complex legal document that should be reviewed by an attorney. After the attorney has had the opportunity to review the document in detail, schedule a meeting and ask all the "what if" questions. Examples might be: What if I lose my license? What if I do not like one member of the group? What if I disagree with a basic philosophy of the group? What if I get sued for professional malpractice? What if I lose my staff privileges or a given surgeon refuses to work with me? What if I become disabled? What if the group breaks up? What if the group loses its contract? What if I want out in 5 years? Write down questions before the meeting and write down the answers the lawyer gives.

After the buy/sell agreement, the next most important document to be considered is the employment contract. An employment contract for a group practice is not significantly different than an employment contract for any other employer. It should define the benefits of employment, including salary and fringe benefits, as well as the duties and responsibilities of the practitioner. It is advisable for all practitioners to have a carefully drafted employment contract to avoid later disputes regarding availability and responsibility of the practitioner. These provisions are even more important in the group practice setting because the employer is also the employee. This is particularly true of the availability provisions of the employment contract, which should spell out the call duties and coverage responsibilities of all member/employees of the group.

If there is any major difference in the employment contract with a group practice, it involves tying the employment contract into the buy/sell agreement and the employees participation as a group member. By way of example, it would not be wise to have an "at will" employment contract (either party can terminate the agreement at any time with or without cause) and have no requirement in the buy/sell agreement for active participation in the group as a requirement to maintain group membership. The result would be that the group could fire a member/employee they believed was not professionally competent, but they could not force that member out of the group. As a member of the group, that member would retain all voting rights and the right to share profits. This is not the position in which to place a disgruntled employee.

The primary disadvantages of the group practice setting are generally the result of a failure to plan ahead. If the practitioner has never been involved in a group, whatever its structure, it is difficult to appreciate and anticipate possible conflicts that can arise. As a professional health care provider highly educated in anesthesia, CRNAs are not likely to have the formal preparation or background to anticipate these potential conflicts. It is advisable to seek the counsel of experts experienced in group practice and corporate and partnership law before becoming a member of a group. In that manner the practitioner will more fully understand the concept of group practice and the structure and constraints of the practice about to be formed or joined. This will effectively eliminate the major disadvantage of poor planning and allow the advantages of sharing professional knowledge and responsibilities with other anesthesia providers. The result is frequently increased financial rewards, job satisfaction, and job security.

Institution-Based Practice

The professional CRNA often considers employment with a large group, such as a hospital, clinic, or HMO. The majority of anesthetists have had vast experience with this practice setting working as a registered nurse and additional experience within the hospital environment during the time of educational preparation. This experience and the support of an often large anesthesia department make a traditional hospital setting a comfortable first practice experience.

In addition to the comfort and security of prior experience, the large group or hospital setting offers the practitioner other advantages. The most commonly cited advantage of the large group or hospital setting is a steady paycheck. This is an important consideration; however, as discussed later, it can be both an advantage and a disadvantage. The next most commonly cited advantage is the opportunity for professional challenge and growth through participation in hospital-sponsored education programs and through exposure to more complex anesthesia cases. Larger hospitals are frequently in possession of the newest equipment and involved in the latest techniques of anesthesia practice. It would be a mistake to assume that other practice settings do not enjoy the same opportunities, but the large hospital setting is almost guaranteed to offer these opportunities.

Teaching, as well as learning opportunities, are an often-cited factor in selecting this practice setting. In addition to these professional considerations, the large group or hospital offers the security of size and the ability to be "lost in the crowd." Many people, and anesthesia practitioners are no exception, prefer this work environment and the anonymity it offers. The inevitable insulation from the impact of the business of anesthesia allows the practitioner to concentrate on the practice of anesthesia without worrying about the business aspects until contract negotiation time. Finally, it would be inappropriate to fail to consider geographics and opportunity as a motivation to select this practice setting. As a practical matter, larger groups and hospitals are located in metropolitan areas that are also the home of large numbers of anesthesia providers. That is not to say that independent group practices and sole practitioners do not practice in the same geographic area; it is not necessary to abandon metropolitan areas or large hospitals to fulfill one's career goals.

For all the advantages of the large group or hospital practice there are also disadvantages. One of the most common is the anesthesia practitioner's isolation from the economic realities of anesthesia practice. All practice settings are ultimately impacted by the general economic climate and reimbursement issues. This is true for both the sole practitioner and the largest hospital. The hospital, however, has multiple sources of income, all of which comprise the hospital's budget. The overall effect of these sources can insulate the hospital, at least in the short term, from fluctuations in income generated from anesthesia services. The hospital often uses excess anesthesia income to cover shortfalls in other departments, but consistency in this practice is open to the vagaries of changing reimbursement schedules.

This concept is the greatest source of frustration at contract negotiation time. Anesthesia providers are convinced that the hospital generates a profit from its anesthesia department, but the hospital's position is that overall the budget is tight, and cost-related benefits are unavailable. The hospital's ability to attenuate the effect of changes in the economic climate may mislead the anesthesia practitioner into a false sense of not being personally impacted by those changes. The result may be that the anesthesia practitioner who practices in a large group or hospital setting fails to see the urgency in hospital projects or interest groups that concentrate on political and economic issues. Also, the result of this insulation from the economic realities of anesthesia practice may be a CRNA unprepared to assess and value alternative practice opportunities.

One potential disadvantage of the large group or hospital practice setting lies in the concept of what is often termed being a "cog in the wheel." While there is a certain comfort in anonymity and routine, there can also develop a sense of frustration and "sameness" in regard to the CRNAs continued learning and acquisition of new experiences, which is restricted by hospital routines. CRNAs often fall prey to this situation and frequently fail to maintain skills and experiences for which there is little or no opportunity to participate.

Finally, it should be remembered that in the absence of contract stipulations to the contrary or representation by collective bargaining units, most group-employed CRNAs are considered "at will" employees. As mentioned earlier, this means that the CRNA can be terminated without cause. Although this termination prerogative is offered to both parties, this can be especially problematic for the CRNA who finds other employment opportunities in the area limited. The CRNA should always understand clearly, via policy review, what his or her rights are in these situations prior to signing an employment agreement or contract.

Each of the three major practice settings enjoys certain advantages and disadvantages. It should be evident that there is no ideal practice setting that offers only advantages. However, there is a common thread that runs through all of the practice settings discussed: the preferences and goals of the anesthesia practitioner. There are almost unlimited opportunities but no perfect setting. The conclusion to this review of practice settings must be that the anesthesia practitioner is in a unique and enviable position, to consider preferences and goals and select the practice setting that best meets those choices. In reviewing options, bear in mind that it is not possible to consider every advantage or disadvantage of a particular practice setting. This review has not mentioned the important factors of friendship, mutual and professional respect, trust, and common goals. Simply stated, people are as important a consideration as the environment within which individual interaction takes place.

EMPLOYMENT CONTRACTS

Having considered the benefits and selected a particular employment setting, the only remaining items, before going to work on the first day, are the duties and obligations of each party and the contract itself.

The contract is the beginning of the employment setting whether it be as an employee of a facility, an employee of an independently practicing group, or an independent contractor. It is beyond the scope of this chapter to delve into the duties and obligations of each party; however, the importance of these provisions should be emphasized. Often the contract for anesthesia services, be it an employment contract or any other form of contract, is written by the employer. Frequently the contract is lengthy regarding the CRNA's duties and obligations but says very little about the employer's duties and obligations.

Frequently the anesthetist may be exposed to a standard employment contract prepared by the facility where the anesthetist is considering employment. There is often little opportunity to negotiate the terms and conditions of the contract, because the facility may prefer that all contracts for similar services be uniform. This is also the case when there is an organization such as a union in place. In these circumstances the anesthetist will have limited ability to negotiate the terms and benefits of the contract. A standardized contract should not be signed as a matter of routine. The contract is every bit as enforceable as the contract negotiated after hours of effort and deserves careful evaluation and consideration.

When confronted with a standard or required employment contract, the anesthetist should look beyond salary alone and pay particular attention to the benefits and the obligations of the contract. Frequently, such a contract will reference other documents such as professional liability insurance policies, pension and profit sharing plans, health insurance plans, and policy and procedure manuals. These documents are incorporated into the contract by reference and should be examined. CRNAs not only have the right but also the obligation to review any such referenced documents before signing the employment contract. Pay equal attention to obligations under the contract. Note any grievance requirements, availability and response minimums, termination provisions, and performance minimums, including their evaluation.

Also note the hierarchy or chain of command, if any. Ask questions if any of these important areas of the contract are missing or unclear. In seeking clarification be aware that if the contract is in writing, verbal comments, clarifications, and agreements are unlikely to be enforceable. Write the clarification on the contract and have each party initial the additions. CRNAs should be prepared to sign the contract only when confident they understand their obligations and the hospital or facility's obligations as well as the benefits conferred on both. Prior to signing a contract, it is advisable to confer with an attorney or at least with an experienced colleague who does not work for the facility offering the contract.

Contract Law

After considering salary, fringe benefits, and the duties and obligations of both parties, it is time to consider the contract itself. Contract law is one of the oldest forms of law and is governed by traditions and rules that predate the discovery of America. Many of those rules still apply today in drafting, interpreting, and enforcing a contract. The idea of a contract seems simple enough; it should amount to nothing more than expressing, either in written form or by verbal agreement, what the parties intend. Problems develop when another person reads or listens to this contract and has a different interpretation. The first step in any contract negotiation involves discussing the contract in the first place. While CRNAs should seek all the advice available, they are the ones who must ultimately decide what the goal of the contract will be. Even if CRNAs employ an attorney to assist in drafting a contract, they must know what they want that contract to accomplish.

Four Corners Doctrine

As mentioned earlier, contract law is one of the oldest forms of law, steeped in tradition. The interpretation of ambiguous language is the first place that tradition applied. In an effort to place the burden of interpreting the contract on the party who wrote it rather than on the court who may have to interpret the contract, several important concepts of contract law have developed. The first of these concepts is called the *Four*

Corners Doctrine. The Four Corners Doctrine provides that the court interpreting a written contract can look only at the contract. That is to say, they look only at what is written in the agreement. They do not consider comparable contracts. They do not consider what is usual and customary. They do not consider the advantages or disadvantages of one party over the other unless those advantages or disadvantages are unconscionable. They do not consider the negotiation process that went into the contract. They consider only the written contract.

Construed Against the Drafting Party

The next traditional rule that impacts the written contract is that if, when looking to the Four Corners Doctrine, the court is unable to establish the meaning of any particular words of phrases or is unable to define the duties or obligations of any party, then the contract is *construed against the party who drafted it.* Simply stated, if one drafts an anesthesia contract or has a contract drafted for them, and there is a question about the meaning of any part of that contract, it would be interpreted in favor of the other party.

Parole Evidence Rule

Finally, the last general rule impacting the interpretation of a contract dates to feudal England and arose because of land ownership disputes between the lords. That rule is known as the *Parole Evidence Rule* and it remains an integral part of modern contract law. What the Parole Evidence Rule means today is that when the court interprets a written contract and applies the Four Corners Doctrine, they cannot consider anything that was said between the parties in drafting that particular agreement. In other words, they cannot consider any of the negotiation process. They cannot consider the prior performance or arrangement between the same parties. They cannot consider an argument or a statement to the effect "that's not what we intended to say." The only exception to the Parole Evidence Rule is if the contract language itself is ambiguous and even when construing the contract against the party who wrote it, the court is unable to ascertain the intentions of the parties. It is reasonably rare to have that happen, however, because the last traditional rule of contract law is that the courts cannot rewrite the contract for the parties.

It is a good idea to get many contracts and look them over. There are a number of sample anesthesia contracts available from colleagues, advertisements in the back of journals, and sometimes even from hospitals. In this manner CRNAs can get an idea of how other parties are addressing concerns that are probably very similar to personal ones. While it is wise to gather all the available information before beginning negotiations, there are risks associated with "borrowing language" from contracts. All the language in a contract is read together and with the presumption that the parties intended it to say what it says. In keeping with the Four Corners Doctrine there is the presumption that the language of the contract encompassed all the concerns the parties had when they drafted it. It is a bad idea to copy language from one agreement to another agreement unless the language is clearly understood, fits within the total agreement to be signed, and accomplishes what is intended.

Contract Negotiation

The negotiation of the contract is entirely dependent on obligations of the parties and the benefits each party is to obtain as a result of the performance of their respective obligations. Exercise caution because contracts and contract laws are complicated. All the effort put into negotiating the contract is ultimately merged in the contract. The contract is the final document, and the efforts gone through to get the contract are rarely considered in interpreting its meaning. This is the area where an attorney with experience in anesthesia service agreements can be very helpful, as can other anesthetists with personal experience in contract negotiations.

A contract has been defined as an agreement, on sufficient consideration, to do or not to do a particular thing. Contracts are divided into express contracts and implied contracts. For purposes of this text, only express contracts will be considered. An express contract may be defined as one in which the terms are openly stated at the time of the making of the contract. In other words, in an express contract, the parties have generally negotiated to reach a final agreement. A promise, the basis of a contract, is an expression of the intention that the promisee will conduct himself or herself in a specified way or bring about a specified result in the future, communicated to the promisor in such a manner that he or she may justifiably expect performance and may reasonably rely on it.

The central elements of a contract are parties competent to contract, a proper subject matter, legal consideration, mutuality of agreement, and mutuality of obligation. Be careful here; competent does not mean sane, it means authorized. There must be, among other things, an offer and an acceptance, as well as consideration. Mere discussions and negotiations, or even unaccepted offers cannot be substituted for the formal requirements of a contract. A contract is not made as long as, in the contemplation of both parties, something remains to be done to establish the contractual relationship. The law neither makes a contract when the parties intend none, nor regards an arrangement as complete until the parties regard it as being complete.

A word of caution about verbal contracts is in order. The obvious difficulty with the verbal agreement for anesthesia services arises when there is a dispute as to the exact obligations of the agreement. These difficulties are frequently unknown until a dispute actually arises. For purposes of brevity, however, the only thing to specifically say about a verbal agreement or verbal contract is that it is an enforceable agreement between the parties.

What are some "essential elements" of an anesthesia contract? Anything the parties may care to put into a contract is acceptable, but specific goals should be kept in mind. Written anesthesia contracts range in length from one paragraph to dozens of pages. As long as that one paragraph has the essential elements of a contract, it is enforceable.

The following minimum essential elements in an anesthesia contract should be included:

- The parties to the contract must be clearly defined.
- The duties of *each party* should be clearly defined.
- The consideration or benefit to be received by each party should be clearly expressed.
- The length of the contract and termination provisions should be clearly defined.

In negotiating contracts, the CRNA traditionally looks at his or her own personal considerations. It can be a mistake not devoting equal time viewing the other party's considerations.

Before there can be a contract, there have to be negotiations leading to a "meeting of the minds." Under general principles of contract law, negotiations are not part of the contract, and all negotiation efforts are merged in the final contract. Often contracts contain a clause (known as the *merger clause*) which specifically states that all negotiations, promises, discussions, and representations are contained in that agreement and superseded by the agreement. If a contract is signed that contains a merger clause it is very important to read that clause carefully. Merger clauses are often overlooked because they are considered "boilerplate" clauses or legalese. If one drafts a contract or has one drafted, pay particular attention to language like merger clauses, because the courts will.

A contract must establish a mutuality of obligation. Contracts cannot arise when there is no mutuality or when one party has no intention of binding himself or herself and is not even supposed by the other party to be making himself or herself liable. However, getting as close to the line of not binding oneself while still achieving a mutuality of obligation is generally the starting point of the parties in negotiations. The easiest way to visualize this concept is to envision a line or continuum with the number 1 at one extreme and the number 10 at the other. Let us call the employer's position number 1 and the anesthetist's position number 10. Each party will attempt to negotiate contract provisions that are as close as possible to their number on the continuum. The ideal contract negotiation would result in an agreement binding each of the parties exactly the same and converging at the midpoint, or the 5 position. That would be highly unusual. An agreement or contract at the 1 or the 10 position would be unenforceable for failure of mutuality. The idea is to negotiate for a position as close to your end of the scale as possible. Of course, that is also the other party's goal.

The best way to envision this goal-oriented approach to drafting an anesthesia contract is to contrast language involving the same right. The following sample language was taken from two different anesthesia contracts. Note that the negotiating positions of the parties is significantly different in these contracts.

> The Corporations shall establish subject to the Hospital's approval, a schedule of fees to be charged to all patients furnished by or in the Hospital's Anesthesia Department. This schedule may be amended by mutual agreement, in writing, between the hospital and the corporation.

> As consideration for the services to be provided by the Corporation, the Corporation shall have the exclusive right to bill patients or third party payers for all anesthesia services rendered at the hospital and to collect from such parties all amounts owed for such services. The Corporation's fees shall be in general accord with customary fees for comparable services.

Read the first paragraph carefully. This is the language the employer would most prefer in pursuing its goal-oriented approach to negotiations. On the continuum, this language would probably be at the 3 or 4 position. Note that the fee schedule to be developed for all patients is subject to the employer's approval. There are no restrictions whatsoever on the employer granting or withholding that approval. The language does not address what would happen if the employer withheld its approval or if the corporation continued to bill at its current rates while the parties were mutually discussing amending the fee schedules.

By contrast, consider the second paragraph. Obviously this language would be preferred by the anesthesia provider. On the continuum this language would probably be around an 8 or 9 position. We are assuring the employer that fees will be "in general accord with customary fees for comparable services"; however, nothing in the language specifically says what the fees will be. Also the employer has no input in enforcement of this provision. However, there is something else very good in this provision. It gives the corporation the exclusive right to bill for all anesthesia services rendered at the hospital whether rendered by the corporation or any other anesthesia provider. The exclusive right to bill is the consideration for the agreement. If any one else has the right to bill for anesthesia services, the consideration for the contract fails, at least in part, and the corporation could be released from any obligation to perform any of the duties or obligations required by the agreement. This paragraph was the only place where consideration was mentioned in the contract. Note that billing the patient is the consideration for providing anesthesia service. The exclusive right to bill is the sole consideration for providing the anesthesia services to the hospital. In addition to these consideration provisions there should be, and there was, a provision for the exclusive right to provide anesthesia services. That provision, however, should be one or two lines long. The significance of this language does not end with consideration. Look at the word "or" in the third line. The anesthesia provider can bill the patient or third-party payers. This is a "nonparticipating" agreement at the anesthetist's option. It is important to retain the right to bill patients for your services. The contract can specifically include a nonparticipation clause or it can treat this important provision in this way. Often the emphasis placed on a term or condition dictates its content in the final contract. If this contract contained a specific nonparticipation provision, this language should be changed. The most important thing to remember is that a contract must be read as an entire document and not as one isolated line by one isolated line or as one isolated provision by one isolated provision. It all must fit together in the end.

Frequently anesthesia providers seek staff privileges or membership on the medical staff. There are many advantages to membership on the medical staff. By way of example, there may be specific appeal provisions in the event privileges will be amended or revoked. Membership may also impose additional duties and obligations.

Therefore, if the contract will provide for membership on the medical staff, read the Bylaws of the Medical Staff and The Rules and Regulations of the Medical Staff. These documents must be considered in preparing the anesthesia contract. The contract should specify what will happen if there is a conflict between the staff privileges and the contract.

BENEFIT PACKAGES

Benefits are an integral part of the negotiation process and often involve substantial noncash compensation. Depending on the type and range of benefits, this can amount to between 5 and 40 percent of the total annual cash compensation (average considered about 20 to 25 percent). Consequently, the CRNA should try to determine as closely as possible the value of these benefits, in order to determine the equity of base salary. That is, a single anesthetist without children may receive substantially fewer benefits than the married CRNA with a family, potentially justifying an increase in base pay.

Benefits can be considered in three groups. The first group involves money and includes salary, professional liability insurance premiums and coverage, pension and profit sharing plans, third-party billing and nonparticipation provisions, life, health, and disability insurance, tax-sheltered annuities and related tax-deferral tools, and reimbursement of expenses arising from the performance of the contract. The second group of benefits involves time and includes vacation, personal leave, continuing education leave, call schedules, availability of the anesthetist, and exclusive service provisions. The third group of benefits involves employment security and future growth. These benefits include grievance provisions in employment contracts, noncompetition provisions, chain of command in decision making, options to gain shareholder status (become a partner), advancement and promotion guidelines, and termination provisions.

There is a long list of potential benefits that should be considered at the earliest stages of contract negotiations, and yet many anesthetists are concerned primarily with the salary provisions. Obviously, salary is very important and frequently starts the negotiation process; however, it should never be allowed to overshadow the equally important and often more valuable remaining benefits.

It is beneficial to approach contract negotiations with specific goals in mind. Each anesthetist's goal regarding fringe benefits will necessarily be slightly different. Therefore, it is highly recommended that fringe benefits be individually valued before entering into contract negotiations. The advice of a CPA for assistance in this area is strongly advised. A CPA can assist in tax planning and in projecting actual costs to the potential employer of the benefits desired by the potential employee, as well as the replacement cost of each such benefit if the potential employer declines any requested benefit. It is only in this manner that one can enter the negotiations being fully aware of the benefits package offered. It may be advantageous to accept a lower salary and a better benefits package. This arrangement may provide tax savings and job security. Keep in mind that the potential employer also has goals for the final contract.

Health and Medical Insurance

The following is an example of health insurance provisions in an anesthesia service contract. The proposed language allows the anesthetist the opportunity to opt out of the coverage and receive additional compensation. Note that the language does not specify who the health insurance carrier is nor does it specify coverage to be provided. This information is routinely provided in the certificate of insurance for individual carriers and the anesthetist should review these documents carefully before signing a contract with language such as the following.

> *Health and Medical Insurance:* Anesthetist shall be provided full family health insurance coverage, Corporation being responsible for any deductible associated therewith. Anesthetist may elect, on an annual basis, not to participate in such program and in that event shall be entitled to receive an amount equal to Corporation's actual cost of obtaining and maintaining such insurance during the period Anesthetist elects not to so participate.

Life Insurance

Life insurance benefits are often overlooked or relegated to a lower position on the goal-oriented approach to benefit negotiations. This is unfortunate because whole life and annuity insurance provisions can offer significant tax and estate benefits. Prior to valuing this benefit, it may be helpful to speak with an attorney and accountant regarding this potentially valuable benefit and to consult with an insurance agent regarding existing insurance. The following is an example of very simple language regarding only term insurance. Note, however, that in this language the employer (corporation) is surrendering any claim it may have on the insurance proceeds, notwithstanding the fact it is paying all the premiums. Such is not always the case.

> *Term Life Insurance:* Corporation shall purchase and maintain on behalf of Anesthetist a Term Life Insurance contract in the amount of $50,000 and shall have no claim upon said insurance proceeds as a result of said premium payments. Anesthetist shall name the beneficiary thereof and upon termination of this contract Anesthetist shall be entitled to assume the payment of any premiums of said insurance policy.

Disability Benefits

Perhaps some of the most important fringe benefits involve disability. The disability provisions are critical to both parties because not only do they provide a source of income for the disabled anesthetist, but in the event of disability they provide the terms on which the employer may terminate its relationship with the anesthetist. Not all disability provisions include insurance, though. The careful anesthetist should negotiate for insurance protection. In the event one has an individual disability policy, the anesthetist should still consider a disability provision in the employment contract. Pay particular attention to payment of concurrent benefits in the event of disability and of the definitions of disability in the insurance policies themselves. Alternatively, CRNAs may wish to negotiate payment of their disability premiums by the employer. Discuss possible tax considerations regarding these options with a tax advisor or attorney. Ideally the language in the contract defining disability should refer to the language in the disability policy, but *only* if the CRNA is completely familiar with that language. The following sample language is an attempt to incorporate the language of an existing disability policy and to add a rather ambiguous definition of "substantially prevented from performing her duties hereunder." Note, however, that the proposed language can work against the anesthetist if the insurance policy does not include a given disability and the employer considers the disability to substantially prevent the anesthetist's performance of duties. In that event the corporation could pay 60 days of compensation and benefits and thereafter terminate the anesthetist's employment. Of course, the disability insurance would not pay disability benefits because under the policy definition no disability exists.

> *Disability:* In the event Anesthetist should become incapacitated due to illness or injury, and substantially prevented from performing her duties hereunder, anesthetist shall receive her full compensation and benefits as provided herein during the first Sixty (60) days of such incapacity, less any amounts paid over to her under a disability income insurance policy, the premiums for which have been paid by Corporation. In the event Anesthetist shall be incapacitated for a period exceeding Sixty (60) continuous days, such incapacity shall, at the option of Corporation, constitute a termination of this Agreement.

Pension and/or Profit Sharing Plans

Perhaps one of the most difficult fringe benefits to value is participation in a pension and/or profit sharing plan. Seek the advice of experts in this area to discuss vesting schedules, contributions, and tax benefits of the proposed plan. Generally, contract language regarding participation in any such plan is simple once the plan itself is reviewed.

Professional Liability Insurance

The final sample language offered for consideration involves professional liability insurance coverage as a fringe benefit. Once again the insurance policy itself is of primary concern. If an employer is self-insured, as many are, review the insurance coverage to be sure there are no subrogation provisions. Subrogation is the right of the insurer to seek reimbursement of any losses that may incur as a result of a claim from the insured. Certain subrogation clauses also include the right to seek reimbursement of legal expenses and losses even if those expenses were occasioned as a result of a settlement. The sample language governs those circumstances where the employer provides an insurance policy in the name of the anesthetist. In this event the Optional Reporting Endorsement is a critical provision because such options can be very expensive.

> *Professional Liability Insurance:* Corporation shall secure, at Corporation's sole expense, professional liability insurance for Anesthetist in the minimum amount of $1,000,000 per occurrence and $3,000,000 in the aggregate. In the event this Agreement is terminated for any reason or upon completion of this Agreement Corporation shall secure and pay for an Optional Reporting Endorsement (tail) on behalf of Anesthetist.

When reviewing each of the sample contract provisions, remember that all sample language is just that: sample language. Use sample language as a starting point to negotiations and not as an insert or substitute for consulting with qualified individuals. With a carefully drafted contract, CRNAs can provide professional services for the benefit of patients, the community, family, and dependents for years to come. One's degree of success in these endeavors depends in large part on that contract. Treat it accordingly.

RESUMES AND INTERVIEW TECHNIQUES

Job opportunities for nurse anesthetists are excellent today even in the face of a competitive job market with other anesthesia professionals. Nurse anesthetists can choose to be "choosy." It is imperative, however, that anesthetists market themselves in a professional, competent, and informed manner.

Many times the first chance to make a good impression is with a well-constructed, printed resume, and the last chance is during an interview. Working from this premise, it is the objective of this section to help assess one's job goals, learn tips to compile an effective resume, and successfully interview. It is not possible to cover the many styles of resumes or interviewing strategies in this section alone. A more comprehensive discussion on resume writing and interviewing may be found in any of the Bibliography entries following this chapter.

Getting Organized

First, take a sheet of paper and make a list of places to apply. Write down what is perceived as the employer's goals, and then write down one's own goals for employment. This exercise will sometimes help focus attention to long-term job satisfaction rather than a short-term means to an end.

Second, analyze personal achievements and list them. This helps to refresh one's memory about possible accomplishments that may have been forgotten. Listing accomplishments may help during the interview process. Focus on strengths, but consider weaknesses. Be realistic without being overly critical; remember, we are generally our own worst critic. This exercise may seem simplistic, but a commonly asked question by an interviewer is "Why should I hire you?" This list will help provide confident answers to that question.

Drafting Your Resume

After having taken a personal inventory of education, skills, experience, strengths, and goals, the next step is to draft the resume. A resume is not autobiographic or a lengthy description of life accomplishments; rather, it is an advertisement or promulgation. It is how one sells oneself, or at the very least kindles interest in a perspective employer. The function of the resume is to get an interview.

Choosing a resume format may sound easy, but on investigating the various styles, the vast multiplicity to choose from becomes apparent. Despite numerous variations, there are three basic formats: chronologic resume, functional resume, and combination resume. Below is a brief description of each.

The *chronologic resume* is the most widely accepted and most familiar format. It is true to its name. First list employment and education history in reverse chronologic order, beginning with the last job held and latest educational achievement. Chronologic resumes are easy to write and to read. They are particularly good for people with an excellent work history without gaps in employment.

A *functional resume* downplays gaps in employment or frequent job changes. This format simply lists the years of employment (e.g., 1965 to present) with a brief description of what has been done during that time, emphasizing certain skills or titles held. This section is followed by an educational history only inclusive of the schools, degrees, and years degrees were granted.

A *combination resume* combines both the chronologic and the functional formats. The only variation, which comes after the brief description as explained under the functional format, is that this resume is inclusive of a reverse chronologic listing of places of employment.

It is important to do first and second drafts when compiling the resume. This allows opportunity to critique what has been written, make additions and deletions, and strive for brevity. It is important to remember that even an accomplished professional should be able to limit his or her resume to two or two and one-half pages (the curriculum vitae required for academic positions is excepted). Figure 11–1 shows an example of a Harvard-style resume. It is a combination of the various styles of resumes and is an excellent format for use by anesthesia providers.

For those CRNAs applying for academic positions, there is considerable variation in the form of the curriculum vitae (CV—academic resume) required. Usually, there is no initial objective statement. The CV starts with a biographic listing similar to the example in the appendix. This is followed by list of professional licenses and certifications, dates of expiration, and license numbers. Next is a listing in reverse order of academic and clinical degrees, date obtained, name of degree, institution, and concentration. The balance of the CV should list, in order, teaching experience, clinical experience, research experience, funded or written grants obtained, publications, and presentations. Whether preparing a resume or CV, the CRNA should omit any excessively informal narrative and listings of hobbies, interests, and so on. Under no circumstances should there be spelling errors or inconsistency in format. Many CRNAs take advantage of professional firms to collate and print their resumes or curriculum vitaes.

Writing a Cover Letter

Once satisfied with the resume, a cover letter is written to accompany it. The cover letter personalizes and directs the resume toward the interviewer and provides a brief statement of the applicant's purpose and why he or she is interested in the employer's particular employment setting. This letter also initiates communication between the potential employee and the interviewer. It is important to arrange the letter in an appropriate business style and avoid typographic or grammatic errors. This is the first professional impression the CRNA will make in addition to his or her resume. If guidance is required, published reference texts on writing business correspondence are available. This reference is commonly found in most bookstores in the reference section and is fairly inexpensive.

Preparing for the Interview

Thorough preparation prior to an interview may well determine the benefit and success of the interview. While a potential employer is interviewing the potential employee to form some basis on which to judge him or her, the interview is also the employee's opportunity to learn more about the employer. The interviewer has researched the employee through the CV, letters of reference, and other documents provided in the application process. Similarly, a potential employee should research the employer. It is advisable to learn as much as possible about the work setting and employer prior to the interview. This knowl-

Jane Smith CRNA, MSN
1529 Lane Avenue — Phone: 615-361-9951 (H)
Nashville, TN 37203 — 615-342-3405 (O)
SSN # — Digital Beeper: 615-923-6045

Professional Objective
To work with a progressive anesthesia group in a teaching facility that encourages CRNAs to be autonomous practitioners in all facets of anesthesia practice, including regional anesthetic techniques.

Experience
My nursing career began in 1971. I worked as a professional registered nurse in a variety of capacities including (from staff nurse to nurse manager) in critical care as well as postanesthesia care. In 1981, I began my certified nurse anesthesia practice in a combined CRNA/MDA practice in Nashville at a level I trauma center. Recently, I have been working locum tenums based out of my home in Nashville.

Chief CRNA
Duties included active recruitment of CRNA professionals, CRNA scheduling, and case assignments. 1989-1991.

Anesthesia Research Assistant
Collected data for research project conducted by six members on staff and helped conduct research in the clinical area. Research findings published in the AANA Journal in 1991. Copy of work available for review. 1990.

Journal Club Instructor
Facilitated journal club meetings once a week for 20 students from a local school for two semesters during the 1987 to 1988 school year. Currently serve on their obstetric advisory committee.

Staff CRNA
Worked 50 plus hours in an active level I trauma center, which was inclusive of in-house call twice a week. A variety of general, vascular, neuro, obstetric, and pediatric cases were done. Regional skills were not only encouraged but required. 1981-1989.

Education

MSN in Critical Care Nursing
Vanderbilt University, 1987

Certificate in Nurse Anesthesia
Erlanger Medical Center, 1981

Baccalaureate in Nursing
Belmont College, 1985

Diploma in Nursing
St. Thomas Hospital, 1971

Professional Membership and Involvement
American Association of Nurse Anesthetists member 1981 to present
Tennessee Association of Nurse Anesthetists member 1981 to present
American Nurses Association member 1971 to present
Advanced Cardiac Life Support Instructor 1984 to present
Advisory Committee member local school 1987 to present
Practitioner Committee member to the AANA education committee 1990

References available upon request

Figure 11–1. Sample resume.

edge provides background information and allows one to establish areas to pursue in detail. There are many sources for this information. Most hospitals and clinics have information and public relations material available describing their size, services, goals, philosophy, and financial track record.

If the interview is in a different community, use the interview to learn about the area. Prior to the visit, obtain information about the community through the local chamber of commerce, small business association, or visitors bureau. Set aside some time to experience (or "interview") the community. Use every resource available. The potential employee can establish himself or herself as someone who is sincerely interested by showing initiative in preparation. Research will help avoid spending most of the interview with the litany of facts and information about the institution and focus on more productive conversation. Most importantly, background research helps establish goals prior to entering the interview. Use the research to establish what information is desired in the interview process and as the basis for directed questioning.

Prior to the interview, list strengths and weaknesses in an honest, personal evaluation. Enlist the help of a candid (but not brutal) friend or co-worker in this self-assessment exercise. Anticipate potential questions and have a general idea of responses so that the subsequent answers are well thought out. Construct a list of questions to be answered during the interview. Salary and benefits may be stated or open to negotiation in an initial interview but often are reserved for the second meeting. Determine benefits and salary requirements prior to the meeting and negotiate from this premise.

Interviewing

Interviewing is an essential skill for a professional. It is possible to establish rapport with the interviewer by speaking clearly and openly. The potential employee will find that many interviewers are capable of setting the applicant at ease quickly while others elect not to. Be conscious of your personal behavior and physical movements while assessing the work situation and personnel of the potential employer; they are in turn making their own assessments. Put the best foot forward but always be honest. Avoid demanding or arrogant posturing. Interviews can be an enlightening experience, one which teaches sponteneity, self-discipline, and facility at developing written and verbal skills.

Also be aware that physician and CRNA groups and hospitals often conduct business on an "as needed" basis. In other words, they do not start interviewing personnel until a crisis in human resources has developed. Consequently, the tendency is to obtain "a warm body." Do not allow potential employers to gloss over questions you feel are critical to your success and satisfaction while in their employ. If your questions are evaded or answered with more rhetoric than substance either restate the question or graciously terminate the interview. It is likely the behavior you experience from the employer during the interview will be the same after you are employed. If you are making considerable effort to act in a professional manner and with integrity, require your interviewer to do likewise.

Miscellaneous Tips for Interviewing

On the morning of the interview take out the resume and pertinent information regarding the group with which you will be interviewing. This is also the time to review the strengths and weaknesses lists. Bring a typewritten list of references with their addresses. Most resumes generally state references available on request, and references will be requested. Bring to the interview any publications or abstracts regarding research involvement. This is particularly important if the position applied for is in education or research.

Every interviewer sets dress standards in their mind. Dress is a very powerful, nonverbal statement; plan attire in advance and double-check before going to the interview. Take the opportunity to tour the anesthesia department and operating rooms. Talk with the staff and look to these sources to provide additional information. Be advised that anyone may have input relevant to the employment decision.

Last, if they do not have a contractual agreement listing salary and benefits, then ask that they compile something in writing. If you are truly interested, schedule a second visit to spend time in the work area. This follow-up maintains contact but prevents making a hasty decision.

Resume writing and interviewing allows the CRNA to view himself or herself and accomplishments in an organized manner and presents an opportunity for self-evaluation, change, and growth. Interpersonal skills may be enriched, and the process allows comparison between present employment and potential employment. Remember, you are your own best marketing tool.

BIBLIOGRAPHY

Bostwick, B: Resume Writing, ed 4. John Wiley & Sons, New York, 1990.

Catalyst Staff: Marketing Yourself, ed 6. Bantam Books, New York, 1986.

Delton, J: Most Common Writing Mistakes, ed 1. Writers Digest Books, Cincinnati, OH, 1985.

Gratus, J: Successful Interviewing, How to Find and Keep the Best People, ed 1. Penguin Books, London, 1988.

Hizer, D and Robenberg, A: The Resume Handbook, ed 2. Bob Adams, Holbrook, MA, 1990.

FIVE

Legal Aspects of Anesthesia Practice

12

The Legal System in the United States

Gene A. Blumenreich

OUTLINE

THE GOALS OF THE LEGAL SYSTEM
STATE VERSUS FEDERAL COURTS
State Courts
Federal Courts
Lawsuits Arising Under Federal Legislation
Federal Property
Diversity
SOURCES OF LAW
Legislature
Courts
Common Law
Executive Branch
Administrative Agencies
DEFERENCE TO THE HEALTH CARE PROFESSION
THE ROLE OF THE LEGAL PROFESSION
NATURE OF THE COURTS
Conflicts Among Courts
Civil/Criminal Matters
Civil Litigation
TORT LIABILITY
Standard of Care
Failure to Comply with Law or Regulation
SPECIFIC TOPICS
Vicarious Liability
Misrepresentations Concerning Vicarious Liability
Damages
Res Ipsa Loquitur

OBJECTIVES

On completing this chapter, the reader will be able to:

1. Demonstrate knowledge of the goals and organization of the federal and state court systems in the United States.
2. Describe the various sources of law including the legislature, courts, common law, executive branch, and administrative agencies.
3. Describe the nature and role of the legal profession and its traditional relationships to the health care professions.
4. Discuss tort liability as it relates to standards of care and concepts of negligence.
5. Demonstrate knowledge relative to the issues of vicarious liability, damages, and the concept of *res ipsa loquitur*.

---

*Some of the material in this chapter is based on articles appearing in the Legal Briefs section of the *Journal of the American Association of Nurse Anesthetists*. The author would like to thank Betsy L. Wolf for her assistance with the material on negligence per se, which appeared in the *Journal of the American Association of Nurse Anesthetists*.

Nurse anesthesia is a legally recognized specialty of the nursing profession, defined by licensing statutes with a great body of law and decisions arising out of litigation in the courts. It is important for any health care professional to have an understanding of the legal system because the system has a profound effect on the way all professions are practiced. Unfortunately, it is especially important that nurse anesthetists understand the legal system because many of the challenges to nurse anesthesia practice have been based on misinformation concerning the legal status of nurse anesthetists. Consequently, an understanding of the legal system and the nurse anesthetist's relation to it is crucial.

The legal system affects the scope and method of nurse anesthesia practice. Practice is directly regulated by state licensing statutes and boards of nursing. Within limits set by federal and state constitutions (concerning such matters as equal protection and due process of law), states may permit or prohibit virtually any aspect of professional practice. As we will see, state legislatures and the legal system as a whole have deferred to the health care community to permit the health care system to develop in ways the community believed best.

In addition to direct regulation, the legal system indirectly governs practice through decisions arising out of malpractice litigation. Nurse anesthesia is a profession. The hallmark of a profession is its ability to set its own standard of practice. The courts learn of the standards of practice through expert testimony. Experts may disagree, however, and the courts may have to choose between conflicting testimony. Consequently, the courts play a major role in the development of the standards of practice.

THE GOALS OF THE LEGAL SYSTEM

The U.S. legal system was largely inherited from Great Britain. In making decisions, the judicial system has taken as its goals: fairness, consistency, predictability, and the effectuation of public policy. While the system may make unpopular decisions, it must appear to be fair in its process. It must be predictable as well. Those who are governed by the system must be able to understand what the system expects and how the system will operate. The system must also be consistent. It would be unfair to award damages for negligent operation of a vehicle in one case and not award damage for the same negligent act in another. A system that lacks consistency is neither predictable nor fair.

An additional goal of the legal system is to encourage actions that benefit society as a whole and to discourage actions that harm society. Consequently, the legal system inherited from England had at its heart that all members of society must act as reasonable people would act and when they do not, they are responsible for any damage they cause.

While individual court decisions may be difficult to justify, these decisions must be judged by whether they carry out the goals of fairness, consistency, predictability, and effectuation of policy. Sometimes, to carry out its ultimate goals, the legal system may produce decisions that seem incorrect. Truly difficult decisions arise when the courts find fundamental principles to be in conflict. Sometimes the system simply yields incorrect decisions, as does any human system.

STATE VERSUS FEDERAL COURTS

The U.S. legal system is divided into two separate and largely independent systems—a legal system belonging to the federal government and legal systems belonging to each of the 50 states and the District of Columbia. While there is some overlap in jurisdiction, the federal and state governments have their own laws, traditions, judges, courtrooms, rules, and body of law. Certain areas have been reserved exclusively for the federal system, including matters affecting interstate commerce. Over the years, the level of impact that legislation must have on interstate commerce to justify federal regulation has been more and more liberally interpreted so that today the federal government has numerous programs affecting the health, safety, and welfare of citizens of the United States that the courts have held are proper because of their impact on interstate commerce.

State Courts

Matters affecting the health, safety, and welfare of citizens generally come within the "police" powers of states and are reserved for state government. This includes not only the states but also cities, towns, and other local governments. As part of their police powers, states have primary jurisdiction in licensing the health care industry. Disputes between people arising out of agreements or contracts are decided by state laws as are claims by one person that he or she may have been damaged by the negligence or actions of another.

Federal Courts

Litigants have only limited rights to choose between federal and state courts. The jurisdiction of the federal courts is limited to actions brought under federal statutes, actions involving federal property, and actions between citizens of different states (diversity). The perception (which may or may not be accurate) is that plaintiffs get bigger awards in federal courts.

Lawsuits Arising Under Federal Legislation

Lawsuits based on federal statutes may be brought in federal courts, and if there are related state issues to be decided, the federal courts may decide them. Federal laws take precedence over state and local laws. If both the federal and state governments enact legislation in a particular area, the federal act prevails. Under the Doctrine of Preemption, once the federal government has enacted legislation in an area, state laws may no longer be enforced unless the federal government specifically permits states to enact legislation in the area. The Doctrine of Preemption ensures that the purpose of federal legislation will be carried out and not be affected by inconsistent state laws.

Sometimes Congress determines that state acts would promote and not interfere with federal policy. In such cases, Congress may permit states to adopt their own regulation. For example, in the field of antitrust law, the federal government has indicated that states may also adopt legislation prohibiting constraints of trade. Numerous states have adopted "baby antitrust statutes."

Federal Property

The second area of jurisdiction of the federal courts is that of disputes relating to federal property or to which the federal government is a party. In feudal England, a person could not have a dispute with the king. The king was immune from suit. Under the Doctrine of Sovereign Immunity, government cannot be sued by its citizens without its consent. Today, most citizens would be very unhappy if they were to suffer damage because of the negligence of a government worker and could not be compensated because of "sovereign immunity." The federal government permits lawsuits to be brought against it under most circumstances, but these lawsuits must be brought in federal courts.

Diversity

Finally, the federal government is committed to protecting interstate commerce. Because of the founding fathers' concern that state courts would give unfair advantage to citizens of their own states, the third area of federal court jurisdiction consists of situations in which a citizen of one state sues a citizen of another. Even though a matter may involve only a state issue, if the plaintiff is a resident of one state and the defendant is a resident of another, the lawsuit may be brought in the federal court if the matter involved in the controversy exceeds $50,000.

Until 1938 the federal courts applied their own common law doctrines in diversity cases. Outcomes of cases could be different depending on whether suit was brought in state or federal court. Since 1938, federal courts have applied state law to diversity cases as best they can. In diversity cases, federal courts are now obligated to decide legal issues as would the state court.

SOURCES OF LAW

Each of our three branches of government has its own effect on the legal system.

Legislature

The legislature passes laws. Its legislative powers are limited only by constitutional restrictions and the political control of the voting public. Statutes become effective after signature by the executive or by legislative action if vetoed by the executive. Statutes are forward looking; they affect actions taking place after their effective date. When legislation is passed, courts interpret it by trying to determine what the legislature intended. The courts must interpret existing law. Court decisions state what the law is and, theoretically, always has been; not what the law will be. Only the legislature has the authority to change the law. Only the legislature can say that after a specific date the law will be something else. The legislature can reverse decisions made by the judiciary. The legislature is limited by constitutional restrictions such as limitations on enacting legislation that makes something that has already happened a crime or taking property or imposing punishment without following "due process" (a process designed to allow persons to present their side of a dispute and have a fair hearing). The judiciary interprets the constitution. Judicial interpretations of the constitution cannot be overruled by the legislature.

Courts

Courts do not make law the way the legislature does, stating that after a certain date the law will be changed. Rather, the courts interpret existing laws. Court decisions are applicable to actions that occur both before and after their decisions. A court interpretation of a statute affects all actions subject to the statute, whether the action occurred before or after the decision.

Even though courts interpret what the law always was, the fact is that society changes, and its institutions change. Consequently, statutes and the constitution are constantly reexamined and reinterpreted by the courts in the light of modern day events and situations. For example, when the antitrust laws were passed in 1890, they were intended to prevent the excesses of the robber barons of the late 19th century who manipulated prices of oil, steel, and other products. Probably very few people in 1890 could have imaged that the antitrust laws would ever be applicable to services, especially professional services. It was not until 1942, 52 years after the passage of the original legislation, that the Supreme Court held that the antitrust laws applied (and had always applied) to restraints of trade in the health care field. Today, the antitrust laws are often applied to matters involving the health care professions.

Common Law

In some countries, the judicial system is entirely based on the interpretation of statutes. In feudal times in England, the courts were called on to decide disputes between persons when there were no statutes or legislation. The courts decided these matters using the goals of the legal system: consistency, fairness, predictability, and effectuation of policy. These decisions eventually resulted in a large body of "common law," legal principles and precedents the courts used to make individual decisions in areas not governed by statute. The English system, including the tradition of common law dating back to feudal times, forms the basis of law in every state of the United States except Louisiana. At the time of its acquisition by the United States, Louisiana had a thriving commercial port with important commercial transactions. Fairness and consistency required that Louisiana continue its system based on the continental system of statutory interpretation rather than common law.

In feudal times, the king rode from location to location resolving disputes between his subjects. These disputes often involved the ownership and use of land. It was important to the feudal economy that there be quick and consistent resolution of these disputes; land represented wealth and capital. If land was properly used, the kingdom would prosper, but if land was unused, the kingdom would suffer. Determination of disputes between individual citizens was an important function for the king. Over time the process of dispute resolution became institutionalized. The king's assistants who became better at dispute resolution than others became judges. The tradition (largely oral) of these judges became the basis of common law. Eventually, persons seeking justice in the king's legal system were allowed to confer with other persons with experience in the system. Thus, the profession of law developed.

Executive Branch

The executive branch enforces laws made by the legislature and interpreted by the courts. Before the American Revolution, the executive was the monarch. Now the executive is the president or the governor.

A part of the executive branch of government is the attorney general, who serves as the lawyer for the government. The attorney general serves two functions: first, as the government's lawyer bringing lawsuits and representing the country or the state in court. Second, the attorney general interprets the law for various branches of the government. Interpretations of the law by the attorney general do not have the force of law. They are important, however, because they tell you how the attorney general's client, the government, will act.

An example of an attorney general interpretation important to nurse anesthetists is the opinion of the California attorney general regarding whether nurse anesthetists could administer regional anesthetics. The attorney general is often asked to give opinions when there is very little authority or precedent to go on. In 1972, the attorney general of California was asked if it was legal for nurse anesthetists to give regional anesthetics. The attorney general searched the case law and found an isolated statement by the California Supreme Court in the case of *Magit v. State of California* (57 Cal. 2d 74, 1961). In *Magit*, three foreign anesthesiologists were administering anesthesia without medical licenses. The chief anesthesiologist who employed them was prosecuted for aiding and abetting the unauthorized practice of medicine. His defense was based on the case of *Chalmers-Francis v. Nelson* (6 Cal. 2d 402, 1936), one of the fundamental cases upholding nurse anesthetist practice. In particular, the chief anesthesiologist claimed that since California courts permitted Dagmar Nelson, who was a nurse, not a physician, to administer anesthesia, California should permit the nonlicensed anesthesiologists to provide anesthesia as well. The California Supreme Court noted the special position that nurses have to the health care system, and pointed out that the *Dagmar Nelson* case had been decided at a time when California did not have a Nurse Practice Act. A Nurse Practice Act had since been enacted. Therefore, as precedent, the *Dagmar Nelson* case was limited to its facts—a nurse anesthetist administering a general anesthetic was not illegally practicing medicine.

From the simple statement in *Magit* that the *Dagmar Nelson* case was limited to its facts—a nurse anesthetist administering a general anesthetic was not illegally practicing medicine—the California Attorney General developed a theory that under California law nurse anesthetists could only administer general anesthesia and could not administer regional anesthetics. While the ruling was patently absurd, nurse anesthetists in California were uneasy that the decision would be enforced by the board of nursing. Very few nurse anesthetists continued to administer regional anesthesia, although most believed that the attorney general's decision was incorrect. In 1976, the California Association of Nurse Anesthetists went back to the attorney general and asked for a reversal of his prior decision. The attorney general agreed that the *Magit* case was not authority for his ruling. Unfortunately, the attorney general now found a new problem. The legislature had passed a bill to specifically give nurse anesthetists the ability to administer regional anesthetics, but the bill had been vetoed by the governor. The attorney general decided that the California legislature must have believed that nurse anesthetists required additional statutory authority to give regional anesthetics or the legislature would not have passed the bill. Since the bill had been vetoed, nurse anesthetists did not receive the additional authority and must still lack the power to administer regional anesthetics. In fact, the California governor had vetoed the bill because he thought it was unnecessary.

The attorney general's ruling stood for 8 more years until, in 1984, he finally issued an opinion that there was no prohibition against nurse anesthetists giving regional anesthesia. As can be seen, the attorney general rendered two incorrect decisions that were not subject to review or correction. The decisions were troublesome because they were binding on administrative agencies. Although they did not have the force of law, nurse anesthesia practice was harmed in California in the years the ruling stood.

Administrative Agencies

A special form of executive function is the administrative agency. The administrative agency is a part of the executive branch of government, but it combines elements of all three branches of government. An administrative agency such as the Interstate Commerce Commission (ICC) has a legislative function in that it adopts regulations that have the force of law, an executive function in that trucking firms that violate the regulations are prosecuted by the ICC, and a judicial function in that the agency hears the charges and determines guilt or innocence. Regulations issued by an administrative agency must be consistent with enabling acts and other legislation. While an agency may clarify unclear or ambiguous terms, it cannot reverse the clear language of legislation. Licensing agencies such as boards of nursing, boards of medicine, and boards of pharmacy are administrative agencies and combine functions of each of the branches of government in their own functions. The area of licensing is an interesting example of the power of the legislature.

DEFERENCE TO THE HEALTH CARE PROFESSION

The legal system defers to the health care system. Regulation of health care differs significantly from regulation of other industries, such as banking. Bank regulation clearly and specifically sets forth powers, duties, and procedures. However, in medical and nursing regulation, there is a large degree of deference to the health care community by both legislatures and courts.

This deference is expressed in the California Nursing Act (Cal. Business and Professions Code, Chapter 6):

> In amending this Section at the 1973–74 session, the legislature recognizes that nursing is a dynamic field, the practice of which is continually evolving to include more sophisticated patient care activities. It is the intent of the legislature in amending this section at the 1973–74 session to provide clear legal authority for functions and procedures which have common acceptance and usage (Cal. Business and Professions Code 2725).

Law school students learn very early that during a trial, "law" is determined by the judge, whereas "facts" are determined by the jury, if there is one, or by the judge if there is not. Evidence is offered by the parties to help determine the facts. In some cases involving the health care field, judges appear to be relying on expert testimony for much more than mere facts. For example, in *Chalmers-Francis v. Nelson* (6 Cal. 2d 402, 1936):

> There was much testimony as to the recognized practice of permitting nurses to administer anesthetics and hypodermics. One of the plaintiff's witnesses testified to what seems to be the established and uniformly accepted practice and procedure followed by surgeons and nurses, and that is that it [nurse anesthesia practice] is not diagnosing nor prescribing by the nurses within the meaning of the Medical Practice Act (6 Cal. 2d 404).

Note that the Court relies on expert factual testimony to determine the meaning of the California Medical Practice Act.

In the case of *Bentley v. Langley* (249 S.E. 2d 481, N.C. 1978), a deposition was introduced in which an anesthesiologist was permitted to testify that a doctor who supervised a nurse anesthetist was responsible for the anesthesia services administered. Legal responsibility is a question of law, not a question of fact. Again, it is very unusual for a court to accept expert testimony from an anesthesiologist as to matters of law the court should be deciding. The parties objected to the affidavit and to the fact that the case did not discuss whether this portion of the anesthesiologist's testimony could be relied on.

In the area of health care as in very few other areas, licensing statutes describe rather than define practice. Statutes defining the powers and functions of banks are strictly enforced. If a bank attempts to carry out a power that is not permitted by its statute, the bank will be prohibited and even penalized for the unauthorized act. In the area of health care, state statutes tend to be interpreted in a manner as to permit practices the health care community believes are safe, even if the legislature has not considered them.

This special position the courts give to health care can sometimes be taken advantage of. In the case of *Sermchief v. Gonzales* (660 S.W. 2d 683, Missouri 1983), the Missouri legislature had amended the Missouri statute on nursing so as to permit advanced practice nurses to give routine examinations and dispense medications within a medical protocol without being under the direct supervision of a physician. The Missouri Medical Board, known as the Board of Registration for the Healing Arts, threatened criminal prosecution of nurses carrying out these activities, claiming that the nurses were engaged in the illegal practice of medicine. A group of nurses sought protection against the Board of Registration for the Healing Arts. Both the nurses and physicians presented the case in such a manner as to ask the court to draw what the court referred to as "that thin and elusive line that separates the practice of medicine and the practice of professional nursing in modern day delivery of health services." Instead, the court pointed out that what the nurses were doing was, in fact, exactly what the legislature intended them to do. Because licensing is the prerogative of the legislature, the fact that the legislature had authorized nurses to do something that physicians thought might have been the practice of medicine was irrelevant. If the legislature said that nurses could do it, it was the practice of nursing and the physicians had no right to interfere with their practice of it.

In the context of the legal system it is strange that one regulated group would even dream of challenging the authorization of another group to do something. It is an indication of the deference that the legal system has given to the health care professions that the physicians were tempted to do so.

THE ROLE OF THE LEGAL PROFESSION

Who does the lawyer represent? The case of *Trementozzi vs. Safety Insurance Co.* (Massachusetts Suffolk Superior Court Civil Action No. 90-1017B, June 26, 1991) stated that the duty of a lawyer provided by an insurance company to represent an insured is to represent the insured and not the insurance company even though the insurance company may pay the bills. Both the lawyer and the insurance company are obligated to act in the best interests of the insured.

Kerry Trementozzi was one of four passengers in a car driven by Paul Whooten involved in an accident. As a result of the accident, Kerry became a quadriplegic. Paul Whooten's insurance company appointed a lawyer to defend him. Kerry Trementozzi's lawyer demanded the policy limit of $10,000 for bodily injury per person and that the insurance company pay Trementozzi's medical bills under the policy's personal injury protection portion. When the insurance company failed to pay the demand, Kerry Trementozzi's lawyer claimed that the insurance company's refusal to settle violated Massachusetts' consumer protection statutes.

The insurance company's claims adjuster conferred with the lawyer the company had appointed to represent Whooten. However, Whooten and the insurance company had totally different exposures. The insurance company's exposure was limited by its policy limits, but Whooten's liability was unlimited; he was liable for whatever damages a jury might award. Instead of trying to reach a settlement with Trementozzi, the insurance company, under the guidance of the lawyer it appointed to represent Whooten, settled with the other passengers, paying the policy limit and ending its liability. Whooten claimed that the lawyer should have tried to enter into a settlement with the most injured passengers, which would have given Trementozzi most of the recovery because she had been the most injured. If they would have settled with Trementozzi, even if they left the smaller claims unresolved, Whooten would have been better off.

Lawyers are not supposed to represent clients with different interests at the same time. The Model Code of Professional Responsibility (1980) prepared by the American Bar Association has been adopted by many states. It provides that

> The professional judgment of a lawyer should be exercised within the bounds of the law,

> solely for the benefit of his client and free of compromising influences and loyalties. Neither his personal interests, the interests of other clients, nor the desires of third persons should be permitted to dilute his loyalty to his client. . . . Maintaining the independence of professional judgment required of a lawyer precludes his acceptance or continuation of employment that will adversely affect his judgment on behalf of or dilute his loyalty to a client. This problem arises whenever a lawyer is asked to represent two or more clients who may have differing interests, whether such interests be conflicting, inconsistent, diverse or otherwise discordant (Model Code of Professional Responsibility EC5–14).

Nurse anesthetists must be aware of and involved in their legal defense. Even knowledgeable health care defense attorneys may not be familiar with the capabilities of nurse anesthetists. Second, the insurance companies may find themselves with multiple defendants. Nurse anesthetists must be vigilant that their interests are being protected. Nurse anesthetists should know that they are entitled to a defense that protects their own best interests.

The attorney/client privilege protects one of the oldest confidential relationships in society. It grows out of the need of attorneys and their clients to have open, full, and frank discussions. What happens to this privilege when the attorney is representing conflicting clients? The attorney/client privilege only protects documents and disclosures that are not disclosed to third parties. If someone discloses information to persons with whom there is no privilege, then the information is not confidential and it is no longer privileged even if disclosed to his or her attorney.

NATURE OF THE COURTS

Courts are either trial courts or appellate courts. *Trial courts* are where cases are brought and facts are presented. The trial court makes determinations of the facts of the case as well as the applicable law. In certain circumstances, the trier of facts is not a court but a jury. The Seventh Amendment to the Constitution preserves the right of a citizen to trial by jury. Over the years, the Seventh Amendment has been interpreted to mean that in those matters in which a trial by jury was provided when the Bill of Rights was adopted, citizens still have rights to trial by jury. In other cases, litigants can choose trial by jury, but it is not guaranteed.

For example, historically, trial courts were divided into two types: courts of law and courts of equity. Courts of law decided disputes under existing laws, whereas courts of equity granted special kinds of relief such as injunctions (a court order that someone must or must not do something). A court of equity may also correct documents and otherwise give equity. Courts of equity did not have juries. Therefore, if you believed that someone was about to publish an article defaming your character, you might bring suit and seek an injunction prohibiting the publication of the article. At the hearing for the injunction, you would not be entitled to a jury because, historically, injunctions were granted by courts of equity in which juries were not available. If the court refused to grant the injunction, the article may be published and you might sue for damages. You will be entitled to a jury trial in your suit for damages because, historically, trials for damages were heard by courts of law in which there were juries.

Conflicts Among Courts

Trial courts are required to make decisions quickly, in the heat of litigation. Mistakes frequently occur. In both federal and state systems, decisions of trial courts can be appealed to appellate courts. The appeals process provides time for consideration and research. In some states there may only be one appellate court, which would be the highest court in the state. In other states, in which the volume of litigation is much larger, there may be a series of appellate courts. In the federal system, decisions of the trial or district courts are appealed to a U.S. court of appeals for the region in which the state is located. Decisions of the court of appeals may be appealed to the Supreme Court of the United States although in some circumstances cases may be appealed directly from the trial court to the Supreme Court. (There are some matters for which the Supreme Court may serve as the trial court but these are so unlikely to occur that their main value is for trick questions in trivia contests.) The Supreme Court has the right to set its own agenda. That is, many more cases are appealed to the Supreme Court than the Supreme Court can hear. Consequently, the Supreme Court is given the right to decide which cases it will hear.

In general, decisions by the trial court as to facts either made by the judge or jury are accepted because the judge or jury has had the opportunity to see the witnesses and to determine their credibility. Testimony that is reproduced in written form does not give a reader the chance to make observations: Did the witness look people in the eye, squirm, appear uneasy, or otherwise indicate that the testimony was unreliable? Consequently, the appellate courts often defer to the fact finding of lower courts unless it is clear from the record that the finder of fact was erroneous or prejudiced.

In matters of law, appellate courts are free to review any decision made by a trial court and to come to their own conclusion. The decisions of the appellate court are binding on all courts within its jurisdiction. Consequently, many of the decisions of the appellate courts are collected and published so that people will have a chance to see what the law is as it has been adopted by the court.

Each state is free not only to adopt legislation that differs from that of other states but also to have its courts make their own interpretation of nonstatutory common law. While states may be interested in what other state legislatures and courts may have done in addressing common problems, they are not obligated to follow their lead. Obviously, because of common backgrounds and restraints, there is more uniformity than diversity among states, but diversity does exist.

Civil/Criminal Matters

The judicial system distinguishes between civil and criminal matters. A *civil matter* is a dispute between two parties. *Criminal matters* are proceedings in which criminal statutes have been violated. Legislatures enact criminal penalties consisting of jail or monetary punishments for violation of the basic fundamentals of societal living (murder, robbery, etc.). Another common use of criminal punishment is to facilitate the enforcement of regulatory matters. In order to give administrative agencies authority, the legislature provides that violation of regulatory acts or rules are criminal and can be punished by monetary penalties or incarceration. For example, in *Chalmers-Francis v. Nelson*, one of the fundamental cases upholding nurse anesthetist practice, Dagmar Nelson was prosecuted under a criminal statute for illegally practicing medicine.

In a civil case, the courts are more concerned with compensating people for damages they have suffered because of the improper actions of the other than with punishment. It is difficult to provide absolute distinctions between criminal and civil matters, however, because legislatures have recognized that private litigation may also play an important role in public policy. To encourage private litigation, some statutes provide that litigants are entitled to multiple damages. If the behavior of the defendant is reprehensible or careless, the courts sometimes impose punitive damages to discourage the defendant. In the antitrust area, Congress recognized that the attorney general did not have the budget to bring every possible antitrust suit. To encourage private parties to bring antitrust actions, Congress provided that private litigants could recover not only their damages but three times their damages and receive attorneys' fees as well.

Civil Litigation

The two basic forms of civil litigation are disputes over contracts and claims for negligent or intentional infliction of injury, known as *torts*. The law of contracts allows private parties to create their own legal framework governing their behavior. When parties enter into a contract, both parties are expected to perform their obligations. If one of the parties fails to perform that obligation the court will award damages based on the value of the performance the injured party did not receive. Tort liability, on the other hand, recognizes that each of us has a duty to act in a reasonable manner and that where our failure to act in a reasonable manner hurts or damages someone, and the damage was reasonably foreseeable, the court will award a monetary payment intended to equal the damages caused.

An illustration of the difference between contracts and torts can be seen in the case of *Hawkins v. McGee* (84 NH 114, 146 A. 641 New Hampshire, 1929), where a physician told a patient that the physician would transplant skin to replace damaged skin on the palm of the hand. The physician promised that he would make the hand perfect. In fact, the physician transplanted skin from a hairy part of the body to the palm with the result that the plaintiff had a hairy palm. The patient sued. In this classic case, which many law schools use to illustrate the difference between torts and contracts, the question was not whether the physician was negligent for using skin from a hairy part of the body but only whether the physician had promised to give the patient a perfect hand and had carried out his contract. The court held that the physician had not made good on his promise and awarded damages. Damages were not based on the damage the physician had caused—the tort standard—but on the difference between a hand with hair on the palm and one that was perfect (the damage resulting from the physician's breach of contract).

TORT LIABILITY

Standard of Care

The law of contracts governs many things concerning nurse anesthetists, including their employment contracts, their relationships with hospitals and physicians, purchases of drugs and equipment, and numerous other matters. Tort liability affects nurse anesthetists as it affects any member of society. When engaged in activities in which it can reasonably be foreseen that our failure to act in a reasonable manner will result in harm, each of us owes a duty of care to others to act the way a reasonable person would act. For example, careless operation of an automobile can kill or severely damage other people. We are expected to drive our automobiles as reasonably prudent men and women would drive their vehicles.

Because the courts do not understand what nurse anesthetists do, they designate nurse anesthesia as a profession. In the professional area, the expectation of the standard of care becomes slightly more complicated. The professional must render care with the same degree of skill and care as a reasonable member of that profession in similar circumstances would render. A nurse anesthetist has expertise and education that ordinary members of society do not have. A nurse anesthetist has an obligation to render care to patients that is not merely the same care a reasonably prudent member of society would render but which other nurse anesthetists would render. This gives members of the profession the ability to determine the quality of care to be rendered by the profession. When a patient questions whether the nurse anesthetist has rendered appropriate care, the court hears expert testimony as to what that standard is.

Normally, only members of the profession are competent to testify as to the standard of care for their profession. In the area of anesthesia, the courts have not distinguished between the type of care rendered by nurse anesthetists and the type of care rendered by anesthesiologists. Consequently, there are cases when courts have permitted anesthesiologists to testify as to the standard of care to be followed by nurse anesthetists and cases where nurse anesthetists have been allowed to testify as to the standard of care of anesthesiologists. In some health care areas, the quality of health care may vary from community to community and area to area. In those cases, practitioners are only held to the standard of care within their community. In specialty areas, such as anesthesia, there is a nationwide standard of care that does not vary from community to community.

Some people erroneously assume or question whether there is a dual standard of care in the anesthesia field, one for anesthesiologists and one for nurse anesthetists. In fact, because of the nature of anesthesia and the fact that attention and proper monitoring of patients is the overwhelming consideration in the practice of anesthesia, there is a single standard of care. The single standard of care is reflected not only in the "reality of practice" but also in the decided cases that discuss the standard of care.

Standard of care is closely related to the quality of care. A profession that renders care at a lower standard than another will necessarily have a different quality of care. In the anesthesia field there is a rather uniform quality of care between nurse anesthetists and anesthesiologists, and that is further evidence that the "standard of care" is the same.

The standard of care for nurses is "to apply that degree of skill and learning in treating and nursing a patient which is customarily applied in treating or caring for the sick or wounded who are suffering in the same community." The case of *Whitney v. Day* (100 Michigan App. 707 1980) is interesting because it was claimed that nurses were not entitled to a shortened statute of limitations available for professionals sued for malpractice. The charge was made that nurses had to be examined on the same negligence standard as the general population. In *Whitney v. Day,* the court specifically discusses the profession of nurse anesthetists. The court said

> . . . nurse anesthetists are licensed as nurses and then they are certified after an 18 month period of study [this has, of course, been increased] in their specialty. Thus, they are professionals who have expertise in an area which is akin to the practice of medicine. Because a nurse anesthetist possesses responsibilities greater than those possessed by an ordinary nurse, and because those responsibilities lie in an area of expertise in which some physicians receive full residency training, we conclude that it was not error for the trial court to set forth a standard which . . . [incorporates the malpractice standard]. (Page 711)

The court pointed out that the Michigan statute had been amended so that malpractice limitations were made specifically effective to all nurses.

Since nurse anesthetists have been recognized as a separate professional group that establishes its own standard of care, it is understandable that the uninformed would assume that this standard of care would be different than that of an anesthesiologist. For example, in another Michigan case, *Theophelis v. Lansing General Hospital* (366 N.W. 2d 249, 1985), there had been a suit against a hospital where both the nurse anesthetists and the anesthesiologist had been released from liability prior to trial. In what really amounted to legal maneuvering in the absence of any factual information, the hospital argued that a release of the nurse anesthetist and the anesthesiologist implied that the hospital was innocent as well. The court, attempting to justify the trial court's determination to let trial proceed against the hospital, wrote

> . . . we note for example that it would have been possible for the jury to determine that Nurse Palmer, given her limited training, was not negligent in failing to use a precordial stethoscope but that the hospital was negligent in not requiring the use of one. (Page 252)

This is sheer speculation on the part of the court and not in any way a determination that there is a different standard of care for nurse anesthetists. It does, however, illustrate what can happen when laypersons (who unfortunately include judges) are allowed to speculate, in the absence of information, about the nature of nurse anesthetists and nurse anesthesia.

More typical is the case of *Webb v. Jorns* (473 S.W. 2d 328 Texas, 1971). In this case involving a cardiac arrest during the course of administering the anesthetic preparatory for an operation, the court turned its attention to whether the nurse anesthetist had been negligent; whether the patient had received an overdose of halothane. The expert testimony that was introduced was that of a physician. The testimony did not concern what a nurse anesthetist would have done or would not have done under the circumstances but rather whether in the physician's judgment there had been an overdose of halothane. The physician had testified that a mixture in excess of 1.5 percent halothane would have been an overdose, but the facts supported the position of the nurse anesthetist that the mixture had never exceeded 1.5 percent. Thus, the standard by which negligence was judged was a general standard based on what happens in the anesthesia area and not one that focused on whether nurse anesthetists follow different standards than anesthesiologists.

In *Aubert v. Charity Hospital of Louisiana* (363 So. 2d 1223 Louisiana, 1978), anesthesia was administered by a first-year resident in anesthesiology and a student nurse anesthetist. The chief of anesthesiology at another local hospital testified that there had been a negligent intubation. There was no discussion as to whether the nurse anesthetists had a different standard of care in intubating a patient than did anesthesiologists. There is a right way to intubate a patient, and the failure to properly intubate, whether by nurse anesthetists or anesthesiologists, is negligence.

A Louisiana statute requires that health care professionals, in a recognized field of specialty, render professional services using a degree of skill ordinarily employed under similar circumstances by the members of that specialty. In another Louisiana case, *Mohr v. Jenkins* (393 So.2d 245 Louisiana, 1981), the question was whether Valium had been injected at too quick a rate. The nurse anesthetist had not used a watch to time the injection. The court pointed out that expert testimony revealed that the use of a watch was not the standard of practice and that "specialists do not follow manufacturers' inserts concerning the administration of Valium or any other medicines strictly or literally." Again, the court is referring to a standard of care in the anesthesia field, rather than a standard of care applicable solely to nurse anesthetists.

In *Parks v. Perry* (68 NC App. 202 No. Carolina, 1984), the question was whether numbness and weakness in a patient's hand resulted from the negligent administration of an anesthetic. There was no direct testimony that the acts of the nurse anesthetist were negligent. The trial court had submitted the case to the jury under the doctrine of *res ipsa loquitur* based on expert testimony that the damage would not have occurred in the absence of negligent administration of an anesthetic. Again, the testimony that was admitted did not refer to the standard of care by nurse anesthetists and anesthesiologists but to what was common in the anesthesia field. In fact, the expert testimony was given by a physician and not by another nurse anesthetist.

In the case of *Yoos v. Jewish Hospital of St. Louis* (645 S.W. 2d 177 Missouri, 1982), the question, on appeal, was whether the expert's testimony was sufficient to establish that damage occurred because of negligence. The defendant claimed that the expert testimony was conflicting because the medical expert had testified that it was his "feeling" that the accident occurred, at least in part, because of technical error. On the other hand, the expert had previously written a book in which he had written "failure due to technical errors cannot be wholly excluded even in the most skilled hands." Nevertheless, the court accepted the expert's "feeling" as an expression of expert opinion. The court upheld the jury verdict based on the expert's "feeling" that the accident should not have occurred. The expert could not definitively point to a particular action that violated the standard of care. The courts do not look at separate standards of care; they are concerned with what should and should not occur in the field of anesthesia.

Why is there only one standard of care in the anesthesia field? Because there is only one quality of care. Studies have shown that anesthesia incidents tend to occur because of human error or failure, not because of lack of education. Care and attentiveness are not attributes that depend on whether the practitioner is a nurse or a physician. Therefore, the standard of care in anesthesia is to be as careful and attentive as the human mind will permit.

The issue of the standard of care is a factual matter because it depends on the testimony of expert witnesses. What the expert testifies to and what the jury believes can vary from case to case. Disquieting though it may be, as a practical matter it must be recognized that the standard of professional care is determined on an individual basis for each case. Thus, to discuss whether something is or is not required by the standard of care is really to make a prediction as to what experts will testify to and what will be believed by both jury and judge at a malpractice trial.

This point is illustrated by the case of *Washington v. Washington Hospital Center, et al.* (579 A.2d 177, District of Columbia Court of Appeals, 1990, herein referred to as the *Washington* case). Expert testimony as to what constitutes the standard of care cannot be based on mere speculation or conjecture but should have an adequate factual basis. "While absolute certainty is not required, opinion evidence that is conjectural or speculative is not permitted" (*Washington v. Washington Hospital Center* quoting from *Sponaugle v. Pre-term, Inc.*, 411 A.2d 366, District of Columbia, 1980). The testimony must show what the standard is as practiced by the profession. What a single practitioner would do does not establish the standard of care. Similarly, the testimony should not be what the expert would have done under similar circumstances but what members of the profession would do.

In the *Washington* case, the plaintiff was a healthy 36-year-old woman who underwent elective surgery at the Washington Hospital Center on November 7, 1987. The endotracheal tube was inserted into the esophagus rather than the trachea. It was not noticed until it was too late and the plaintiff suffered catastrophic brain injury. The nurse anesthetist and anesthesiologist settled and the case proceeded only against the hospital. It was claimed that the hospital was negligent in failing to provide an end-tidal CO_2 monitor which would have allowed early detection of insufficient oxygen, arguably in time to prevent the brain injury. After a jury verdict in favor of the plaintiff, the hospital asked the trial court to rule that the expert testimony offered was insufficient and that judgment should have been entered in the hospital's favor, notwithstanding the jury verdict. The trial court refused and the hospital appealed the decision to the District of Columbia Court of Appeals.

The plaintiff's expert had testified that the hospital deviated from the standard of care by failing to supply a CO_2 monitoring device. Among other things, the hospital claimed that the plaintiff's expert lacked an adequate factual basis for his testimony. The court noted that the standard of care was

> the course of action that a reasonably prudent [professional] with the defendant's specialty would have taken under the same or similar circumstances. . . . Thus the question for decision is whether the evidence as a whole and reasonable inferences therefrom, would allow a reasonable juror to find that a reasonably prudent tertiary care hospital . . . at the time of [plaintiff's] injury in November 1987 and according to national standards, would have supplied a carbon dioxide monitor to a patient undergoing general anesthesia for elective surgery.

The plaintiff's expert had testified that the standard of care in November 1987 required a hospital to provide an end-tidal CO_2 monitor. The hospital claimed that the plaintiff's expert based his opinion on inadequate facts. Even though the expert gave no testimony on the number of hospitals having end-tidal CO_2 monitors in place in 1987 and never referred to any written standards or authority as the basis of his opinion, the court concluded that his opinion, combined with other evidence concerning the standard of care, was sufficient to create an issue for the jury.

The plaintiff's expert had based his testimony on his practice at the Los Angeles County Hospital and from "What I have read where [the monitors were] available in other hospitals." The expert's testimony was also based on standards for basic intraoperative monitoring approved by the American Society of Anesthesiologists (ASA) House of Delegates on October 21, 1986, which encouraged the use of monitors. The expert also mentioned an article entitled "Standards for Patient Monitoring During Anesthesia at Harvard Medical School," published in August 1986 in the *Journal of the American Medical Association.*

The hospital argued that these statements were indications that end-tidal CO_2 monitors were not the standard of care. The ASA policy was only a recommendation, and the Harvard standards referred to CO_2 monitors as an "emerging" standard. The court indicated nonetheless that the expert's testimony should be allowed to stand based on other testimony introduced at trial. The question is what a reasonably prudent hospital would do and "Hence, care and foresight exceeding the minimum required by law or mandatory professional regulation may be necessary to meet that standard." Thus, the fact that neither the ASA nor Harvard Medical School recognized CO_2 monitors as a standard of care was irrelevant if a reasonably prudent hospital would have provided them.

Other testimony introduced in the *Washington* case included a 1986 alumni newsletter from the Department of Anesthesia at the University of Pennsylvania that indicated CO_2 monitors were then in use at that institution's hospital and the defendant's expert testified that not only had his hospital installed CO_2 monitors by early 1986, but by 1987 many hospitals were in the process of converting to CO_2 monitors.

Finally, the court was clearly impressed by evidence from the defendant hospital's own chairman of anesthesiology. In December 1986, or January 1987, the chairman had submitted a requisition to the hospital to acquire end-tidal CO_2 units stating that if the monitors were not provided the hospital would "fail to meet the national standard of care." If the request had gone through, the monitors would have been fully operational in July 1987, 4 months before the unfortunate incident that gave rise to the case. The court concluded that the jury had sufficient evidence from which it could determine that the standard of care required an end-tidal CO_2 monitor.

It is interesting to note the limited role the court permitted a professional organization to play in setting standards of care. While the organization's determinations are evidence of the standard, what both the jury and the court really want to know is not what the professional organization says but what is customarily followed by members of the profession.

The significant issue in the case was not whether CO_2 monitors were part of the standard of care, which the court clearly accepted as true, but only if having monitors was part of the standard of care in 1987 when the accident occurred. To someone not familiar with anesthesia, the principles underlying the *Washington* case seem straightforward. The proof that was offered in the *Washington* case to the judge and jury that CO_2 monitors were the standard of care seems pretty thin. The only real evidence was that the University of Pennsylvania hospitals, Los Angeles County Hospital, the hospital of the defendant's expert, and *some* Harvard hospitals had CO_2 monitors. Arrayed against the experts' opinion were contemporaneous writings and statements of professional organizations that end-tidal CO_2 monitors were not widely used in 1987 and were not part of the standard of care. The *Washington* case glosses over serious questions of accuracy and seems to stretch the facts to justify leaving the jury's verdict.

Even though the standard of care is set by practitioners, it must be found and applied by courts who are subject to pressures and their own emotional contexts. Standards set by professional organizations may be evidence of the standard of care, but they are not necessarily accepted as the standard of care. In addition, the courts reserve the right to determine that the level of care practiced by an entire profession may be inadequate, although this has been rare in the health care field.

Failure to Comply with Law or Regulation

There are two companion issues worth noting. First, the doctrine of negligence per se—the failure to follow a standard of care set forth in a statute—is evidence of negligence.

Central Anesthesia Associates, P.C., et al. v. Worthy, et al. (254 Ga. 728, 333 S.E.2d 829 1985) demonstrates the legal principle of *negligence per se:* the violation of a statute that creates a standard of conduct is sufficient evidence, by itself, to establish negligence. To apply, the person injured must be someone the statute was trying to protect. The principle of negligence per se is helpful to a plaintiff because the plaintiff does not have to offer expert testimony on the standard of care.

In the *Worthy* case, anesthesia was administered by a registered nurse enrolled as a student nurse anesthetist in a school operating at the hospital. The student nurse anesthetist was under the supervision of a physician assistant. During the tubal ligation procedure, Ms. Worthy suffered cardiac arrest, resulting in brain damage.

During the cardiac arrest, only the obstetrician gynecologist, the physician assistant, and the student nurse anesthetist were in the seventh floor operating room where the surgery was being performed. At the time, Georgia had a statute that required that a CRNA administer anesthesia "under the direction and responsibility of a duly licensed physician with training or experience in anesthesia."

The *Worthy* court held that the Georgia statute created a standard of conduct for those who are authorized to administer anesthesia and that the standard of conduct was created to protect patients from unreasonable risks associated with the administration of anesthesia. The court held that under the statute, the role of supervising a nurse administering anesthesia could not be delegated to a physician assistant. As a result, the court concluded that the defendants had violated the statute and they were, therefore, negligent per se.

The defendants argued that a Georgia Board of Nursing regulation provided that a registered professional nurse holding a temporary permit or a current license to practice nursing, enrolled as a student in a nurse anesthesia program, may administer anesthesia as long as the practice of anesthesia is confined to the educational requirements of the program and the student nurse anesthetist is under the direct supervision of an anesthesiologist or a CRNA. The Georgia Supreme Court stated that even if the regulation applied, the student nurse anesthetist still was improperly supervised because supervision by a physician assistant was not supervision by a physician or CRNA as required by the regulation. Consequently, the regulation had no bearing on the case. The Georgia court raised but did not answer whether the regulation was valid under the Georgia statute.

The requirement that the supervising physician have "training or experience in anesthesia" is unusual: state statutes requiring supervision only require that the supervisor be a physician. Whatever Georgia's statute means, it does not mean that a physician assistant can supervise student anesthetists.

What role do hospital rules play in establishing negligence? Courts are unwilling to expand the principal of negligence per se beyond its application to statutes and governmental regulations. The courts defer to the legislature's determination of what constitutes a standard of conduct as a matter of public policy. The courts do not recognize nongovernmental rules as rising to the level of public policy. For example, in *Williams v. St. Claire Medical Center* (657 S.W.2d 590 Ky. Ct. App. 1983), the issue presented to the court was whether a hospital owed a duty to its patients to enforce its policies and bylaws and if so, whether a violation of these policies and bylaws constituted negligence per se. The patient suffered permanent brain damage while being administered an anesthetic by an uncertified nurse anesthetist.

The hospital's policy required that anesthetics be administered by a CRNA or a qualified physician. In addition, CRNAs were required to be supervised by the chairperson of anesthesia services and be in communication with an anesthesiologist and surgeon or obstetrician, except in emergency procedures when an anesthesiologist was not available. At the time of the incident, the hospital, contrary to its own policies, did not have an anesthesiologist on staff and the nurse anesthetist had graduated from school 1 month prior to the incident, had not yet taken the examination for certification, and was not a CRNA.

The court held that when a patient consents to and authorizes an operation, he or she thereby accepts all the rules and regulations of the particular hospital at which the operation is performed. The court further held that while a patient must accept the hospital's particular rules and regulations, the patient should be able to rely on the hospital to follow its rules and regulations, ostensibly established for the patient's care. The plaintiff in this case argued that the hospital's violation of its own policies constituted negligence per se. The court, however, refused to extend this principle to the hospital's policies and allowed the policies to be admitted only as evidence of negligence.

In *Castillo v. US* (406 F. Supp. 585 N.M. 1975), a federal court rejected the argument that violations of a hospital manual governing psychiatric services constituted negligence per se. The manual required notification of patient's guardians and/or next of kin when the staff discovers that a patient is missing. The plaintiff sued the hospital for the staff's failure to notify her of her brother's departure from the hospital's psychiatric ward prior to his suicide. The plaintiff claimed that the violation of this policy was negligence per se and that the hospital, therefore, was liable for her brother's death.

The court noted that the principal of negligence per se did not apply. The court held that this principle only applied to cases in which a New Mexico state statute or municipal ordinance had been violated. The court did say that the regulations should be considered as a relevant factor in determining the extent of the duty owed to the patient and whether the duty was breached. The manual was only evidence of negligence.

While courts refuse to extend the principle of negligence per se to hospital regulations, the courts are willing to allow hospital regulations to be admitted as evidence of negligence.

SPECIFIC TOPICS

Vicarious Liability

As hospitals evolved in the later part of the 19th century, the courts were confronted with some unusual situations. Their approach to these situations gives us an opportunity to examine decision making in the legal system. One of the goals of the legal system is to effectuate public policy. Part of the public policy that is carried out by the courts in the area of tort liability is to discourage dangerous conduct. First, persons held liable should be able to adjust their conduct to avoid situations that cause damage. Second, persons liable should either be able to afford the damage or should be in a position to pass the risk of the damage on to other users of the products or services.

How do the courts address damage caused by nurses employed by hospitals but assisting independent contracting physicians? While nurses could be liable for their own negligence, this was little comfort to patients since the nurses were often not capable of paying for the damage their negligence might have caused. At the same time, the nurses were employees of hospitals that frequently were charitable institutions. Hospitals seldom made sufficient profit on the services to absorb the cost of negligent care. Much of a hospital's operating budget consisted of charitable contributions. Holding hospitals liable for the negligence of the nurses they employed really meant asking contributors to the hospital's charitable drives to pay patients for the damages incurred. Consequently, the courts developed the concept of "charitable immunity" whereby hospitals would not be liable for the negligence of their employees.

The Doctrine of Charitable Immunity can be traced back to 1876 and the Massachusetts case of *McDonald v. Massachusetts General* (*Hospital* 120 Mass. 432 1876). In *McDonald,* a patient claimed that he had been damaged by the actions of a doctor on the staff of Massachusetts General Hospital. The patient was receiving free care at the hospital and the physicians and surgeons were also providing free services. Moreover, the funds for Massachusetts General Hospital were derived primarily from grants and donations. Patients paid only according to their ability and not according to the services that they received. The Massachusetts court reasoned that the hospital was acting in a similar way to a government agency. Just as a government has sovereign immunity (meaning neither the king nor his government can be sued), the court held that a charity had *charitable* immunity. If the grants and donations the charity solicited from the public were used to pay malpractice claims, the court worried that the public would not support the hospital, and a very worthwhile activity would be denied the public. The result of this determination was apparently that patients themselves would bear the risk of negligence. However, the courts were not willing to agree that patients who were injured at charitable hospitals had *no* recourse.

One of the principles of negligent actions was the Doctrine of Respondeat Superior: let the master answer. When damage is caused by a servant (later an employee), the master (later an employer) should be held responsible for it. It was the employer who controlled the way things were done and was in the best position to see that the action giving rise to negligence was avoided or was done in a more careful manner. It was the employer who sold the product, set the price, and earned the profit. When respondeat superior was applied to hospitals, the idea of holding the hospital responsible was not appealing. Who served in the role of "master" with regard to the negligence that occurred in hospitals? The answer was the surgeon. It was the surgeon who attracted patients to a hospital, the surgeon who profited from the services of the hospital and its nursing employees, and the surgeon who had the apparent authority to be responsible to see that negligent actions were controlled and did not cause damage. Although the surgeon was not the employer in a strict sense, the surgeon stood in the same position as the employer for purposes of tort law.

In a number of cases, one of which is *Schloendorf v. Society of New York Hospital* (211 N.Y. 125, 105 N.E. 92 1914), the courts held that physicians who were on the hospital's staff were not employees of the hospital for purposes of liability. Similarly, nurses engaged in treating patients, even though paid by the hospital, were not acting for the hospital but as servants of the surgeon. From this developed doctrines known as "Captain of the Ship" (once the surgeon assumes control of the operating room, the surgeon is responsible for any negligence that occurs) and the "Borrowed Servant" rule (which holds that a doctor may be held liable for the negligence of a hospital employee who is subject to the doctor's control).

Consideration had to be given to the fact that hospitals had administrative employees who were not engaged in patient care. Nurses did not spend all of their time on patient care; time was also spent on administrative matters. Despite the doctrines of "Captain of the Ship" and "Borrowed Servant," there were some activities of hospital employees for which only hospitals should be liable. In some states, persons damaged by "administrative" acts of hospital employees were unable to recover. In other states, the courts attempted to deal with this problem by developing exceptions to Charitable Immunity and "Captain of the Ship." In those states, when a nurse negligently injured someone while engaged in "administrative" activities the hospital was liable, but when a nurse injured someone while engaged in "medical" duties, a physician was liable.

This led to any number of seemingly inconsistent holdings on liability of nurses and hospital employees, and, because there were some activities of their employees for which some hospitals were liable, hospitals began to purchase liability insurance. In 1957, New York began to roll back its support of the doctrines of Charitable Immunity and "Captain of the Ship" in the case of *Bing v. Thunig* (2 N.Y. 2d 656, 143 N.E. 2d 3 1957). The court in *Bing v. Thunig* emphasized the inconsistent results of Charitable Immunity. Although the court did not base its decision on the presence of insurance, you can see that the presence of insurance did have a major impact on the court's outcome.

When Charitable Immunity died, one would have expected its companions, "Captain of the Ship" and "Borrowed Servant," to die with it. However, the courts were unwilling to place innocent victims in a position where they could not fully recover for their injuries. When the persons who cause damage are unable to compensate victims, victims actively pursue relief against persons whose wrongdoing is more remote.

As the "Captain of the Ship" doctrine unfolded and was further perfected by the courts, the courts realized that what was important about the relationship of the surgeon to the hospital staff was not the legal status of employer/employee but the nature of control established by the surgeon. Where the surgeon actually controlled the negligent act, the nurse or other assistant was acting as the surgeon's agent, and the negligence of the nurse or other assistant should properly be imputed to the surgeon. Because anesthesia is a specialized area requiring additional education, surgeons do not normally control the actions of nurse anesthetists. "Captain of the Ship" and its fellow travelers such as "Borrowed Employee" have fallen out of favor in recent years. Increasingly, surgeons are held liable only when they actually control the action that gives rise to the negligence and not when they are deemed to have assumed the "helm" of the operating command or are deemed to satisfy other nautical or military analogies.

Misrepresentations Concerning Vicarious Liability

In the early part of the 1980s, the number of anesthesiologists in the United States increased dramatically. It had been a tenet of faith of certain anesthesiologists that when there were a sufficient number of anesthesiologists, the health care community would turn to physician anesthesia and the practice of nurse anesthesia would die out. When that did not happen, some anesthesiologists took it on themselves to warn surgeons of the so-called significant risks that surgeons took when operating with a nurse anesthetist rather than an anesthesiologist. This risk was based in large part on the "Captain of the Ship" theory of legal liability even though it had largely died out long before.

In holding physicians liable for the negligence of anesthetists, the courts, except in states still following "Captain of the Ship," do not look at whether the anesthesia administrator is a nurse or a physician but at the degree of control the physician exercises over the anesthesia administrator—whether that administrator is a CRNA or an anesthesiologist. The issue in each case is the extent to which the physician has control over the anesthesia administrator. Thus, a court may render different conclusions for cases that involve a physician working with a CRNA—or, for that matter, a physician working with an anesthesiologist—if the physician controlled the anesthetist in one case but not in another. A physician or authorized provider is neither automatically liable when working with a CRNA, nor is the physician immune from liability when working with an anesthesiologist. In *Schneider v. Einstein Medical Center*, 390 A.2d 1271 (Penn. 1978) and *Kitto v. Gilbert*, 570 P.2d 544 (Colo. 1977), the court found surgeons liable for the negligence of anesthesiologists because the surgeons were in control of the anesthesiologist's actions. The question, as in cases of a physician working with CRNAs, is whether the physician was in control of the acts of the anesthesiologists. This is a factual inquiry and not a conclusion of law. There are many cases in which courts have found that the surgeon was not in control of the CRNA and, therefore, not liable for the negligence of the CRNA: *Cavero v. Franklin Benevolence Society* (223 P. 2d 471, California, 1950); *Fortson v. McNamara* (508 So. 2d 35, Florida, 1987); *Hughes v. St. Paul Fire and Marine Insurance Company* (401 So. 2d 448, Louisiana, 1981); *Kemalyan v. Henderson* (277 P. 2d 372, Washington, 1954); *Parks v. Perry* (68 N.C. App 22, North Carolina, 1984); and *Sesselman v. Mulenberg Hospital* (306 A. 2d 474, New Jersey, 1954).

Even in cases in which the surgeon was held liable, there is often evidence of individual wrongdoing on the part of the surgeon. Moreover, numerous cases hold that mere supervision or direction of a CRNA is insufficient evidence to hold a physician liable for the CRNA's negligence. See, for example, *Baird v. Sickler*, 69 Ohio St. 2d 652 (1982); *Foster v. Englewood Hospital*, 19 Ill. App. 3d 1055 (1974); *McCullough v. Bethany Medical Center*, 235 Kan. 732 (1984); *Elizondo v. Tavarez*, 596 S.W. 2d 667 (Texas, 1980); *Parker v. Vanderbilt* 767 S.W. 2d 412 (Tenn., 1988); *Whitfield v. Whittaker Memorial Hospital*, 210 Va. 176 (1969). It is clear from the case law that in order for a physician to be liable for the acts of the anesthesia administrator, the physician must be in control of the administrator's actions and not merely be supervising or directing the administrator.

Consequently, court decisions concerning liability of surgeons for the negligence of nurse anesthetists have varied depending on the facts of the particular case. Where surgeons have been held to be in control they have been held liable, and where they have not, they have not been held liable. The same principles govern liability of surgeons for negligence of anesthesiologists, and there have been cases where surgeons have been held liable for the negligence of anesthesiologists.

Damages

It is unusual for punitive damages to be awarded against nurse anesthetists. In many malpractice cases in the health care area, the amount of damage is a major area of dispute. In the case of bodily injury, monetary damages are awarded to compensate people for damage that has no monetary value. What is the value of a chipped tooth? How do you compensate for the loss of eyesight or death with a monetary award? Some lawyers have been quite successful refining techniques maximizing jury awards for damage to the body. Awarding damages when harm results from a failure to meet the standard of care compensates the individual who was damaged and encourages practitioners to be careful. Damages based on the "value" of the injury caused, even if it is difficult to value, are called "compensatory."

If the wrongdoing has been intentional or gives a sense of outrage, courts have permitted the jury to award "punitive" or "exemplary" damages. Something more than mere negligence is required for punitive damages. There must be circumstances of aggravation, spite, or "malice"; a fraudulent or evil motive; or a conscious disregard of the interests of others (Prosser, *Handbook of the Law of Torts*, Page 9). Punitive damages are private fines imposed to punish reprehensible conduct and to deter its future occurrence.

An important element of punitive damages is lack of insurance protection. Many malpractice insurance policies do not insure against intentional acts. Punitive damages are imposed for intentional actions and therefore are not covered by malpractice insurance policies. Critics of the legal system contend that, in the health care field, when juries award punitive damages they merely multiply their award. Since awarding "compensatory" damage for bodily damage has little basis in reality anyway, "compensatory" damage already punishes the defendant and awarding "punitive" damages is just another opportunity to assess large awards.

Cases imposing punitive damages against nurse anesthetists are rare. The Georgia Court of Appeals, in a close, 5:4 split, reversed the award of punitive damages. Apparently, the anesthesia machine ran out and had to be refilled during the operation. Running out of an anesthetic agent in the middle of surgery is, obviously, a violation of the standard of care.

Four of the nine judges would have upheld the award of punitive damages. They reasoned that the jury had determined that the anesthesia machine had run out of anesthetic agent; it would not have run out if it had been checked, and the failure to check the level of anesthetic was similar to failing to check the level of gas before flying an airplane. It shows such a "conscious indifference" to the patient's well-being that the jury was entitled to award punitive damages. On the other hand, the majority of the Court of Appeals held that there was no evidence of an intentional disregard of the rights of the patient nor was there any evidence that the anesthesia providers knowingly or willfully disregarded the rights of the patient so as to authorize a finding of conscious indifference to consequences (200 Ga. App. 788; 409 S.E. 2d 572, 1991).

Another case involving punitive damages arose in Arkansas, where a jury assessed $3 million in punitive damages against the manufacturer of a ventilator. There was evidence that the manufacturer of the ventilator was aware that anesthetists using a selector valve could easily place hoses on the wrong unmarked valves with disastrous results. In the Arkansas case, someone had incorrectly put a hose where only a bag should have been connected. When the nurse anesthetist decided to change bags, she attached a hose to the wrong port. The effect of the improper connection was to permit the anesthesia machine to continue to pump air into the patient's lungs, with no way for the air to escape. The ensuing buildup of pressure and lack of oxygen resulted in damage to the patient's lungs and brain. The manufacturer claimed it was not at fault because separate acts of negligence had to occur for the accident to result. Many witnesses testified that the accident was foreseeable. The unmarked valve had been criticized in premarket tests, and other incidents involving the machine had been reported.

The standard for imposing punitive damages in Arkansas is that the defendant must have known, or ought to have known, in the light of the surrounding circumstances, that its conduct would naturally or probably result in injury and that the defendant continued such conduct in reckless disregard. The court upheld the jury award of punitive damages because the manufacturer knew that the patient's life always depended on the artificial breathing supplied by the ventilator (*Airco, Inc., Appellant, v. Simmons First National Bank, Guardian,* 276 Ark. 486, 638 S.W. 2d 660, 1982).

Because of the great risks involved in anesthesia, nurse anesthetists are aware that the smallest moment of carelessness can have disastrous consequences. This situation may lead to malpractice attorneys seeking punitive damages when bad consequences result from lapses. Nurse anesthetists can avoid the imposition of punitive damages by being able to prove that they followed procedures, such as the use of checklists, designed to minimize the possibility of lapses and by being able to document that they acted in the best interest of their patient, even after an incident may have occurred.

Res Ipsa Loquitur

A key element of the law of negligence is fault; the defendant must have caused the damage. The theoretic basis of negligence or malpractice is that the defendant should pay for damages caused to the plaintiff because, between the two parties, the one at fault should bear the damage. In terms of *prevention,* the knowledge that one can be held liable for malpractice or negligence is supposed to make people more careful and avoid negligent actions in the future.

In cases involving anesthesia, how does the patient show that the anesthetist was at fault? The field is too complicated for the average patient to understand, and sometimes the patient is unconscious when the actions that cause the damage, if any, are taken. As a result, many cases involving malpractice of anesthetists involve the legal principle of *res ipsa loquitur.*

Res ipsa loquitur, literally translated as "the thing speaks for itself," had its basis in a case decided in 1863 in which a barrel of flour rolled out of a warehouse window and fell on a passing pedestrian (*Byrne v. Boadle,* 1863, 159 Eng. Rep. 299). Although the pedestrian had not personally observed whatever went wrong on the upper floor of the warehouse, it was clear that this type of accident would not have happened without *someone's* negligence and whoever caused it must have been under the control of the warehouse owner (see *Law of Torts,* William L. Prosser, page 217).

The Doctrine of *res ipsa loquitur* depends on three things: (1) the injury must occur under circumstances such that in the ordinary course of events, the injury would not have occurred if someone had not been negligent; (2) the injury must be caused by something within the exclusive control of the defendant; and (3) the injury must not have been due to any voluntary action or contribution on the part of the plaintiff.

Classic examples are exploding boilers, defective food in sealed containers, and various types of falling objects including not only barrels of flour but elevators and, in one case, a 600-pound cow.

Anesthesia accidents almost invite the application of the Doctrine of *res ipsa loquitur.* In an anesthesia accident, the third requisite, that the plaintiff did not contribute to the accident, is almost always true, especially where the patient is unconscious. Similarly, if an anesthesia injury has occurred, the instrumentality that caused the damage will be within the exclusive control of the anesthetist. It is the application of the first requisite, that the event must be of a kind that ordinarily does not occur in the absence of someone's negligence, that has caused whatever theoretic disputes there may be over the application of the doctrine to anesthesia.

The basis of the law of negligence is *fault.* Many accidents can occur without anyone being at fault. Someone slipping and falling, a blowout of a tire, skidding cars, and fires of unknown origin have all been held to be situations where the Doctrine of *res ipsa loquitur* would not apply because it could not be said that the injury could not have occurred without negligence (see Prosser, page 220).

Theoretically, laypeople are supposed to understand that anesthesia is an area where accidents can happen without anyone being at fault. Realistically, however, it is a tribute to anesthetists that anesthesia accidents occur so infrequently that there is a common tendency, albeit incorrect, to believe that the accident would not have occurred without *someone* being negligent.

There is also a great economic incentive for the patient to base the case on *res ipsa loquitur.* Lawsuits can be very expensive and they can be made even more expensive by having to hire expert witnesses to testify as to the standard of care. The major benefit to a patient of the Doctrine of *res ipsa loquitur* is that it throws the burden of proof on the defendant.

How can a defendant-anesthetist defend a case of *res ipsa loquitur?* The defendant must introduce the defendant's own proof that (1) whatever instrumentalities were in the defendant's exclusive control during the operation were not those that caused the injuries; and/or (2) there were ways in which the incident could have occurred other than the anesthetist's negligence. Thus, in anesthesia cases, the role of the jury becomes one of choosing to believe the defendant's expert witnesses or the plaintiff's expert witnesses as to whether the injury would have occurred without negligence.

One issue the courts often address is the question of whether the doctrine can be applied when the plaintiff has *some* proof of how the injury occurred. In *Kemalyan v. Henderson,* 277 P.2d 372, the court pointed out that when the plaintiff's evidence establishes how an injury occurs, the plaintiff cannot rely on the Doctrine of *res ipsa loquitur.* In the *Kemalyan* case, the hospital alleged that because there was some testimony (one of the doctors testified that the accident was likely to have occurred because of a negligent intubation), the plaintiff should not be allowed to rely on the Doctrine of *res ipsa loquitur.* Nonetheless, the court held that the doctrine could still be used by the plaintiff.

In *Marrero v. Goldsmith* (486 So. 2d 530 Florida, 1986), the plaintiff complained of numbness, weakness, and pain in her left arm. The plaintiff produced expert medical testimony that this type of injury is one that ordinarily does not occur in the absence of negligence and that it was probably caused by incorrect arm positioning during surgery. The court noted that a plaintiff could still rely on *res ipsa loquitur* even if some direct evidence of negligence had been introduced. The court agreed, however, that there comes a point when a plaintiff can introduce enough direct evidence of negligence to eliminate the justification for the doctrine.

The court said

> It is quite clear that under traditional *res ipsa loquitur* analysis, the defendant doctors in this case cannot be said to have each possessed exclusive control at all times when plaintiff's injury may have occurred. Yet the patient is in no position to prove which defendant or combination of defendants caused her injury to an area of her body remote from the site of surgery, because she was unconscious when it occurred. We are persuaded that the fairest route to take under these particular circumstances is to allow the plaintiff to go to the jury with the benefit of *res ipsa loquitur* instruction.

In a case involving similar facts, the defendant argued that a patient could begin to rise out of an appropriate level of unconsciousness despite the exercise of due care. However, the court pointed out that the damage in the case was caused by disconnection from the anesthesia equipment and there was "no testimony that this disconnection could have occurred without negligence" (*Kitto v. Gilbert,* 570 P.2d 544 Colo. 1977).

In *Morgan v. Children's Hospital* (480 N.E.2d 464 Ohio 1985), the expert witnesses agreed that the patient suffered brain damage as a result of oxygen deprivation. The plaintiff requested that the jury be instructed on the application of *res ipsa loquitur* and was refused, and the jury returned a verdict in favor of the defendant anesthetist. On appeal, the court held that the jury should have been instructed on *res ipsa loquitur.* A dissent in the case pointed out the difficulty in establishing whether there was evidence sufficient to prove that the injury would have occurred in the absence of negligence.

In a California case, there was a verdict against both the surgeon and an anesthesiologist who apparently failed to communicate how long each expected the operation to take. The anesthesiologist had given a spinal anesthetic which became ineffective prior to the completion of the operation, and although he testified that he could have extended the spinal anesthesia if he had known the operation would have taken longer, the surgeon became uneasy as the effects of the anesthetic wore off and quickly terminated the operation. The court noted that there was sufficient evidence to support a conclusion of negligence against both doctors, but nonetheless determined that an instruction on *res ipsa loquitur* should have been given to the jury (*Clark v. Gibbons,* 66 Cal. 2d 399 Apr. 21, 1967).

SUMMARY

The legal system is imperfect, as are all human systems, in its attempts to resolve disputes in a fair, consistent, and predictable manner. Nurse anesthetists should be aware of their status as professionals and the principle that the system expects them to act as other nurse anesthetists would act.

13

Understanding Malpractice Litigation

Janet M. Simpson

OUTLINE

OBJECTIVES

On completing this chapter, the reader will be able to:

1. List and discuss the components of medical negligence including duty, breach and causation, and assessing standards of care.
2. Discuss issues and factors that are operative in negligence allegations and tort justice.
3. List procedures and a general course of events to be followed or experienced by the CRNA if named in a negligence suit.
4. List "tips" for avoiding litigation.
5. Discuss general trends in the evolution of tort reform in the United States.
6. Discuss the role of professional liability insurance as it relates to litigation.

Throughout the course of any active clinical career, most Certified Registered Nurse Anesthetists (CRNAs) are likely to come in contact with the civil justice system. It is to be hoped that it will not be a personal involvement where the anesthetist is a defendant. However, if such an occasion does arise, it is incumbent on the nurse anesthetist to understand in detail the course of malpractice litigation and how best to defend oneself in that event.

In this chapter, the reader is introduced to the most common sources of claims and lawsuits filed against anesthetists. Details are presented regarding the frequency of suits, assertions of negligence, causes of injuries, types of injuries, and amounts of money paid in damages to the plaintiff. By studying this data, one can draw some general conclusions regarding the prevention and defense of medical negligence actions.

The chapter also helps acquaint the reader with the process of a medical negligence lawsuit and educates the CRNA about what to expect during the proceedings, including guidance from an insurance company and attorney, depositions and trial testimony, acting as an expert witness, confidential and privileged communications, and settlement and trial considerations. Also discussed are the purchase of professional liability insurance, coverage benefits, tort reform, and the long-term effects of changes in malpractice legislation of the 1980s.

Finally, the reader will come to understand the importance of communication with families as a primary defense against malpractice litigation. Even as the trend nationally has demonstrated a decrease in the number of anesthesia mishaps and complications, the severity of injury from complications is still devastating. Since the anesthesia profession is still the highest-risk area in which nurses practice, it is paramount for CRNAs to appreciate the fact that effective, attentive communication with families and patients helps to attenuate litigation risk but only when accompanied by comprehensive and legible documentation of perioperative events.

FACTORS IN NEGLIGENCE ALLEGATIONS

The ever-present threat of a medical negligence lawsuit greatly influences the day-to-day delivery of health care in this country. Reasons include the fact that there is general consumer dissatisfaction and frustration with the health care system at large. The system appears insensitive and generally fails to consider the effects of its actions or nonactions on the patient and patient's family.

In addition, adequate health care is priced beyond the means of many. Today in the United States there are nearly 38 million people who cannot afford health insurance. We spend over $800 billion a year on health care yet provide no universal coverage for all. With these statistics, it is no wonder that many citizens hold great contempt for the system in general as well as the providers of health care.

Often patients and their families have unrealistic expectations of the health care system and of providers. Complicated medical and surgical procedures that do not produce desired outcomes often reinforce the public's perception that failure to guarantee medical results rightly constitutes negligence. Often, however, litigants have unrealistic expectations both of the monetary awards that can be secured in negligence cases and of the total cost of litigation itself.

These facts often overshadow the fact that, over the past decade, anesthesia mishaps have been on a steady decline for both nurse and physician providers of anesthesia. As is consistently shown, there is no statistically significant difference between CRNA and anesthesiologist rates of injury and death attributable to anesthesia-related causes.[1]

STATISTICS OF MORBIDITY AND MORTALITY

Generally, injuries associated with an anesthesia mishap are severe. Death is most commonly the result. Nerve damage is the second most common result, with brain damage a close third. This assessment corroborates a study performed by the National Insurance Commissioners.[2] Injuries are associated with all ages of patients yet are more common with generally healthy American Society of Anesthesiologists (ASA) I or II patients.[1] Death attributable directly to anesthesia-related incidents has been reported at

3.7 per 10,000 anesthetics for the years 1948 through 1952. Over the next 30 years the death rate dropped dramatically, varying between 0.7 and 2.2 per 10,000 anesthetics, depending on the source consulted. A British study covering a 1-year period in 1985 to 1986 found the death rate solely attributable to the anesthetic to be 0.054 per 10,000 anesthetics.[3]

The Committee on Professional Liability of the American Association of Anesthesiologists reviewed 1541 negative outcomes beginning in 1985. Three serious results accounted for the majority of the outcomes; death 565, nerve damage 227, and brain damage 188. In evaluating the cause of these injuries it is clear that respiratory management is the key element accounting for 34 percent of the adverse outcomes. Results can be summarized as follows. Inadequate ventilation and oxygenation account for 13 percent, esophageal intubations 6 percent, difficult intubations 6 percent, airway obstruction 2 percent, bronchospasm 2 percent, aspiration 2 percent, premature extubation 1 percent, inadvertent extubation 1 percent, and inadequate inspired oxygen concentration 1 percent.[4]

A large insurance company analyzed all anesthesia-related claims that it was involved with from July 1, 1985 through June 30, 1990. Two thousand three hundred and eighty-eight operating room and recovery room claims were evaluated. Of those, 239 were determined to be anesthesia-related. There was only slight variation on the cause of injury when compared with ASA closed-claims data. The frequency of causes is categorized as follows. Problems with intubation or extubation account for 38.1 percent, improper technique 19.2 percent, adverse reaction 15.1 percent, positioning 10 percent, monitoring during and after the case 6.3 percent, intravenous (IV) technique 3.3 percent, anesthetic overdose 2.1 percent, equipment problems 1.7 percent, misadministered medication 1.3 percent, and miscellaneous problems 2.9 percent.[5]

At least one research team has attempted to evaluate outside the litigation arena whether or not the appropriate standard of care was met in a set of anesthesia-related closed-claims.[1] They determined that the standard of care was met in 54 percent of the claims. In cases in which they believed the standard was not met, payment was made to the plaintiff 84 percent of the time; 10 percent of plaintiffs received no compensation. Action in the balance of the cases could not be determined based on the records available. This team determined the standard of care was not met if the anesthetist used a short-cut methodology, did not continuously or appropriately monitor the patient, made a serious error in judgment, or made a poor choice of method for conducting the anesthetic. In some instances, payment was made in cases the research team determined met the appropriate standards. However, there was a significant difference in the dollar amount paid on claims where the standard of care was met and those where it was not.

As an example, in cases of severe injury where standards were met, the average payout was $93,000. Compare this with an average payment of $463,000 in cases from the same injury category where the standard of care was not met. In cases involving death, using the same analysis, the comparison was $115,000 to $200,000, respectively. In instances of low severity of injury, claims paid were $10,000 and $15,000, respectively. One must remember that this analysis considered only investigator interpretations of the appropriate standard of care.

Another research team attempted to determine on a retrospective basis whether or not additional monitoring would have prevented the anesthetic complication.[6] In analyzing 1437 closed-claims where such a determination could be made, they found additional monitors probably would have prevented the problem in 484 cases, or 33.7 percent. The median payout in these cases was $225,000. The median payout in the remaining 953 cases where additional monitoring would probably have had no effect was $30,000. A combination of end-tidal CO_2 and pulse oximeter monitors would likely have prevented 239 of the preventable complications, or 49 percent. A pulse oximeter alone may have prevented 196 of the complications, or 41 percent. An end-tidal CO_2 monitor alone could have prevented 15 complications, or 3 percent; other types of monitors could have prevented 34 complications, or 7 percent.

Mishaps following esophageal intubations are a fairly manageable subgroup of the anesthetic closed-claims analysis. In reviewing the closed-claims materials available from a variety of insurance companies, it is apparent that in the majority of cases (77 percent) the anesthetist never mentioned that the intubation was difficult.[7] This leads one to conclude that the endotracheal tube was placed easily. It has often been stated that to place a tracheal tube in the esophagus is not medical negligence. However, failure to recognize misplacement in a timely manner is negligence. In this study, only 3 percent of the esophageal intubations were recognized in less than 5 minutes. One can assume that in most instances, where this is recognized promptly, there is no patient injury and the case never makes its way to an insurance company's closed-claims file. Sixty-one percent of these claims were detected within 5 to 10 minutes of placement, and 36 percent were recognized more than 10 minutes after intubation.

In these cases of esophageal intubation, breath sounds were noted by the anesthetist 63 percent of the time. In only 5 percent of these cases did the auscultation lead to a correct diagnosis of esophageal intubation. The remaining 58 percent concluded incorrectly that the tube was properly placed. A hemodynamic derangement ultimately preceded the detection of the esophageal intubation in 65 percent of the cases. The documented derangements included bradycardia 57 percent, asystole 55 percent, hypotension 49 percent, arrythmia 10 percent, tachycardia 5 percent, and ventricular fibrillation 1 percent.

This barrage of statistics and closed-claims analysis offers several general conclusions. Although anesthesia mishaps have fortunately declined over the last 40 or 50 years, when injury occurs it is often serious. Some may argue that recently applied minimum standards of monitoring may simply be a formalization of practice patterns already in place. However, the advent of pulse oximeters and end-tidal CO_2 monitors affords the anesthetist the benefit of early warning of patient misadventures. Even if a lawsuit ensues, the anesthetist's chances of a defendant's verdict or of paying far less are significantly enhanced when these monitors are used.

ANATOMY OF MEDICAL NEGLIGENCE

Often one hears the term "medical malpractice" used more frequently in popular jargon than the term "medical negligence." The former is technically incorrect as there is no legal theory of malpractice, be it medical, legal, architectural, or related to any other discipline. There is, however, a legal theory of negligence about which the CRNA must become familiar.

Components of Medical Negligence

Legal theories are comprised of elements, much like chemical compounds. The first element in negligence is "duty." The plaintiff has the burden of proof on all elements. The plaintiff must prove that a duty to exercise reasonable care existed between the plaintiff and the defendant, in this case the anesthetist. Any time an anesthetist undertakes patient care, he or she must exercise reasonable care. There is no debate on the latter part of the element. If debate arises on this element it generally involves whether or not the anesthetist ever entered into a professional relationship with the patient.

As an example, if two anesthetists with the same last name work in a single hospital and a plaintiff sues the one who did not provide anesthetic care, the claim fails because there is no duty to exercise reasonable care flowing from the anesthetist sued to the plaintiff. No patient-anesthetist relationship was ever established. Taking a less obvious example, if an anesthetic is planned for 1300 hours, and the patient was visited preoperatively by the anesthetist at 0900 hours, can the patient prevail in a suit against the anesthetist if her appendix ruptures between 0900 and 1300 hours? Does a duty exist between the two? The simple answer is "probably." However, circumstances involving other elements will likely arise to make that case defensible as well.

The second element involves a "breach" of the anesthetist's duty to exercise reasonable care with the patient. This is the negligent act, error, or omission part of the formula. The anesthetist must act within the appropriate standard of care in providing anesthesia services to the patient. The patient's petition or complaint filed to initiate the lawsuit generally sets out the allegations of negligence. A plaintiff asserts that several actions were carried out improperly or were omitted. The plaintiff claims that these actions, errors, and/or omissions constitute negligence on the part of the anesthetist.

For example, the plaintiff may claim the defendant should have performed a regional anesthetic rather than a general technique. This allegation involves negligent professional judgment. A plaintiff may allege the anesthetist improperly placed an endotracheal tube in the esophagus and failed to recognize its misplacement. This involves an allegation of technical error and a judgment or diagnostic error.

In all instances, the breach must have caused physical injury to the plaintiff, or the plaintiff's decedent, as the case may be. This represents the third element, causation. The anesthetist may have negligently administered the anesthetic, but the patient has no injury. For example, if the CRNA anesthetized the patient with a general anesthetic agent, turned on the ventilator, and left the room, this would constitute improper care. Yet, if the patient awoke at the end of the case without sequela, a lawsuit based on these circumstances would fail for lack of a causation element. There was no physical injury.

Assume the same conduct by the anesthetist, but this time the patient is injured. The surgeon nicked a ureter. Still, the case of medical negligence fails as to the anesthetist because the nicked ureter and the anesthetist leaving the operating room are not linked. Again, there is no causation element. The plaintiff must prove he or she was injured as a result of the negligent conduct.

As mentioned earlier, the burden of proof rests with the plaintiff. An unfortunate result, in and of itself, does not raise the question of negligence. In fact, law is to the contrary. The plaintiff must prove all elements of the claim of medical negligence. In most jurisdictions the health care provider is entitled to exercise his or her best judgment. The public and courts understand that medicine is not an exact science. In some jurisdictions, if the health care provider exercises the required degree of skill, he or she is not liable for any honest error in judgment.[8] This assumes that the action carried out was an action that a reasonable health care provider might elect as an option of treatment.

ASSESSING STANDARDS OF CARE

For a plaintiff to proceed to a point where a jury can consider the case, he or she must establish what the appropriate standard of care is in relation to the alleged negligent acts or omissions. The *standard of care* can be defined as that level of care generally practiced by members of the profession in the same or similar circumstances, a deviation from which represents a risk of injury to the patient/plaintiff. The same or similar community is also referenced by many when describing the appropriate standard of care. Be aware that the definition of community has expanded dramatically because of continuing education requirements and availability, and because national practice groups have promulgated standards and goals for safe practice. The professional groups publishing and endorsing such standards hope that, by reducing patient injury, the number of medical negligence claims and lawsuits will decrease through improved practice techniques, focusing the issues and merits for attorney consideration before suits are filed, and shortening the time and expense associated with litigation.[9] No firm results are yet available on this subject; not enough time has passed since the endorsement of the standards and the evolution of practice techniques, claims, and lawsuits.

There are a variety of means available to establish, for a jury's consideration, the appropriate standard of care. These include but are not limited to textbooks, authoritative treatises, professional journal articles, facility policy and procedures, standards or policy statements of professional organizations, expert witnesses, state or federal statutes, and prior case law.

Textbooks, treatises, and journal articles, however, may not be sufficient by themselves to override the professionals' general practice patterns. This evidence often must be supported with expert testimony.[10] An individual facility's policies and procedures are really self-imposed standards. They make a statement of the standard of care that is expected of its health care providers.

The rationale for these standards is generally patient safety. Therefore, if an anesthetist fails to follow anesthesia departmental policies and procedures, and an adverse result occurs, there is little justification for the deviation. Such cases are difficult to defend successfully. State or federal statutes and prior case law come into effect somewhat less frequently. However, consider the statute enacted in Massachusetts, which requires that end-tidal CO_2 monitors and pulse oximeters be used in all general anesthetics. An anesthesia mishap that can be tied to a failure to use one of these legally required monitors would be devastating from a defense standpoint. Legal cases that have been appealed through the appellate courts sometimes make blanket statements of what the court considers the appropriate standard of care to be. This statement can be translated into law in future cases.

Damages

To collect money for negligent conduct, the plaintiff must establish damages. Damages may be of several forms: economic (sometimes called compensatory), noneconomic, or punitive. The petition or complaint also sets out in general terms the damages claimed in the lawsuit. Economic or compensable damages include all things lost to the plaintiff as a result of the alleged negligence and resultant injury that can be measured through economic calculations. Economic damages may include medical expenses attributable to the injury, both past and future. Economic damages may include lost wages due to time off work to recover from the injury and future lost wages. If the patient has died, heirs may be entitled to recover the patient's projected lifetime wages through a claim filed by the deceased's estate.

Loss of household services are routinely compensated as economic damages. Some courts allow economists to testify for the plaintiff as to the economic value of more esoteric functions such as the loss of guidance a parent provides to a child. If the parent has died as a result of medical negligence, that person's minor child may be able to recover the economic loss associated with the parent's guidance and counseling. The precise calculation of economic damages varies considerably among jurisdictions. Calculations change dramatically depending on the circumstances of the parties as well. Look to your attorney for specific information on the calculation of economic damages if you are a defendant and compare this calculation with the amount of professional negligence insurance coverage you have available.

Noneconomic damages are the intangible elements of life. They include pain, suffering, loss of enjoyment of life, and disfigurement. As between a husband and wife, noneconomic damages also include loss of consortium, or loss of sexual or other marital relations, between the two. Some jurisdictions rule that loss of affection, guidance, and counseling to an injured party's minor child fall within noneconomic damages. It is the noneconomic damage portion of awards that the plaintiff has historically tried to inflate. By injecting a medical negligence case with extreme sympathy for the injured party, the plaintiff's attorney seeks to inflate the verdict far in excess of the actual economic damages. Some courts have recently placed caps, or maximum recovery limits, on the amount of noneconomic damages a plaintiff may recover. The jury is generally allowed to render any verdict it selects. The court then applies the cap, if appropriate, to reduce the noneconomic portion of the verdict.

Occasionally a defendant's conduct will be such that the plaintiff will seek punitive damages. The key words generally found in a petition or complaint that indicate punitive damages are requested include gross, willful, and/or wanton. A specific request or prayer for punitive damages may or may not be articulated in the petition or complaint. Seldom does a claim of medical negligence rise to a punitive level. Generally a court must decide whether the evidence is sufficient to allow a jury to consider awarding punitive damages. Circumstances when a court might allow punitive damages include a patient who is under a general anesthetic, on a mechanical ventilator, and the anesthetist leaves the hospital without concluding the anesthetic. Habitual negligent conduct may also give rise to punitive levels. As the word indicates, punitive damages are meant to punish the offending defendant. These damages are not covered by professional liability insurance and cannot be discharged through bankruptcy proceedings. The defendant is obligated to pay them personally.

ISSUES OF TORT JUSTICE

The original purposes for the tort justice system were to provide compensation and deterrence. In recent years the system has come under more frequent attack for several reasons. Critics lodge the system affords variable and unpredictable compensation for injuries. Because a jury determines the dollar award, if any is to be awarded, plaintiff's with similar injuries may receive vastly different awards. Another criticism proposes that too much of the professional liability insurance premium does not reach the injured party. Rather the premiums are used in defense costs, operating the company and profit for the company's shareholders.[11] Finally, critics of the current system assert that too much of the jury award goes to the plaintiff's attorney in fees, generally 33 to 50 percent. Deterrence can more readily be handled through effective risk management and quality assurance efforts.

There are strong justifications for leaving the basic tort system in place, however. If inequities exist, adjustments in the law can compensate. Allowing a jury to consider evidence on an individual's injuries provides compensation, if deserved, in an amount appropriate for the plaintiff's circumstances. A no-fault compensation system would likely decrease the costs of defending medical negligence claims, but the number of claims would likely rise dramatically, thereby saving no money because of the increased overall payout. There are certainly inequities and abuses in the current no-fault worker's compensation system, but without it, the health care provider would have no opportunity to defend his or her reputation, and providers in high-risk health care areas might decide to leave practice. Also, checks in the current system make portions of the award paid to a plaintiff's attorney subject to court approval in some jurisdictions.[12] This at least prevents the plaintiff's attorney from blatant overcharging.

THE EXPERT WITNESS

The most commonly considered evidence of whether or not an appropriate standard of care was upheld comes from the expert witness. The court makes the determination of whether a proposed expert witness qualifies as such and may testify. Some states have statutory limitations on who may testify. For instance, Kansas requires that the expert testifying on liability issues must practice in the same profession at least 50 percent of his or her time within 2 years of the incident in question.[13] This is meant to prevent physicians from retiring and spending their golden years in the courtroom supporting or criticizing the actions of others. This does not prevent a retired professional from giving an opinion on causation. All testimony must be offered on the standard of care in place at the time of the incident. This is difficult at times, as several years may pass between the incidents and the filing of the lawsuit. Additional years may pass before the case comes to trial. This is especially true in cases where minors are involved and the statute of limitations, in some states, allows filing lawsuits up to 19 years after the alleged negligent conduct.

An expert witness must testify in terms of medical probabilities or events that are more likely than not. An expert may not speculate to establish the alleged deviation. An expert must also indicate a familiarity with the standard of care. To simply advise a jury, "I administer anesthesia this way" is not sufficient. One individual's practice does not comport with the definition of appropriate standard of care. Expert witness testimony is generally required to show both liability and causation. Causation testimony deals with what medical injuries have been incurred to date as a result of the negligent act and what will likely be suffered in the future.

An expert witness serves the purpose of informing the jurors on specialized areas not within the knowledge of laypersons. Occasionally medical negligence cases are filed that can be analyzed without the assistance of medical expert testimony. As an example, if a patient falls from the operating room table and is injured, a jury could well assess whether this could occur absent negligence on the part of the professionals attending the patient in the operating room. Another common example involves the retained sponge or instrument. A jury can assess without expert testimony whether or not items should be left in a body cavity following surgery. Jurors are encouraged to rely on their own common sense and life experiences when making such judgments. As medical negligence actions often involve more than one defendant, and patient care generally involves more than one provider, comparative fault becomes a critical issue. Strict comparative fault means the plaintiff collects the percentage of the award assessed against each defendant. Variations apply; for example, some states do not allow the plaintiff to collect at all if that plaintiff is judged to be 50 or 51 percent negligent. Instances where the plaintiff's fault may be compared include failure to return for follow-up treatment, smoking with knowledge that the same causes lung cancer, or failure to follow rehabilitation instructions. The rules also vary on whether nondefendant health care providers' fault can be compared. Some states allow this, and some do not. However, if a party settles with the plaintiff before trial, his or her negligence can be compared unless the remaining defendants have agreed to the contrary.

WHAT TO DO IF NAMED IN A SUIT

It has been suggested that every anesthetist will be sued one time for every 10 years of practice. This author believes this often-quoted figure is too high to truly represent an anesthetist's chances of being named in a medical negligence lawsuit. Regardless of the incidence, a lawsuit can be an intimidating process. It is helpful to have some idea of how to proceed and what to expect over the ensuing months.

Process Service

The first involvement with a new lawsuit is service of process, meaning the delivery of the lawsuit petition or complaint to the provider. This is the document filed by the plaintiff with the court setting out the complaint of negligence or other wrongdoing alleged. This document may be served personally. A court representative actually locates you, generally at home or work, and personally delivers the petition or complaint along with information indicating when you must respond to the allegations to avoid a default judgment. A default judgment results when the defendant has failed to respond in a timely fashion to the petition or complaint. The plaintiff's allegations are therefore deemed admitted and judgment in the amount requested by the plaintiff is entered. As one can see, the appropriate response or answer to the service of process is very important.

There are other means of receiving notice of the lawsuit, including delivery via certified mail. This too is an appropriate way to effect service on a defendant in most jurisdictions. Occasionally service of process is improper. The precise rules dictating proper and improper service and remedies for improper service vary among jurisdictions. Generally, if the plaintiff is trying to carry out personal service and someone leaves the documents with an office or hospital employee who is not designated with authority to receive such documents, that service is invalid. However, if the court representative leaves the documents with someone of "suitable age" at your home, service is valid.

There are two important points to keep in mind when one is served with process. First, make a note of the date, time, and manner in which the documents were delivered and the date and time you received the documents if that is different from the former. An attorney will need this information. Second, notify your professional liability insurance carrier immediately that you have been named in a lawsuit and served with process. Notify your carrier initially by telephone and follow this notice with a letter advising the company of the new lawsuit and enclose a copy of the suit papers received. Next, open a personal records file to keep copies of documents, letters, and other papers that will be generated during the course of litigation.

One should not ignore the service of process, as a default judgment can be entered following the time allowed for your answer to be filed with the court. In addition to the risk of default judgment, ignoring service of process places your professional liability insurance coverage at risk. Most policies contain a clause requiring you to notify the company of a claim or lawsuit so that a defense can be undertaken. Failure to comply with this requirement may void your coverage. Above all, the CRNA should speak to no one about the allegations or the case. The plaintiff's attorney may ask in deposition or trial who you have spoken with about this case. By talking about the lawsuit with others, you may be involving them unnecessarily in the litigation process.

Some professionals want to undertake an immediate and independent investigation of the facts. Avoid this urge until you have consulted with the attorney that your insurance company appoints to the case. Certain privileged status attaches to investigation undertaken at the direction of your counsel. Embarking on an independent investigation before conferring with counsel regarding your intended efforts may result in your work ending up in the hands of the plaintiff and plaintiff's counsel.

In summary, when served with process advise your insurance carrier of this fact. Do not speak with others regarding the lawsuit. Do not undertake an investigation of the matter without first speaking with and clearing your proposed action with your appointed attorney.

Selection of Counsel

Once advised of the lawsuit, a claims adjustor with your professional liability carrier will appoint an attorney to defend you. Selection of counsel is obviously an important aspect of defense. Some professionals in seeking a level of comfort with the whole process will request that a friend, neighbor, or relative be appointed to handle the case. Most adjustors resist this suggestion with good reason. Attorneys, similar to health care providers, specialize in their practice area. It takes years to acquire the knowledge of medicine necessary to defend medical negligence actions. Likewise, it takes years to develop networks with potential experts around the country. It is not in your best interest for the insurance company to accede to your request and appoint an attorney friend or acquaintance.

One should feel comfortable with inquiring into the proposed attorney's background and qualifications. Professional liability carriers generally have a limited list of attorneys who they have previously investigated relative to qualifications and past work performance. These attorneys generally limit their practice to medical negligence defense. You may want to inquire in some general areas such as an attorney's prior experience with medical negligence cases and anesthesia cases in particular.

Often more than one defendant is named in a medical negligence action. Often, one attorney represents more than one defendant. If you find yourself being represented by an attorney who also represents a codefendant in your lawsuit, you can question this arrangement with your adjustor and the attorney if the arrangement seems inappropriate to you. The analysis made in this situation is twofold. First, do you and the co-defendant have the same interests, that is, are you both employed by the same hospital or professional group and did you both provide care to the allegedly injured party? Second, do you have conflicting interests that could result in compromising the defense of one to bolster the defense of the other, that is, did the two of you disagree regarding the method of anesthesia used with the allegedly injured party?

CRNA Responsibilities in Tort Action

Professional liability insurance finances your defense and provides coverage in case of monetary settlement or verdict. However, in addition to paying premiums, you have other duties under the terms of the insurance contract. As mentioned earlier in this section, you have a duty to report notice of receipt of a claim or lawsuit so that an investigation and defense can be set in motion. You also have a duty to assist and cooperate in preparing your defense. This includes being available to meet with your attorney to discuss the facts of the case, plan a defense, and prepare for your deposition and trial. Failure to make yourself reasonably available may result in a warning that your company will no longer finance your defense and will not be responsible for a settlement or judgment. Continued failure to cooperate and make yourself reasonably available will result in the warning being carried out.

Generally, nurse anesthetists are interested in being involved in the progress of discovery and in assisting with the defense. Early in the relationship, you should enter into an understanding with your attorney regarding your level of involvement. Always feel free to contact your attorney with questions or comments. You may wish to limit your involvement to periodic reports from the attorney of discovery schedules, important court dates, and settlement discussions. You may wish to assist in selecting expert witnesses, by attending many depositions or by suggesting demonstrative ways to explain the technical aspects of the case to the jury. Your attorney will welcome your interest and participation.

Certain privileges attach once your attorney becomes involved in the litigation. As with the privilege of confidentiality, often called the physician-patient privilege, there is a privilege of confidentiality between an attorney and client. In order to qualify under the attorney-client privilege, there must be true confidentiality of communications. Therefore, when you meet with your counsel, do not take your spouse or best friend along for moral support. As your attorney does not represent this person, the confidential nature of the attorney-client communications would be destroyed. A plaintiff's attorney could later ask your spouse or friend what was said during the meeting. Also do not describe the content of the communications between yourself and your attorney to third persons later. This too destroys the confidential nature of the communication and subjects them to the possibility of disclosure to the opposing side.

A second privilege that attaches after your attorney is appointed to represent you deals with attorney work product. This means that all efforts undertaken by the attorney or someone under his or her direction and acting on the attorney's behalf are privileged and cannot be discovered by the opposing side. Therefore any investigation that you assist with should be specifically requested by your attorney in order to remain protected and thus confidential. Investigation you may assist with includes literature searches on relevant standards of care or causation issues, review of the patients' lifetime medical records, or review of literature authored by plaintiff and defendant experts.

Peer review, quality assurance, and risk management activities may or may not be protected from discovery, depending on the state and jurisdiction. However, if these activities are to be protected under the laws of any jurisdiction, they must be handled in a confidential manner. If you participated in a peer review activity or know that one was conducted on your case, advise your attorney of this fact to allow him or her an opportunity to deal with the issue before it becomes a problem.

The Process of Planning for Litigation

Within the time allowed, your attorney will prepare an answer denying the plaintiff's allegations of negligence and file this with the court. This document is general in nature and requires little, if any, input from the defendant to complete. As soon as practical, your attorney will want to meet with you to discuss the case. Be prepared to review the anesthetic record with your attorney in detail. Even experienced medical negligence attorneys have difficulty deciphering the symbols and abbreviations used on an anesthetic record. Also be prepared to discuss other parts of the patient record that contain your notations or to which you refer when preparing for or administering an anesthetic. If you have the opportunity, review the entire patient record before the initial meeting. You may be able to isolate events or conditions that explain the patient's condition, that may or may not have to do with anesthetic management.

In addition to the thorough record review, your attorney will want your best recollection of the events at issue. Do not prepare a written chronology unless asked to do so by your attorney. Include as much detail as possible in your oral description. Your attorney may also want a description of formal and informal relationships among all operating room personnel. Laws vary from state to state regarding lines of responsibility and comparative fault principles. The better defense is one with all defendants agreeing there is no liability among themselves. If the defendants point fingers at one another and claim the other is at fault, the plaintiff wins automatically. The plaintiff does not care where the money comes from, only that money is recovered. Therefore, the best defense is a joint defense, whenever possible. Confide in your attorney any suspicions that other health care providers may have been at fault. Discuss this matter thoroughly with your attorney before offering testimony at deposition or trial to this effect.

During the initial interview with your attorney, a preliminary list of the plaintiff's specific allegations of negligence will be discussed. Your input into weaknesses in the case is important. Also, your attorney will ask your opinion of standard of care matters at issue. Sources for supporting your care can be identified. These may include standards from the American Association of Nurse Anesthetists (AANA), ASA, facility policies and procedures, textbooks, articles, and so on. Be certain to point out portions of the patient record that support your defense and refute the plaintiff's theories. This is the time for a frank, open discussion of the case. It is best to make a sound preliminary judgment as soon as practical regarding the likelihood of prevailing should the case proceed to trial.

Your initial interview will also include a discussion of potential expert witnesses. Because of your expertise, you can suggest local anesthetists who are familiar with the standard of care, are articulate, and are not intimidated by direct questioning. Nationally recognized experts may also be considered, depending on the issues to be addressed. Because the standard of care for administering anesthesia is the same for both physician and nurse anesthetists, either CRNAs or physicians may be used as expert witnesses. Friends are generally not preferred as potential expert witnesses, because the jury may discount their testimony as biased. Areas of expertise beyond anesthesia may be required to fully support your patient care in a case. The causation element may be addressed by others such as a forensic pathologist, neuroradiologist, neurologist, and so on.

Finally, in an initial interview, you will probably discuss the course of the litigation. This is a time for you to learn what to expect and over what time frame. Expect delays and cancellations through the discovery process. It is not clear whether these are due to the nature of litigation or the nature of attorneys. Whatever the reason, flexibility is a must. During the pendency of the litigation there will be many occasions to rediscuss and refine the items mentioned thus far. A specific discussion of the discovery process and deposition testimony is found later in this chapter.

Some time during the course of the action the plaintiff makes a demand for settlement, meaning payment of a specific dollar payment will resolve the matter without trial. Settlement discussions can take on many formats, both formal and informal. Formal settlement discussions may be held outside the courtroom through mediation or arbitration. Mediation often takes on a form of shuttle diplomacy. Each side presents the strengths of his or her case and points out the weaknesses in the other side's case. This is generally done through statements of counsel. Clients are generally in attendance, along with a representative of the professional liability carriers. After listening to both sides make a presentation, the plaintiff and defendant sides often separate. The mediator then meets with each side to discuss privately and candidly their chances of prevailing at trial. Demands and offers to settle are made and conveyed by the mediator.

Arbitration is different from mediation in that the independent arbitrator may be an individual or a group. The sides present their arguments and the arbitrator arrives at an opinion regarding the value of the case and proportionate shares of contribution, if any. Arbitration may be binding or nonbinding depending on the agreement made before the process is undertaken. If the arbitration is binding, the parties are agreeing in advance to accept the arbitrator's judgment and forgo a trial. If negligence is found by the arbitrator, money in the amount and proportions suggested by the arbitrator is paid. Nonbinding arbitration is advisory only. It allows the parties to consider how a jury might react to the facts of the case. Both mediation and arbitration are generally undertaken when both parties are genuinely interested in settlement.

Court-managed settlement conferences are mandated in some states. A judge serves in a role similar to the mediator. The judge's status often influences the parties to accommodate and makes the parties feel they have aired their relative positions in open court.

Both are obvious advantages when dealing with the emotions that often charge a party's judgment. Informal settlement negotiations are generally conducted between the attorneys. You have the right to inquire about and be kept advised of this process. You may not have the right to prevent settlement under the terms of your insurance contract.

When considering whether to support settlement efforts or proceed to trial and a jury verdict, there are considerations beyond the merits of the case. Is there a large sympathy factor for the plaintiff? Will trial pose a significant personal expense in terms of time away from employment? Is there a significant chance there could be a verdict in excess of policy limits?

This last item, excess verdict, brings the subject of personal counsel into discussion. Even though your attorney, paid by the insurance company, represents your interests, there may be times when it is prudent to undertake the personal expense of consulting with additional counsel. If punitive damages are claimed or if there is a significant chance that a jury could reach a verdict against you in excess of your policy limits, your personal assets are exposed to said judgment. Punitive damages are generally not covered by insurance and the company may be reluctant to offer the money necessary to settle the case. A personal attorney can make an independent evaluation of these factors and advise you accordingly. You may request that the personal attorney press the insurance company to settle the case so that you avoid exposure of personal assets.

Assuming the lawsuit is moving on to trial, anticipate extensive preparation beforehand. You will need to review the medical records and know their contents thoroughly. Allow time to read depositions of all important witnesses before trials begins. Feel free to take notes regarding aspects of testimony that can be improved or attacked. Note the style of questions posed by plaintiff's counsel. Conduct any final research and review your attorney's research as it applies to standard of care and causation issues.

Assist in gathering anesthesia equipment, anatomical models, or other items that will help educate the jury about your role as an anesthetist. Juries appreciate a witness who takes time and effort to teach them about the subject matter. Your testimony has a much greater impact on the jury when you use demonstrative aids. The jury remembers what you show them longer than what you tell them. This way you demonstrate to the jury that you are knowledgeable about the equipment and procedures. Be absolutely positive all demonstrative aids brought to the courtroom function properly.

Make yourself available for extensive conferences with your attorney before trial as your attorney will want to prepare you for testimony before the jury. Generally this includes actual practice situations where you are asked to respond to questioning. All of the exhibits and means to use each will be reviewed. Preparation is a key element to success at trial. Spend the time necessary to prepare adequately. Know the medical record and listen to your attorney.

Personal attendance is required every day of the trial and it is important for you to assist your attorney with the defense. Attendance also shows the jury that you care about the outcome of the litigation. Depending on the complexity of the issues and the number of parties, an average medical negligence case may last 1 to 4 weeks. If you do not live in the city where trial will be conducted, discuss your personal expenses associated with room, meals, and so on ahead of time. Your policy of insurance probably does not cover these items. They will likely be your responsibility.

Dress professionally for the trial. This means a jacket and tie for the men and suits or dresses for the women. Avoid flashy clothing and jewelry. Avoid driving an expensive car to the courthouse. Jurors can become offended by an obviously expensive life style. Always conduct yourself professionally in the courtroom. Appear interested in the proceedings. Remember that the jurors are constantly evaluating you, whether you are testifying or not.

After a verdict is rendered, the losing side may take an appeal to a higher court. The specific circumstances and implications of an appeal are so individual that we cannot speak to them here. Should an appeal be taken in your case, look to your attorney to explain all possible results and ramifications.

DEPOSITIONS AND TRIAL TESTIMONY

Types and Purposes of Depositions

Depositions are used by attorneys in the discovery process of any major piece of litigation. Specific rules governing the procedure are set out in every state and vary somewhat among the jurisdictions. Generally, depositions are conducted outside the courthouse, by agreement of the parties. The witness swears to tell the truth. A certified court reporter takes down every word spoken during the deposition. Attorneys ask questions and the witness, or deponent, answers. The stress of these proceedings is most often relieved by adequate study and preparation prior to the event.

The deponent may provide valuable information to a medical negligence case for several reasons. First, the deponent may have been present when the events in question occurred. The deponent may have treated the individual at another time, making him or her knowledgeable about the plaintiff's condition. In these types of situations, the deponent is a "fact" witness. There is no anticipation on anyone's part that the anesthetist will become a defendant in the lawsuit. A fact deposition is limited to questions involving who, what, when, and where.

A second form of deposition involves the "defendant" who has knowledge about the facts, but also a rationale for decisions, treatment, judgments, and so on as carried out with this patient. As a defendant, your answers to questions are the crux of the case. You will spend a significant amount of time preparing for the deposition before it occurs. Tips for depositions included in this section are particularly applicable to the defendant deponent.

In a third type of deposition, the deponent may be an "expert" witness, someone with no actual knowledge of the facts. The expert witness generally has been selected by a party to testify because of his or her background and education. This makes the person uniquely qualified to offer opinions about the facts of the lawsuit. The expert witness reviews medical records, other deposition testimony, procedural documents, and any other relevant information. He or she then offers opinions on the appropriate standard of care, causation, damages, or other related topics which are beyond the knowledge of laypersons.

Depositions are not always exclusively categorized within one of the three areas mentioned above. For instance, a fact witness may later become a defendant. The fact witness may also have opinions about the appropriate standard of care or causation based on his or her knowledge of the events or experience. A defendant certainly testifies about facts, but may also have opinions about the appropriate standard of care or causation. The expert witness must interpret facts in order to supply the opinion testimony. The boundaries of your testimony should be considered before the deposition begins.

There are multiple reasons for taking depositions and multiple uses for them once they have been completed. Understanding an attorney's intent helps prepare you to offer testimony in the most favorable light. Beginning with the fact witness deposition, the testimony establishes a sequence of events that can later be evaluated. Did the health care providers make appropriate judgments in treating the patient? Did any single act or series of actions lead to the injury? The deposition makes the testimony immortal. If a witness is unavailable for live trial testimony, the deposition can be read to the jury. A witness may be unavailable because of distance from the trial location, death, injury, and so on. If the deponent does appear at trial and changes his or her testimony from the sworn statements given in the deposition, an attorney can point out the changes to the jury. The attorney may suggest a variety of reasons for changing the testimony, such as the deponent has a poor memory, is trying to protect someone, or is simply lying at one time or the other. An attorney may suggest to the jury that the witness is not credible.

Before agreeing to give deposition testimony, a nondefendant anesthetist should fully investigate the possible ramifications of the deposition. Could you become a defendant after the testimony? If the answer is yes, you should advise your professional liability insurance carrier that your deposition has been requested. Tell the insurance representative that you are concerned you may become a party to the lawsuit. Request that an attorney be appointed to prepare you for the deposition and represent you at that proceeding. If there is no chance or likelihood that you will be added to the lawsuit, you will probably work with a defense attorney who represents another health care provider to prepare for the deposition. Note, however, that rules allowing contact between a plaintiff's health care providers and attorneys vary from state to state and must be considered before discussions of a patient's treatment are undertaken.

Documents reviewed in direct preparation for your deposition and relied on for testimony can be reviewed by opposing counsel. Therefore, only review documents before your deposition which your attorney agrees are appropriate. As an example, if your attorney has asked you to provide a narrative of the events at issue and you review this document to refresh your recollection for the deposition, that document may be discoverable by opposing counsel. The same is true for research materials you may locate and review to support your actions and opinions.

If you have an opportunity to attend one or more depositions before yours, it will help you to be comfortable with the process. You will be able to appreciate the attorney's manner of questioning and direction for theories of liability. In general, a deposition is not a time to explain everything that you believe is relevant. Save that detail for trial. Rather, in a deposition, answer only the question that is asked. Answer truthfully, but answer yes or no when possible. Avoid nods of the head and gestures as the reporter can only take down actual words. Explain your answer with detail only when necessary. Any explanation you give will prompt further questions. You are not giving a deposition to help the opposing side. Do not suggest areas of questioning or help the attorney ask the question. If you do not understand a question, say so. Do not answer a question that you do not understand. Ask the attorney to rephrase it. You are not required to answer all questions. There may be occasions when you do not know or remember the answer. Respond accordingly. Do not guess or speculate about an answer. If at the conclusion of the process, you believe the plaintiff's attorney has failed to ask you questions on an important aspect of the case, do not worry. That does not preclude you from commenting on the subject at trial. This is the plaintiff's attorney's opportunity to learn all information that he or she believes is relevant and important to the plaintiff's case. Your deposition is generally not the time for you to win the case. Save your arguments for the jury.

There are three means to testify regarding involvement with a patient. First, you can testify to things you remember. If an event was catastrophic, you may well remember details clearly. If the patient's care was not appreciably different from that of any other patient and a significant amount of time has passed, you may not remember the case at all. Second, you may testify to what is found in the patient care record. While you may not specifically remember that the patient's blood pressure was 120/80 on arrival in the postanesthesia recovery area, the chart indicates that is the fact. Therefore you can say without hesitation what the blood pressure reading was at that time. Similarly, with other aspects of your documentation, you can refer to the record when answering questions. Third, you can testify from habitual conduct. Many things that you do every day are not documented. One cannot document every single aspect of care. However, if you routinely perform a function, you can say you are sure to have performed that act in this case simply because it is your habit. Feel free to testify along those lines. For example, if you routinely follow a check process when setting up your machine for an anesthetic, that fact may not be documented and you may not be able to visualize the process in this particular case. However, if you have followed the same procedure with every case for a long period of time, you can say without hesitation that you checked the machine and equipment in this case. Do not hesitate to testify to facts that fall within your habit, routine, or custom of practice.

Because brain injury or death and other respiratory complications are often the issues when an anesthetist is a defendant in a medical negligence action, a plaintiff's attorney will try to establish events on a minute by minute basis. Discuss with your attorney before the deposition how to approach this subject. Hypoxia and injury occur and become permanent within a very few minutes. Therefore the plaintiff's attorney will attempt to show inappropriate judgments, inattention, or negligent conduct during the critical minutes. Anesthetic records generally provide an accounting of vital signs every 5 minutes. Establishing exactly what occurred between the recorded vital signs is often difficult. Health care personnel use terms that may seem harsh to laypersons. Consider your phraseology and discuss key terms with your counsel before a deposition. As an example, brain-damaged infants are often called "bad babies" in loose conversation. A plaintiff's attorney can make you seem cruel and insensitive for associating a negative term with a helpless infant who has been irreparably damaged due to the negligence of health care providers.

Only parties to the lawsuit, the plaintiff and defendants, their attorneys, the court reporter, and the witness may attend depositions, absent agreement among the parties to the contrary. It is common to take a short break every hour or so. As a witness, you do not want to become overly tired when answering questions. Breaks help refresh you and help keep your mind focused. You can confer with your counsel out of the earshot of all others any time you desire. You have the opportunity to review your deposition after the reporter has transcribed it. Take that opportunity to make *careful and detailed reviews and correct any errors that have been made.*

Your second opportunity to testify is at trial. Needless to say you will spend considerable time with your attorney in preparation. The same cautions apply at trial as in your deposition. In addition to your words, the jury will evaluate your demeanor. You may be called to testify by the plaintiff to establish the events in issue. Seldom can the plaintiff describe to the jury what transpired in the operating room. The health care providers must set the stage for the plaintiff to attempt to prove his or her theories of negligence and show the injury and damage which resulted. Trial testimony is extremely individualized depending on the facts, attorney preference, strengths of the witness, and trial strategy, among other things. This is the main event. Do not spare time in preparation and listen to your attorney's advice.

TIPS FOR AVOIDING LITIGATION

Goals set by every CRNA include helping patients to the best of one's ability, avoiding injury to a patient at all costs, and avoiding involvement as a defendant in a medical negligence action. Avoiding litigation begins with anesthesia education. Attitudes of respect for the patient and caution in treatment decisions set the stage for your career and impact directly on your involvement in situations where medical negligence might occur. One cannot prevent a patient from suing. One can, however, be in the best possible position, should suit be filed. This attitude and manner of conducting oneself may deter some attorney from actually filing the lawsuit.

Communications with Patients and Families

Patients and families should all be treated with respect. Surgery and an anesthetic are significant events in a person's lifetime; consequently, the patient and family deserve time and attention to properly prepare and decrease their anxiety. It cannot be stressed enough that should significant patient complications arise perioperatively, especially those associated with a bad patient outcome, families should be informed immediately. Events can be described in general terms and the CRNA should provide a clear description of what treatments, therapies, interventions, and follow-up care has been planned for the patient. The CRNA should be available periodically throughout follow-up care and should be actively involved in discussions with the family regarding the patient's progress. Often patients and families sue based not on patient outcome alone, but rather on a perceived lack of sensitivity or understanding of the gravity of the situation by the provider.

Obtaining Informed Consent

A patient's memory for details and discussions of informed consent is poor.[2] However, the discussion should go forward, with family members in attendance if the patient desires. The entire process should be documented. List the family members present, for example, husband, aunt, adult daughter, and so on. List the risks of the anesthetic that are discussed. Death, although a rare event, should also be mentioned. List the options of anesthetics discussed. If one option is discarded in favor of another based on patient preference, document this fact. If the option of anesthetic technique selected by the patient is not as advisable as the discarded option, detail this discussion in the patient record. Anesthetic options assume that more than one technique can satisfactorily be accomplished taking into account the patient's condition and requirements of the surgeon. Many institutions are employing a consent form for the anesthetic similar to the one the patient signs authorizing the surgical procedure. The consent form validates that the anesthetist explained the risks and options associated with the procedure and that the patient knew and accepted this information before agreeing to proceed. These forms are proving helpful in defending patient claims of no knowledge of possible death or injury associated with the anesthetic. If an institution provides separate surgical and anesthesia consent forms, both should be signed by the patient. In those cases, the surgical consent alone may not provide sufficiently broad consent for anesthesia.

Documenting Review of Patient Records

The patient's medical history given should be taken carefully and comprehensively and compared with the documented physician history (by surgeon or referral physician). If an anesthesiologist or other CRNA has completed the patient's history and physical, be sure to document on the chart or operating room record that you have been apprised of that information before you administer the anesthetic. By assuming duty for the case, you assume responsibility for all perioperative activities including a competent anesthesia workup.

The respiratory, cardiovascular, and airway examinations are most relevant for anesthetists as failed intubations account for a significant number of anesthetic mishaps. Anticipating potential airway difficulties, via a competent and documented airway examination, will generally result in avoiding patient injury and exposing oneself to litigation. A special anesthesia checklist with blanks for elaborating on information received is an excellent method for documenting the procedure. As always, equipment and machine checks should be documented on the operating room record which attests to proper function and acquisition of baseline physiologic data.

Do not limit your ability to prove that you provided standard of care treatment to a patient by failing to document your actions in the operating room or any other anesthetic setting. Fill out the record completely regardless of whether the case involves sedation and monitoring or a complicated general anesthetic. Sophisticated monitoring of cardiorespiratory status is now commonplace. The information from these monitors must be recorded on the patient record frequently to show you were aware of the readings and that they fell within normal parameters. If the readings are outside normal parameters, a resultant adjustment in the anesthetic should be reflected on the record as well.

In an emergency situation the patient becomes the priority, providing less time for detailed record keeping. During these periods, make short and cryptic notes of vital signs, monitor readings and medications. Once the emergency has passed, complete the anesthetic record as soon as possible. If the patient can safely be left in the care of others, find a quiet place to sit and complete your anesthetic record without distraction. If the timing of events is only approximate, indicate that fact. Review the record carefully to see if all information available has been included. Avoid leaving large gaps in vital sign or monitoring readings. If the original record is illegible, rewrite the entire anesthetic record in clear handwriting immediately after the crisis has passed and place it with the patient record. The legible record should contain the same, but more detailed information than the illegible original. Discard the illegible copy. Do not confuse completing a record with altering an already completed record.

Do not feel restricted to document only on the anesthetic record after a crisis has occurred during an anesthetic. In order to fully document the situation, a dictated or longhand progress note may be indicated. This note should also reflect any conferences with family members after the emergency. Again, list the individuals present for the conference and the general nature of the information you relayed. Note the family response if it seems threatening or out of the ordinary for the circumstances.

Routine Postoperative Patient Follow-up

Crisis or no crisis, you will want to follow-up with your patient after he or she has recovered from the anesthetic. If the patient has a complaint, you may be able to explain why the discomfort was necessary. Your obvious concern for the patient goes far toward avoiding a formal lawsuit. As before, document the substance of the postoperative visit, including all patient complaints and your response. Occasionally a patient complains and files suit much later alleging pain during or a memory of the procedure. However, if the patient voiced no such complaint to anesthesia or hospital personnel, the claim is not likely to prevail. Always make a note of this factor after an anesthetic. Also be sure you have documented that you have transferred care to appropriately licensed individuals in the postanesthesia care unit (PACU) or intensive care unit (ICU) before beginning another case. Remember to maintain continuity in care.

Maintaining and Documenting Standards of Care

At all times, maintain familiarity with standards of care promulgated by anesthesia specialty organizations, the AANA and ASA. These are the academic and clinical constructs against which your performance will be measured. Always pattern your practice in accordance with these standards and fashion your anesthesia record to reflect their implementation. If a patient files a medical negligence action, an attorney will review the case before proceeding to determine its merits. In addition, an expert review before the filing of a lawsuit is obtained by most reputable plaintiff's attorneys, again to assess merit. If the attorney and expert consultant can find no deviation from the appropriate standard of care on your part, based on the patient's record, there is an excellent chance the lawsuit will never be filed.

As a final point in discussing documentation, the question arises as to whether the anesthetist should prepare a set of personal notes describing some crisis event. The better response is "no." The patient record should reflect the patient's condition, treatment provided, and patient's response. A set of personal notes should not elaborate on these items. Generally, an anesthetist considers writing personal notes when disagreement or conflict has occurred. Again the better suggestion is not to undertake the effort of detailing a conflict. Such personal notes prepared without advice and direction of counsel are generally subject to discovery if a lawsuit results. Calmer heads will prevail later. Memorialized conflicts will little serve anyone's purpose at that time.

The Importance of Credentialing

Provider credentialing has become an important issue for hospital administrators and risk managers. Initial credentialing verifies that a health care provider has the requisite licenses, certifications, and education to perform the requirements of the specialty. Repeat credentialing verifies that continuing education and licensure requirements are maintained. This supports the anesthetist's statements that care provided to patients meets appropriate standards and that the anesthetist maintains state-of-the-art techniques and knowledge.

Professional and community participation play a role in one's likelihood of involvement in a medical negligence lawsuit. This is especially true if one lives and works in a smaller community. If one lives a life-style of helping and caring for others, and maintains high personal and professional standards, prospective plaintiffs are less likely to sue, prospective plaintiffs' attorneys are less likely to pursue the case, and prospective expert witnesses for the plaintiff are less likely to agree to testify. Hesitation at any one of the three links in the chain may result in no medical negligence action, or a failed or abandoned action.

TORT REFORM

As mentioned earlier in this chapter, the late 1970s saw a substantial increase in medical negligence cases and plaintiffs' verdicts. Pretrial settlements also increased dramatically as a result of the jury verdicts. Seven of 10 insurance companies that previously wrote policies of professional liability coverage limited that coverage. Some companies quit the market and stopped writing this insurance in any form. Other companies kept their current professional liability clients but took on no new customers. Still others placed limits on the amount of liability coverage that a health care provider or facility could purchase. These actions by the insurance industry resulted in an "availability crisis." There was not enough insurance available to be purchased to provide coverage to all health care providers.

As the jury awards and settlement costs escalated, insurance companies sought to offset losses and protect against future losses by raising premiums dramatically. In some geographic and specialty areas, premiums increased as much as 410 percent.[11] Hence an "affordability crisis" resulted. Even if a health care provider could find professional liability insurance coverage, he or she might not be able to afford the premium charge.

Obviously, the health care profession responded to these dramatic changes. Some of the responses had an adverse effect on the consuming public. Providers near the age of retirement simply left practice. Subsequent to large numbers of early retirements, communities were left with limited or no provider services and other severely limited portions of practice. The high-risk procedures and specialty areas were eliminated from their practice, thus allowing the cost of the insurance premium to decrease to an affordable price. The most common example was the family practitioner who stopped delivering babies. This decreased the family practitioner's premium and allowed him or her to continue the practice of medicine. However, the community was left with fewer or no persons to provide the necessary health care to expectant mothers. Some hospitals closed emergency rooms to avoid exposure to liability in this high-risk setting. Hospitals also reviewed and restricted physician privileges for the higher-risk procedures, decreasing the facility's exposure to liability. This trend also further constricted the availability of health care to the public. Many surgical and obstetrical procedures once performed in the community hospital were restricted and only available in larger institutions.

In response to these crisis situations, legislatures in many states enacted laws that changed the common law system of recovery for negligence. Many states enacted tort reform bills and eventually some general categories of tort reform emerged. For instance, caps were placed on the dollar figure that an injured plaintiff could recover for noneconomic losses. Some states placed a flat amount on this recovery: for example; Kansas limited the recovery to $250,000 per injury. Other states allowed the cap to float based on a complicated economic analysis tied to inflation. Currently, Missouri places this recovery at $450,000 per plaintiff and per defendant. This method encourages the plaintiff to name multiple defendants so that $450,000 in noneconomic losses can potentially be collected from each defendant. Other states that passed laws limiting noneconomic damages include Indiana, Idaho, Virginia, Georgia, and Oregon. The reader should note that the lists of states enacting various tort reform measures mentioned throughout this section are not exhaustive; rather, they give examples of states making the changes referenced.

Traditionally, courts have not allowed juries to consider evidence of collateral sources that may have paid for past or will pay for future economic damages. *Collateral sources* are sources of money outside the plaintiff's personal assets that pay the bills. Collateral sources frequently include insurance benefits, such as health or disability insurance, therapy services available to children in the public school system, and Social Security benefits for loss of a parent or physical disability. The original rationale for excluding this evidence from the jury's consideration went something like this. If an injured plaintiff had been frugal enough to purchase insurance, he or she should not be penalized by this frugality from recovering full damages. This rationale allows the plaintiff a double recovery. First, the insurance company pays the medical bill and second, the plaintiff recovers the amount of the medical bill as part of the judgment in the lawsuit and is able to pocket that money. Defense attorneys have long argued that public sources of benefits and services should not be considered collateral sources and thereby excluded from evidence under the old rule.

Traditionally the courts have not been swayed by these arguments and have excluded all evidence relating to payment of plaintiff's damages by outside sources. Several states have passed legislation to change this rule, Alabama, Georgia, Iowa, Kansas, and North Dakota among them. Generally, under these changes the jury may consider the fact that bills are paid by an outside source. The plaintiff can then introduce evidence of expenses associated with purchasing the insurance that has paid the bill, that is, past insurance premiums as an offset against the actual insurance payment of the plaintiff's incurred expense. The jury then considers all the relevant facts relating to the plaintiff's economic claims and sources available to pay them. From a defense standpoint, this can greatly reduce the value of a plaintiff's economic damage claims, both for past and future damages. This is especially true in the catastrophic cases.

Similarly, several states have enacted laws allowing the defendant to pay the plaintiff's future economic losses in periodic payments, into the future. If the plaintiff claims he or she will incur medical expenses of $100,000 per year for each of the next 20 years, for example, the defendant can pay this amount in the future under the continued supervision of the court. Alabama, Connecticut, Idaho, Iowa, Kansas, Montana, New York, North Dakota, and South Dakota have all enacted some form of legislation allowing periodic payment of a large jury verdict.[14]

Another major tort reform measure involves constricting the statute of limitations. The statute of limitations sets an outside time limit for filing a lawsuit. Shortening the statute of limitations forces a plaintiff to file suit within a prescribed time period or lose the claim altogether. Stale claims are more difficult to defend as records may be lost or destroyed, witnesses move away or die, and the standard of care is more difficult to establish because of the changes in knowledge and advanced technology that have developed in the interim. Witnesses have difficulty remembering exactly how things operated several years prior. Georgia, Kansas, Maryland, Montana, and Virginia have passed laws enacting changes in the statute of limitations applicable to medical negligence actions.

There has been considerable debate over the proportion of the award or settlement paid to the plaintiff's attorney in fees. Some attorney-client agreements call for as much as 50 percent of any recovery to be paid to the plaintiff's attorney. These are called *contingency fee arrangements.* The plaintiff pays the attorney nothing if there is no money recovered. If there is a recovery, the plaintiff agrees to pay his or her attorney a percentage of that amount. The plaintiff's bar of attorneys attempts to justify these arrangements by pointing out that it is the attorney who fronts the cost of the litigation which can easily amount to $50,000. It is actually the plaintiff's attorney who risks this investment if there is no recovery. The plaintiff generally cannot afford to front the cost of litigation or repay the attorney if there is no recovery, or a very limited recovery. However, it is easy to imagine that these fee arrangements hamper settlement negotiations. An offer of settlement that reasonably compensates the plaintiff for his or her losses becomes unreasonable after the plaintiff's attorney calculates his or her fee.

In an effort to control this process several states enacted laws that specifically limit attorney's contingent fee awards, or call on the court to review each settlement or verdict and the attorney fee to be paid from the money recovered. The court may approve the proposed arrangement or order an adjustment, as it sees fit. Some states that have enacted such laws include Connecticut, Hawaii, Kansas, and New Hampshire.

Comparative fault is the comparison of liability among individuals and entities that had a role in the alleged injury. The rules of comparative fault vary significantly from state to state. Some allow comparison of all involved in the injury, including parties and nonparties. Some allow comparison among only those who are parties to the lawsuit. Tort reform adopted in several states enacted a form of comparative fault. It also generally abolished or modified joint and several liability. *Joint and several liability* means that regardless of your percentage of fault, if you have even 1 percent of the adjudged fault, you are responsible for paying the plaintiff's entire verdict. It is then your right to seek indemnity from the remaining defendants who were also judged to be at fault. The protection is for the plaintiff. This increases the plaintiff's chances of recovering his or her verdict in full. The burden shifts to the defendants to recover the disproportionate share of payment to the plaintiff from one another. Joint and several liability encourages the plaintiff to sue several defendants for fear that the most culpable would not have adequate insurance coverage to pay the verdict. Minor defendants, or those with very limited exposure, were added to ensure that adequate funds would be available to pay any award. This made it difficult to negotiate a reasonable settlement on behalf of a minor defendant. States that enacted some form of comparative fault or modified or eliminated their prior system of joint and several liability include Arizona, Colorado, Connecticut, Georgia, Idaho, Louisiana, Missouri, Nevada, New Mexico, North Dakota, and Texas.

In addition, during the late 1970s and early 1980s, there were several large punitive damage awards. It is the rare circumstance that a health care provider intentionally injures a patient. The threat of punitive damages, which are compensable by the individual defendant only, is very intimidating. Legislatures in several states placed significant restraints on punitive damage awards to make them less desirable for the plaintiff to pursue. For example, 50 percent of any punitive damage award in Kansas is paid to the Kansas Health Care Stabilization Fund, a patient compensation fund. Also, the award is limited based on the health care provider's average income over a period of several years. Other states that have modified the punitive damages allowed in a medical negligence action include Alabama, Florida, Georgia, Indiana, Idaho, Iowa, Missouri, Montana, North Dakota, Oregon, Virginia, and Texas.[15]

Several areas of tort reform are of a less dramatic nature and can be quickly summarized with their representative states briefly noted. Some states enact laws to make settlement conferences in medical negligence cases mandatory prior to trial. Examples of these states include Kansas and Ohio. Some states require arbitration of the claims in certain circumstances. A system for operating medical negligence screening panels was devised. These panels, generally made up of health care professionals, determine, by reviewing documents submitted by opposing sides, whether or not negligence has occurred. This is accomplished before expensive discovery is undertaken. States enacting some form of pretrial screening panels include Arizona and Kansas.

As one means of offsetting the legislated limitation on a plaintiff's award or other aspect of proceeding with a medical negligence action, some states require that all health care providers maintain professional liability insurance coverage. Through this requirement an injured plaintiff is assured that money is available to pay a verdict or settlement. During the affordability and availability crisis, some providers "went bare," or practiced without liability insurance coverage. With careful asset management, the health care provider could pay nothing after a jury verdict was rendered. As another means of assuring that compensation is available for an injured party at the conclusion of a medical negligence action, compensation funds were established in some states. Health care providers all contribute to the fund and payments are made to the injured plaintiff according to the specific legislated requirements.[11]

One often-cited problem with our court system, and particularly with medical cases, is the expense of the litigation. Frivolous cases require just as much time, money, and effort to defend as legitimate cases. In an effort to stem the filing of frivolous lawsuits against health care providers, several states enacted provisions that penalize the plaintiff or plaintiff's attorney if the court determines the case is frivolous. Monetary sanctions may be assessed to pay the defendant's court costs and attorney fees, or double these figures. States that enacted variations on these penalty arrangements include Alabama, Connecticut, Georgia, Illinois, Michigan, Minnesota, New York, Oklahoma, Texas, Virginia, and Wyoming.

In addition to making legislative changes in how the injured plaintiff can pursue a medical negligence action and be compensated at its conclusion, some states attempted to improve the practice by establishing quality assurance and risk management procedures in health care facilities. Instances of potential patient injury or potential medical negligence were required to be reported to state agencies, that is, the professional's licensing agency. States that expanded their required peer review system in some manner include Arizona, Indiana, Kansas, Maryland, Oklahoma, and Wyoming.

Because all of the aforementioned statutory changes affect the rights of an injured plaintiff in pursuing a claim of medical negligence, the acts generally apply to incidents occurring after the date the laws are enacted. Therefore, a significant lag time occurs between the enactment of the statutes and their application to specific lawsuits. For instance, if a state enacted tort reform legislation January 1, 1980, it would likely affect only events occurring after that date. There is generally a delay between the medical care that the plaintiff claims was negligent and the filing of a lawsuit, often as much as 2 years. Depending on the jurisdiction, it may take 2 to 4 years for a case to come to trial. Therefore, in this timeline example, the laws passed on January 1, 1980 may not be considered by a court until January 1, 1986. The appellate court process may encompass an additional 2 years. One can see that a definitive court ruling on the validity of tort reform legislation may not be available until 8 years or longer in some states, after the laws went into effect. If the courts strike down some or all of the laws the state legislature must start over and enact additional tort reform laws that the appellate courts will likely uphold.

Generally a trial court follows the laws as enacted by the legislature and leaves it to the appellate courts to determine if the laws "pass muster," or are constitutionally firm or infirm. The most frequent challenges of tort reform legislation claim the laws invade a plaintiff's constitutionally protected rights of equal protection, right to a jury trial, right to free access to the courts, and generally limit the common law rights without providing an adequate "quid pro quo." *Quid pro quo* means something for something. A tort is a common law cause of action. A legislature may alter that common law action when it serves the public good. However, something must be given in exchange. As an example, the legislature caps the noneconomic recovery award but provides for mandatory professional liability insurance so that availability of funds to pay the award is assured.

The equal protection argument generally claims that health care providers are not a special class of citizens, such as minorities or women. Therefore they should not be given special consideration through tort reform laws. The plaintiff claims it is unconstitutional to affect his or her rights of recovery in a medical negligence case in favor of the health care provider. Such special laws generally do not affect personal injury claims caused by a negligently maintained swimming pool, or by a negligent automobile driver. On a similar basis, the plaintiff claims these laws limit his or her ability to have free access to the court and jury. Shortening the statute of limitations, for example, allegedly limits access to the court system. Presenting evidence of collateral sources allegedly limits the plaintiff's right to be fully compensated for his or her damages. Similar arguments are made with regard to noneconomic caps on recovery and other aspects of tort reform legislation.

This author tried a lawsuit in 1991 involving allegations of negligence among anesthetists. This case tested Missouri's tort reform package. Some defendants settled before trial for a total of $6 million. The jury was not made aware of these settlements. A verdict was rendered by the jury for a total of $20 million. If the tort reform package had been held unconstitutional, the anesthetist who proceeded to trial would have been assessed $3.5 million of the award. The tort reform was held constitutional, thereby limiting that defendant's share of the verdict to $1.5 million.[16] A hospital defendant also will pay approximately $1.5 million under the verdict. The plaintiff claims $9 million is insufficient compensation for the injury. How much can be spent on a neurologically damaged individual during a lifetime? How much can our health care system afford in compensation for an unfortunate and sometimes tragic outcome?

It has been estimated that the indirect cost of practicing defensive medicine was $10.6 billion in 1984.[11] There is no reason to believe that figure has decreased in the interim. Indirect costs include increased record keeping, ordering additional treatments and tests, scheduling more follow-up visits than medically indicated, and so on. One prime example of defensive medicine is the high percentage of cesarean sections performed in this country. Defensive medicine also results in negative aspects of patient treatment. Sometimes diagnostic tests are withheld because of the risk of the procedure. A less extensive operative procedure may be selected because there is less risk of patient injury and possible litigation. There are other affects on patient services such as a decrease in the availability of subspecialties and advanced technology in rural areas. The rural health care setting is especially hard hit. Reimbursement is often lower for an identical procedure carried out in a rural setting as compared with the urban setting. Fewer of high-revenue procedures are performed in rural areas. All of this contributes to a disproportionate burden on the rural health care provider who must purchase professional liability insurance coverage.

The appellate courts have reviewed the tort reform measures in most states and in most areas of the reform effort by this time. Perhaps the greatest amount of court activity has focused on legislative limitations on noneconomic or punitive damage awards. Kansas,[17] Indiana,[18] Louisiana,[19] Maryland,[20] Missouri,[16] and Virginia[21] have found these limitations constitutional. Alabama,[22] Florida,[23] New Hampshire,[24] Texas,[25] and Washington[26] courts have struck down such provisions, finding them unconstitutional. Colorado courts applied the laws to specific cases without the parties raising a constitutional challenge. Hawaii and Minnesota have repealed their laws limiting damage awards.

The majority of the courts that have considered a modification of the statute of limitations have found these changes constitutional, including Idaho,[27] Illinois,[28] Indiana,[29] Iowa,[30] Louisiana,[31] Maryland,[32] Minnesota,[33] and Texas.[34] Generally this type of change is easier to justify to the court. The plaintiff's cause of action has not been taken away. The only change is a shortened period of time within which to initiate the lawsuit. However, this view has not been universal. Arizona, New Hampshire,[35] and Oklahoma[36] courts have struck down legislative efforts to limit the statute of limitations. Washington courts have applied the limitation without a constitutional challenge.

The majority of the courts that have considered laws which modify the joint and several liability provisions, implementing a form of comparative fault, have found them constitutional. Colorado,[37] Connecticut,[38] Florida,[39] Missouri,[16] and North Dakota[40] have followed this rule. Several states have applied these provisions without a constitutional challenge: Alaska, Arizona, Georgia, Iowa, Louisiana, New York, Texas, and Washington inclusive.

The elimination of the collateral source rule has sparked a more varied response among the appellate courts that have considered it. Arizona,[41] Illinois,[42] and Minnesota[43] have approved the provisions as constitutional. Georgia[44] and New Hampshire[35] have found them unconstitutional. Florida and New York have implemented the changes without a constitutional challenge. In catastrophic cases where a minor plaintiff is involved, this rule can reduce the plaintiff's damage claim by millions of dollars. It is a very positive benefit for the defense.

The pretrial screening panel does not generally preclude the plaintiff from proceeding with a jury trial after the panel renders an opinion regarding the elements raised by the plaintiff. The format for the panels vary considerably from state to state. All states that considered the constitutionality of pretrial screening panels upheld the laws. These states include Arizona,[41] Florida,[45] Idaho, Illinois,[46] Indiana,[18] Louisiana,[47] Maryland,[48] Michigan,[49] and New York.[50]

The structuring of payment of future damage awards is not an actual limitation on the money the plaintiff recovers. Rather, future damages are paid in the future under court supervision. Florida,[39] Illinois,[42] and Missouri[16] upheld these provisions, while New Hampshire[35] did not. Alabama has applied the statute without a constitutional challenge.

Courts are generally reluctant to interfere

in the contract arrangements between a client and attorney. Few states enacted statutes actually limiting the contingent fees of attorneys. New Hampshire[35] found this provision unconstitutional, as it found all other aspects of tort reform unconstitutional. Illinois and New York have applied the provision without a constitutional test.

Courts have been inclined to uphold provisions which assess penalties against the plaintiff and/or plaintiff's attorney who file a frivolous action. Washington[51] is a prime example. The majority of states have simply applied the legislative provisions without a legal challenge. This is true in Colorado, Georgia, Louisiana, Maryland, New York, and Virginia.

In some instances the legislature has enacted additional laws based on the rulings of the appellate courts. For instance, in Kansas the original tort reform measure limited noneconomic damage awards in medical negligence actions only. The Kansas Supreme Court ruled that the law was unfair because it applied to this limited type of cases. Another statute was then passed which applied to all types of personal injury actions.

It has been difficult to evaluate the overall effectiveness of tort reform. There are various effective dates even within one chapter of statutes in a given state, therefore implementation is staggered. Also, there is a significant delay between enactment of the laws and the judicial review, as mentioned earlier. There is no scientific methodology in place to make the evaluation. Finally, at this point in time, there is a very small database.

Tort reform may limit the financial burden medical negligence lawsuits place on an already overburdened court and health care system. However, this is not the ideal mechanism to check and verify that appropriate standards of care are followed. Other forums such as quality assurance, risk management, and credentialing procedures address these issues, as do state licensing and regulatory boards and impaired practitioner programs. On a national basis, federal peer review organizations and the Joint Commission on Accreditation of Health Care Organizations (JCAHO) require reporting of settlements and judgments. These methods are more likely to have an immediate effect on an individual's practice.

PROFESSIONAL LIABILITY INSURANCE

In general, there are two types of policies written by professional liability insurance companies: occurrence and claims made. Occurrence is by far the preferable type. This type of policy was available generally through the mid- to late 1970s when the medical negligence crisis hit. It is still occasionally available today. However, most sources of medical negligence insurance write only claims made policies at this time.

An occurrence policy covers the insured for all acts occurring within the policy period, regardless of when the lawsuit is filed. If you purchased an occurrence policy for the calendar year 1985 and a minor child filed a negligence claim in 1992, you would be covered under your 1985 policy assuming that is when the alleged negligence occurred. This is obviously favorable to the CRNA. It does, however, make long-range risk and liability planning difficult for the entity that provided coverage. In this circumstance you may have had insurance coverage with this company only one year, 1985. You only paid one premium, in 1985. Yet the company is responsible for defending the lawsuit filed against you in 1992.

A claims made policy is much less favorable for the insured CRNA. Under a claims made policy, you must have coverage at the time of the incident, continuously through the date the claim is made or the lawsuit is filed. To have coverage in the example above, you would have to purchase the insurance in 1985 and maintain coverage continuously with that company through 1992, the time the lawsuit is filed. Obviously the insurance company has several advantages. The early years with an insurance company are relatively low risk. It is not often that an act leading to a lawsuit and the lawsuit occur in the same policy year. Therefore, the company can collect several years of premiums before having to defend a lawsuit. Also, the company's risk begins, as above, in 1985. If you had any anesthetic mishap before 1985, it is not the responsibility of this company. You have no negative history to begin the policy period with. This type of policy also encourages the CRNA to remain with one company over a long period of time, stabilizing the market from the company's point of view. Terminating coverage with the company terminates the company's risk with respect to future claims or lawsuits.

There are ways for a CRNA to change professional liability insurance carriers and maintain continuous coverage. This brings into play two additional insurance terms, retroactive date, often called retro date, and tail coverage. The *retroactive date* is the date for which coverage for incidents begins. One can purchase liability coverage for a time period preceeding the actual date coverage is purchased. For example, if you purchase claims made insurance on January 1, 1992 but have practiced anesthesia since 1990, you may want to purchase coverage for events that may materialize into claims or lawsuits back through 1990. In your policy, the retro date would read January 1, 1990. Any number of years of retroactive coverage is available for a quoted price. The length of time you purchase will depend on a number of individual factors, including your state's statutes of limitation and the length of time you have practiced.

At the other end of the picture is tail coverage. When one is canceling insurance for any reason, it is possible to purchase tail coverage. *Tail coverage* provides insurance benefits in the future for events that may have occurred during the time the insurance you are now canceling was in effect. Using the same years as before, if you maintained claims made insurance with the same company from 1985 through 1992 and canceled, you may be able to purchase tail coverage from that company at the time of cancellation. The tail coverage would provide benefits for a specified number of years into the future, for claims and suits arising from care rendered during the policy years 1985 through 1992. The number of years for which you should have tail coverage varies as with retro dates.

Many people purchase tail coverage on retirement or when moving to a different state where their prior company does not sell insurance. Obviously, one would want to price shop to see if tail coverage or retroactive coverage is the most economical, assuming one is continuing to practice.

Limits of professional liability coverage have two components. The limits are indicated with a slash mark between two numbers, for example, $1,000,000/$3,000,000. This means $1 million in liability coverage is available for any one event in a policy year. Remember, one event may have more than one plaintiff, for example, husband injured and suing for physical injuries and wife suing for loss of consortium. Three million dollars in coverage is available for any number of events in the policy year. These limits concern the payment of verdicts and settlements only. They are not depleted by the expenses incurred in litigation, for example, attorney's fees, deposition and expert charges, and so on.

As you have seen through statistics and examples sited in this chapter, injuries sustained as a result of anesthesia negligence have catastrophic results. Therefore, large limits in liability coverage are recommended. An active practicing CRNA should not carry insurance limits below the $1 million/$3 million example used herein. To carry lower limits exposes your personal assets to attachment and liquidation in order to pay a large judgment.

Your policy details what is and is not covered in your defense. In general, however, all judgments and settlements within the limits are covered. Expenses of litigation are covered. These include fees paid to your attorney, fees paid to expert witnesses, costs of depositions, costs of creating demonstrative exhibits, costs associated with collecting medical records, and numerous other expenses which amount to a significant expenditure when added together. Your insurance covers events occurring within the course and scope of your duties as an anesthetist. Specific exclusions may exist in your policy and you should be aware of these to avoid practicing in a setting where you have no coverage. A policy may cover you while you practice in one state only. This would limit crossing a state line or moving about the nation in a locum tenens arrangement. A policy may cover you while working for your employer only. This would limit freelance arrangements on your spare time. Policies are limited to acts falling within the scope and practice of anesthesia services. While not seen frequently in the anesthesia profession, a claim of improper touching or fondling of a patient may not be covered under your policy.

Professional liability insurance coverage is

available from several types of companies or sources. An insurance company is the most obvious, but not necessarily the most common source, for example, St. Paul Fire & Marine Insurance Company. Many groups of physicians or hospitals have collaborated to form privately owned and operated mutual insurance companies. Some groups with substantial financial backing have self-insured their prospective liability expenses and exposure. These are often health maintenance organizations, hospital chains, or state university facilities. If coverage is not available to a CRNA through one of these means, there may be a patient compensation fund (PCF) in your state. Eleven states operate such funds which assure the public that health care providers in the state will have liability coverage should a judgment be entered against them.

Finally, a joint underwriting association (JUA) may be available. This may be referred to as a high-risk pool. The purpose of a JUA is to provide professional liability insurance for providers who in good faith are entitled to coverage but who are unable to procure even basic insurance from traditional markets.

Availability of medical negligence liability coverage is no longer a problem. Significant changes in the types of insurance policies have prompted claims made policies to replace occurrence policies for all intents and purposes. Deductions have become commonplace, especially with institutional clients. This allows the facility to settle smaller claims and avoid reflections on its premium assessment. The amount of liability limits has also decreased substantially. Limits exceeding $1 million were commonplace in the early 1970s. The cost was low because verdicts had not reached these figures in the past. Lowered limits protect the company in the event of catastrophic cases. Exclusions have been placed in policies and the price or cost to the health care provider for liability coverage has increased dramatically, making the business more profitable for the company.

SUMMARY

It should be obvious to every CRNA and student anesthetist that an in-depth knowledge of the legal system of this country, especially as it relates to malpractice litigation, is mandatory. Both time and care should be taken by the CRNA to meticulously document their standard of care, become familiar with the process of deposition and testimony, and know how to effectively support their attorney's effort to procure a positive outcome for the provider.

REFERENCES

1. Cheney, FW, et al: Standard of care and anesthesia liability. JAMA 261:1599, 1989.
2. Cassileth, BR, et al: Informed consent—why are its goals imperfectly realized? N Engl J Med 302(16):910, 1980.
3. Orkin, FK: Practice standards: The Midas touch or the emperor's new clothes? Anesthesiology 70:567, 1989.
4. Committee on Professional Liability, American Society of Anesthesiologists (ASA).
5. PHICO Insurance Co.
6. Cheney, FW: University of Washington Department of Anesthesia, Seattle, 1988.
7. Caplan, RA, et al: Adverse respiratory events in anesthesia: A closed claims analysis. Anesthesiology 72:828, 1990.
8. *Brown v. United States*, 419 F.2d 337, 341 (1969), Mo. cite - 66C385 (2), E.D., Missouri, E.D.
9. Garnick, DW, Hendricks, AM, and Brennan, TA: Can practice guidelines reduce the number and costs of malpractice claims? JAMA 226:2856, 1991.
10. *Mohr v. Jenkins*, 393 S.2d 245 (Court of Appeals of Louisiana, First Circuit, 1980). K.S.A. 60-3412.
11. Halley, MM, et al: Medical Malpractice Solutions Systems and Proposals for Injury Compensation. Charles C Thomas, Springfield, IL, 1989.
12. K.S.A. 7-1216.
13. K.S.A. 60-3412.
14. Demkovich, L and Morritt, D: State Health Notes, Intergovernmental Health Policy Project, George Washington University, Washington, D.C., Number 78, July-August 1987, p. 1.
15. Tort reform made gains. Independent Agent, January 1988, p. 57.
16. *Adams v. Children's Mercy Hospital*, No. 73867, Slip op. (Mo., May 19, 1992) (en banc).
17. *Samsel v. Wheeler Transport Services, Inc.*, 246 Kan. 336, 337, 789 P.2d 5412 (1990).
18. *Johnson v. St. Vincent Hospital, Inc.*, 273 Ind. 374, 404 N.E. 2d 585 (Ind. 1980).
19. *LaMark v. NME Hospitals, Inc.*, 542 So.2d 753 (1989).
20. *Franklin v. Mazda Motor Corp.*, 704 F.Supp. 1325 (D.Md. 1989).
21. *Boyd v. Bulala*, 877 F.2d 1191 (4th Cir. 1989).
22. *Moore v. Mobile Infirmary Association*, 592 So.2d 156 (Ala. 1991).
23. *Smith v. Department of Insurance*, 507 S. 2d 1080 (Fla. 1987).
24. *Brannigan v. Usitalo*, 587 A.2d 1232 (1991).
25. *Wheat v. U.S.*, 860 F.2d, 1256 (Tx. 1988).
26. *Sofie v. Fibreboard Corporation*, 112 Wash 2d 636, 771 P.2d 711 (Wash. 1989).

27. *Hawley v. Green*, 117 Idaho 498, 788 P.2d 1321 (1990).
28. *Thompson v. Franciscan Sisters Health Care Corporation*, 218 Ill. App. 3d 406, 578 N.E. 2d 289 (1991).
29. *Douglas by Douglas v. Hugh A. Stallings, M.D., Inc.*, 870 F.2d 242 (7th Cir. 1989).
30. *Conner v. Fettkether*, 294 N.W. 2d 61 (1980).
31. *Montagina v. Canale*, 792 F.2d 554 (5th Cir. 1986).
32. *Jones v. Speed*, 577 A.2d 64 (1990).
33. *Willette v. Mayo Foundation*, 458 N.W.2d 120 (1990).
34. *Warner v. Sun Kavalli*, 795 S.W.2d 326 (1990).
35. *Carson v. Maurer*, 120 N.H. 925, 424 A.2d 825 (1980).
36. *Wafford v. Davis*, 764 P.2d 161 (1988).
37. *In re: Air Crash Disaster at Stapleton International Airport*, Denver Co. on November 15, 1987, 720 F. Supp. 1465 (D. Colo. 1989).
38. *Caman v. City of Stamford*, 746 F. Supp. 248 (D. Conn. 1990).
39. *Smith v. Insurance Department*, 507 So.2d 1080 (Fla. 1987).
40. *Kavadas v. Lorenzen*, 448 N.W. 2d 219 (1989).
41. *Eastin v. Broomfield*, 570 P.2d 744 (Ariz. 1977)
42. *Bernier v. Burris*, 497 N.E. 2d 763 (1986).
43. *Imlay v. City of Lake Crystal*, 444 N.W. 2d 594 (1989).
44. *Denton v. Con-Way S. Express*, 261 Ga. 41, 402 S.E. 2d 269 (1991).
45. *Pearlstein v. Malunney*, 500 So. 2d 585 (Fla. App. 2d Dist. 1986).
46. *Deluna v. St. Elizabeth's Hospital*, 147 Ill.2d 57, 588 N.E. 2d 1139 (Ill. 1992).
47. *Seoane v. Ortho Pharmaceuticals, Inc.*, 660 F.2d 146 (5th Cir. 1981).
48. *Robinson v. Pleet*, 544 A.2d 1 (1988).
49. *Brown v. Considine*, 108 Mich. App. 504, 310 N.W. 2d 441 (1981).
50. *Gronne v. Adams*, 793 F.2d 74 (C.A. 2, N.Y. 1986).
51. *Rhinehart v. Seattle Times*, 59 Wash. App. 332, 782 P.2d 1155 (1990).

14

Documenting Anesthesia Care

Cathy A. Mastropietro
Nancy Bruton-Maree

Outline

OBJECTIVES

On completing this chapter, the reader will be able to:

1. List the purposes and goals of perioperative charting.
2. Itemize the essential elements of perioperative documentation for the entire perioperative course, including preoperative note, intraoperative record, and postoperative note.
3. List requisite criteria to appear on the anesthesia record, including the machine check, selection, and implementation of monitoring, drug administration, anesthesia course, relief by other providers, disposition of patient in the PACU or intensive care unit (ICU), general and regional techniques, and untoward clinical events.
4. Recount important legal aspects of anesthesia charting including reference to erasures, record changes, legibility, defensive charting, disposition of records, and common problems associated with record-keeping.

GOALS FOR DOCUMENTING ANESTHESIA CARE

Documentation of anesthesia care had its beginning in 1894 when Cushing and Codman began to record pulse and respiration during administration of ether at Massachusetts General Hospital on early rudimentary records known as "ether charts." Since that time, documentation of anesthesia care has evolved into a complex written account of all aspects of anesthesia perioperative care.[1]

Technologic and pharmacologic advances have necessarily influenced the evolutionary development of complex charting by requiring the anesthetist to devote increasing attention to the myriad of details that need to be included in perioperative records. Therefore, the documents relating to anesthesia care must meet increasing standards for comprehensiveness, legibility, sequence, and information that bears a direct relationship to the complexity of patient management. Anesthesia documentation has become an important medicolegal document that serves a variety of purposes. Among these are:

1. To serve as a basis for planning anesthetic management and care and as a basis for establishing continuity in the evaluation of a patient's condition and treatment
2. To provide permanent, documentary evidence of the patient's anesthetic management
3. To document communication between the anesthetist responsible for the patient and any other health care professional who contributes to the patient's care
4. To assist in protecting the legal interest of the patient, the hospital, and the responsible anesthetist
5. To provide data for verifying compliance with standards of care and institutional policies and procedures
6. To supply an account of care that can be used in peer review procedures, and quality assurance activities, as well as staff education programs[2,3]

SETTING STANDARDS OF RECORD-KEEPING IN ANESTHESIA

The primary tenet that should underlay any philosophy of perioperative documentation is the understanding that written records should reflect the quality of care provided. Such quality, in turn, must be based on current professional practice standards. Standards of care are most appropriately defined by a national professional organization such as the American Association of Nurse Anesthetists (AANA), and adoption of standards of care places the responsibility for their implementation on the provider to know and demonstrate that current standards of practice are met. *Failure to demonstrate compliance with adopted standards of care makes negligence easier to prove in a court of law.* The AANA developed Standards of Nurse Anesthesia Practice in 1974 that guide the certified registered nurse anesthetist (CRNA) in the provision of safe, quality patient care (See Chapter 7). Standard V of that document addresses the anesthesia record.

In addition to those standards previously referenced, student nurse anesthetists and CRNAs alike should be aware that there are other sources of clinical standards. These sources may include certain government entities, such as those that relate to gaseous storage and anesthesia equipment. In addition, local hospital facilities may have standards relating to anesthesia documentation above and beyond those promulgated at a national level. Insurance companies that offer liability insurance are also beginning to introduce practice standards, the adoption of which is mandatory for those insured. Consequently, it is incumbent on all practitioners to survey the variety of clinical standards commonly accepted in practice, in addition to those that address the maintenance of clinical records directly.

Perioperative records are not limited only to intraoperative events. The standard of care is to maintain written preoperative assessment notes; a legal, signed patient consent form; documented equipment malfunction checklist; and a postoperative note, either as part of the anesthesia record or written in the progress notes of the chart. In addition, should an untoward event occur during the perioperative course, the anesthetist should provide a narrative description of events (in addition to those contained in the anesthesia record) that can be maintained as part of the patient's permanent health record.

In every case, the CRNA or other qualified anesthesia provider should begin maintenance of these records during the personal interview with the patient preoperatively. It cannot be emphasized strongly enough that the written record may be the only documentation that can justify the actions of an anesthetist if the case reaches litigation. As memories fade with time, anesthesia-related records become the clearest evidence of compliance with standards of care.

DOCUMENTING THE PREANESTHETIC ASSESSMENT AND INTERVIEW

The preoperative assessment begins with a patient interview and ends with obtaining consent for anesthesia and surgery. A preoperative assessment provides the anesthetist with an opportunity to carefully study the chart, including pertinent medical and social history; converse directly with the patient regarding health-related problems; conduct a physical examination; answer questions; and inform the patient of planned events in the operating room, which may serve to allay the patient's anxiety. Information gathered should enable the anesthetist to determine anesthesia risk factors, American Society of Anesthesiologists (ASA) classification, appropriate preoperative medication, potential intraoperative anesthesia techniques, monitoring modalities and drug selections. The interview should provide the patient with sufficient information to allow informed consent.

Protocols for documentation of preanesthetic evaluations vary among institutions. Many institutions now have a formalized document for such an assessment (Fig. 14–1). Prior to the increase in popularity of outpatient surgery, the preoperative assessment was completed the evening before surgery for all patients; now visits are made the night before surgery for patients admitted to the hospital prior to surgery. Outpatients and "same day" admission patients come to the surgical facility the day of surgery and have little time to be acclimatized to the hospital or to have an unhurried interview and evaluation by the anesthetist.[4] Inventive means for preoperative visits for these patients must be developed. Such methods may include (1) a personal interview conducted during a preadmission testing process by an anesthetist, (2) a mail-in questionnaire that addresses pertinent historical and physical data, (3) a telephone interview conducted by anesthesia personnel, or (4) an anesthesia interview immediately prior to surgery.[4]

Even though methods of preoperative patient interview are diverse, several notations are common to all preanesthesia assessment records. These common notations include (1) patient demographics; (2) a medical, surgical, and pertinent social history; (3) age, height, and weight; (4) baseline vital signs including blood pressure, heart, and respiratory rate; (5) findings of a cursory physical examination by systems review; (6) current medications, including recreational drugs; (7) allergies; (8) prior transfusion history and reactions; (9) pertinent laboratory results, including possible radiologic and electrocardiogram (ECG) analysis; (10) use of dental appliances or contact lenses; and (11) past anesthesia history in self and family. Selections relative to appropriate monitoring should also be documented on the preoperative record. Preoperative recording of all baseline hemodynamic and laboratory data may later assist the anesthetist in identifying significant hemodynamic or biochemical deviations during anesthesia and may also serve to justify treatment.

Once the interview is complete, the anesthetist should make certain that requisite data learned from chart review and patient interview is transcribed onto the anesthesia record (see Intraoperative Documentation, below). The style or format used for documenting preoperative data pertinent to anesthetic management should be thorough yet simple, noting only abnormal or significant findings. Notations should be legible since the interviewer may not be the actual anesthesia provider. In addition, a preoperative note should be made in the patient's

Developed by the American Association of Nurse Anesthetists - 1991

PREANESTHESIA EVALUATION

Age | Sex M F | Height in / cm | Weight lb / kg

Proposed Procedure

Pre-Procedure Vital Signs B/P P R T

Previous Anesthesia / Operations — None ☐

Current Medications — None ☐

Family History of Anesthesia Complications — None ☐

Allergies — NKDA ☐

AIRWAY / TEETH / HEAD & NECK

History From:
☐ Patient ☐ Significant Other
☐ Parent / Guardian ☐ Chart
☐ Communication / Language Problems
☐ Poor Historian

SYSTEM	WNL	COMMENTS
RESPIRATORY	☐	Tobacco Use: ☐ Yes ☐ No _______ Packs / Day for _______ Years
CARDIOVASCULAR	☐	
HEPATO / GASTROINTESTINAL	☐	Ethanol Use: ☐ Yes ☐ No Frequency ________ "Street Drug" Use: ☐ Yes ☐ No Frequency ________
NEURO / MUSCULOSKELETAL	☐	
RENAL / ENDOCRINE	☐	
OTHER		

DIAGNOSTIC STUDIES
EKG
Chest X-ray
Pulmonary Studies
Other

LABORATORY STUDIES
Hgb / Hct / CBC
Electrolytes
Urinalysis
Other

Problem List / Diagnoses

Planned Anesthesia / Special Monitors

PHYSICAL STATUS 1 2 3 4 5 E

Pre-Anesthesia Medications Ordered

Evaluator Signature | Date | Time

POSTANESTHESIA NOTE

Signed ________ Date ________ Time ________

P91-4

Figure 14–1 (A and B). Preanesthetic evaluation forms. Note either form can be used. They differ only in the CRNAs ability to provide documentation in a narrative or checklist form. (From the American Association of Nurse Anesthetists, Park Ridge, IL, with permission.)

Developed by the American Association of Nurse Anesthetists - 1991

PREANESTHESIA EVALUATION

Age | Sex M F | Height in / cm | Weight lb / kg

Proposed Procedure

Pre-Procedure Vital Signs B/P P R T

Previous Anesthesia / Operations — None ☐

Current Medications — None ☐

Family History of Anesthesia Complications — None ☐

Allergies — NKDA ☐

AIRWAY / TEETH / HEAD & NECK

History From:
☐ Patient ☐ Significant Other
☐ Parent / Guardian ☐ Chart
☐ Communication / Language Problems
☐ Poor Historian

SYSTEM	WNL	COMMENTS
RESPIRATORY Asthma, Bronchitis, COPD, Dyspnea, Orthopnea, Pneumonia, Productive Cough, Recent URI, SOB, Tuberculosis	☐	Tobacco Use: ☐ Yes ☐ No _______ Packs / Day for _______ Years
CARDIOVASCULAR Abnormal EKG, Angina, ASHD, CHF, Dysrhythmia, Exercise Tolerance, Hypertension, MI, Murmur, Pacemaker, Rheumatic Fever, Valvular Disease	☐	
HEPATO / GASTROINTESTINAL Bowel Obstruction, Cirrhosis, Hepatitis / Jaundice, Hiatal hernia / Reflux, Nausea & Vomiting, Ulcers	☐	Ethanol Use: ☐ Yes ☐ No Frequency _______ "Street Drug" Use: ☐ Yes ☐ No Frequency _______
NEURO / MUSCULOSKELETAL Arthritis, Back Problems, CVA / Stroke / TIAs, DJD, Headaches / ↑ ICP, Loss of Consciousness, Muscle Weakness, Neuromuscular Dis, Paralysis, Paresthesia, Syncope, Seizures	☐	
RENAL / ENDOCRINE Diabetes, Renal Failure / Dialysis, Thyroid Disease, Urinary Retention, Urinary Tract Infection, Weight Loss / Gain	☐	
OTHER Anemia, Bleeding Tendencies, Cancer, Chemotherapy, Dehydration, Hemophilia, Immunosuppressed, Pregnancy, Sickle Cell Dis. / Trait, Recent Steroids, Tranfusion History		

DIAGNOSTIC STUDIES
EKG
Chest X-ray
Pulmonary Studies
Other

LABORATORY STUDIES
Hgb / Hct / CBC
Electrolytes
Urinalysis
Other

Problem List / Diagnoses

Planned Anesthesia / Special Monitors

PHYSICAL STATUS: 1 2 3 4 5 E

POSTANESTHESIA NOTE

Signed _______ Date _______ Time _______

Pre-Anesthesia Medications Ordered

PATIENT IDENTIFICATION

Evaluator Signature | Date | Time

P91-3

Figure 14–1—continued.

chart, clearly indicating that the interview and assessment have been completed. This note should only include documentation of the patient's ASA classification, preliminary anesthetic plan, acceptance of consent, and pertinent information regarding health history such as allergies or monitoring modalities beyond what is considered usual for the routine case. Information regarding choice of general, regional, or intravenous sedation techniques and plans for airway management should also be noted as part of the preoperative assessment documentation.

OBTAINING INFORMED CONSENT

Administration of health care involves many types of contracts between a patient and a provider. These contracts are based on implied, expressed, constructive, or statutory consent and place certain duties on each involved party. "The health care provider owes each patient five duties: (1) to practice at a professed level of care, (2) to make full disclosure, (3) to protect confidences, (4) to offer continued treatment, and (5) to recognize his or her limitations and seek consultation when indicated."[5] The consent for anesthesia is the contract that binds anesthesia providers to the fulfillment of these duties.[6]

If the consent for anesthesia services is not obtained and followed, the anesthesia provider may be accountable for such acts as abandonment, assault, and/or battery. Although there are many examples of abandonment, one of the more frequent expressions of this tort is substitution of the caregiver. If an anesthesiologist has agreed to personally administer an anesthetic but instead induces the patient and turns the care over to a CRNA, abandonment has occurred.[5]

Patients have the right to be free from any intentional touching of their bodies, and violation of this right constitutes battery. Treating a patient without consent is an example of battery because there has been no permission to "touch" the patient; therefore, anesthesia caregivers must be aware that consent for anesthesia and surgery is a defense for battery.[5] *Assault* is placing one in fear of battery from someone who is capable of carrying out such an act. If a patient refuses certain treatment (i.e., an arterial line), and the anesthetist proceeds to prepare the patient for this procedure and has the needle ready, an assault has been committed.[5]

These possible legal breaches make a significant part of the preoperative assessment one of obtaining appropriate consent. The following quotation emphasizes the importance of informed consent in today's medicolegal climate. The health care provider must disclose the alternatives to and the relative merits of proposed procedures or anesthetics. "The comparative risks between types of anesthetics must be disclosed as part of informed consent. The health care provider's belief that a patient already knows the risks of a proposed procedure is inadequate; valid disclosure must be tailored to the immediate case."[6]

Informed consent protects the caregiver from libelous acts and educates the patient regarding the events surrounding the procedure(s) to be performed. Because the patient needs every opportunity to be aware of the risks and to be able to make an educated decision, consent should be obtained prior to the administration of preoperative medication. The patient needs to be fully aware of his or her commitment. Patients in any stage of sedation or narcosis are generally not considered able to provide informed consent. In those instances, family or legal guardians have to sign consent forms.

Although the most common type of consent is written, there are several ways by which an individual can authorize or consent to a procedure. These consent methods include expressed consent (written versus verbal), constructive consent, and statutory consent (sales versus service contracts).[5]

Expressed Consent

When a health care provider agrees to institute a specific treatment or service, for example, anesthesia, he or she has entered into an expressed contract. Most of the time expressed contracts for health-related services are verbal agreements between the patient and the health care provider, but a contract for diagnostic or therapeutic tests or treatment, particularly those that carry inherent risk, mandates a written contract between patient and provider.[5] Consent for anesthesia and surgery mandates a written contract that must state the procedure, be signed by the patient, and be dated and witnessed. When properly executed and signed, written consent is useful in legal action and should be included as part of the permanent record.[5,7]

A written expressed contract is more commonly deemed to constitute "informed consent." By definition, *informed consent* means that the patient has agreed to undergo a procedure after having had a clear description of the nature of the procedure and any potential side effects. Since a detailed written description is generally not required, informed consent must involve effective communication such that the anesthesia provider has a strong sense that the patient understands to what he or she is agreeing. The use of diagrams or an interpreter may be necessary to ensure an adequate level of understanding. Since laws of informed consent vary from state to state, the anesthesia provider needs to be thoroughly cognizant of state law. Legal counsel should be consulted in the process of drafting consent forms (Fig. 14–2).

A consent form for anesthesia may be either a separate document or may be incorporated as part of the surgical consent form. Regardless of the format, consent for anesthesia (and surgery) should include the patient's name and identification number, authorization for anesthesia, and name of anesthesia provider. In the case of a group employment arrangement, the legal name of the group or legal designee may be used. In addition, it is standard procedure that a note be entered on the preoperative evaluation form stating that the anesthesia technique(s) and risks have been discussed and that there is agreement with the intended anesthesia plan.

For a consent to be valid, the patient must be of legal age and must understand the procedure and the risks involved. If the patient's capacity to comprehend is impaired by language barrier, physical status, medications, unauthorized drugs or alcohol, obtaining consent should be delayed until alternatives to a valid consent are arranged. Only life-threatening circumstances can be an exception in such situations. In the case of minors, the parent(s) or other lawfully designated person must sign the expressed contract. An "emancipated minor," an individual under the age of 18 years who has legal capacity because of marriage, military duty, or who is living away from home and financially responsible for himself or herself, may give his or her own consent.

Constructive Consent

Courts hold health care providers to constructive duty to proceed in the absence of consent in emergency situations that delay life-saving treatment while locating a next of kin. Therefore, "consent may be constructive (construed by the law from the facts of the situation) in nature."[5] Constructive consent, better known as implied consent, carries with it two requirements: (1) the procedure(s) to be carried out is necessary to save a life, preserve a limb, prevent permanent disfigurement, or relieve suffering; and (2) reasonable effort be made, if time permits, to locate next of kin or legal guardian. Constructive consent is also the type of contract in force when parents or guardians of a nonemancipated minor cannot be located in an emergent situation.[2]

Statutory Consent

Statutory consent is consent awarded by state laws that allows care to be given to minors without parental consent in certain situations. One such situation could be the termination of an unwanted pregnancy in a nonemancipated minor.[5]

PREINDUCTION DOCUMENTATION

The preinduction phase of anesthesia care is critical, and most patient interventions during this time warrant documentation. The time prior to induction of anesthesia is when intravenous access is achieved, noninvasive monitors are applied, invasive monitors are inserted and connected, and portions of the patient history reviewed. The anesthetist should remember that minimally acceptable standards for monitoring include use of the ECG, precordial/esophageal stethoscope, blood pressure device, pulse oximeter, end-tidal CO_2 monitor, and temperature

CONSENT FOR ANESTHESIA SERVICES

I, ______________________________, acknowledge that my doctor has explained to me that I will have an operation, diagnostic or treatment procedure. My doctor has explained the risks of the procedure, advised me of alternative treatments and told me about the expected outcome and what could happen if my condition remains untreated. I also understand that anesthesia services are needed so that my doctor can perform the operation or procedure.

It has been explained to me that **all** forms of anesthesia involve some **risks** and no guarantees or promises can be made concerning the results of my procedure or treatment. Although rare, unexpected *severe complications* with anesthesia can occur and include the remote possibility of *infection, bleeding, drug reactions, blood clots, loss of sensation, loss of limb function, paralysis, stroke, brain damage, heart attack or death.* I understand that these risks apply to all forms of anesthesia and that additional or specific risks have been identified below as they may apply to a specific type of anesthesia. I understand that the type(s) of anesthesia service checked below will be used for my procedure and that the anesthetic technique to be used is determined by many factors including my physical condition, the type of procedure my doctor is to do, his or her preference, as well as my own desire. It has been explained to me that sometimes an anesthesia technique which involves the use of local anesthetics, with or without sedation, may not succeed completely and therefore another technique may have to be used including general anesthesia.

☐ General Anesthesia	Expected Result	Total unconscious state, possible placement of a tube into the windpipe.
	Technique	Drug injected into the bloodstream, breathed into the lungs, or by other routes.
	Risks	Mouth or throat pain, hoarseness, injury to mouth or teeth, awareness under anesthesia, injury to blood vessels, aspiration, pneumonia.
☐ Spinal or Epidural Analgesia/ Anesthesia	Expected Result	Temporary decreased or loss of feeling and/or movement to lower part of the body.
☐ With sedation	Technique	Drug injected through a needle/catheter placed either directly into the spinal canal or immediately outside the spinal canal.
☐ Without sedation	Risks	Headache, backache, buzzing in the ears, convulsions, infection, persistent weakness, numbness, residual pain, injury to blood vessels, "total spinal".
☐ Major / Minor Nerve Block	Expected Result	Temporary loss of feeling and/or movement of a specific limb or area.
☐ With sedation	Technique	Drug injected near nerves providing loss of sensation to the area of the operation.
☐ Without sedation	Risks	Infection, convulsions, weakness, persistent numbness, residual pain, injury to blood vessels.
☐ Intravenous Regional Anesthesia	Expected Result	Temporary loss of feeling and/or movement of a limb.
☐ With sedation	Technique	Drug injected into veins of arm or leg while using a tourniquet.
☐ Without sedation	Risks	Infection, convulsions, persistent numbness, residual pain, injury to blood vessels.
☐ Monitored Anesthesia Care (with sedation)	Expected Result	Reduced anxiety and pain, partial or total amnesia.
	Technique	Drug injected into the bloodstream, breathed into the lungs, or by other routes producing a semi-conscious state.
	Risks	An unconscious state, depressed breathing, injury to blood vessels.
☐ Monitored Anesthesia Care (without sedation)	Expected Result	Measurement of vital signs, availability of anesthesia provider for further intervention.
	Technique	None.
	Risks	Increased awareness, anxiety and/or discomfort.

I hereby consent to the anesthesia service checked above and authorize that it be administered by ____________________ or his/her associates, all of whom are credentialed to provide anesthesia services at this health facility. I also consent to an alternative type of anesthesia, if necessary, as deemed appropriate by them. I expressly desire the following considerations be observed (or write "none"):

____

I certify and acknowledge that I have read this form or had it read to me, that I understand the risks, alternatives and expected results of the anesthesia service and that I had ample time to ask questions and to consider my decision.

PATIENT IDENTIFICATION

____________________ *Patient's Signature*	____________________ *Date and Time*
____________________ *Substitute's Signature*	____________________ *Relationship to Patient*
____________________ *Witness*	Developed by the American Association of Nurse Anesthetists - 1991

A

P91-6

Figure 14–2 (A and B). Consent for anesthesia services. This detailed form helps patients to understand risks connected to the particular type of anesthesia selected: general, spinal or epidural, major/minor nerve block, IV regional, and MAC with or without sedation. Form B allows the anesthetist to inform the patient more fully of the risks of blood transfusion and accommodates the patient's authorization for administration of blood or blood products. (From the American Association of Nurse Anesthetists, Park Ridge, IL, with permission.)

CONSENT FOR ANESTHESIA SERVICES

I, ______________________________, acknowledge that my doctor has explained to me that I will have an operation, diagnostic or treatment procedure. My doctor has explained the risks of the procedure, advised me of alternative treatments and told me about the expected outcome and what could happen if my condition remains untreated. I also understand that anesthesia services are needed so that my doctor can perform the operation or procedure.

It has been explained to me that **all** forms of anesthesia involve some **risks** and no guarantees or promises can be made concerning the results of my procedure or treatment. Although rare, unexpected *severe complications* with anesthesia can occur and include the remote possibility of *infection, bleeding, drug reactions, blood clots, loss of sensation, loss of limb function, paralysis, stroke, brain damage, heart attack or death.* I understand that these risks apply to all forms of anesthesia and that additional or specific risks have been identified below as they may apply to a specific type of anesthesia. I understand that the type(s) of anesthesia service checked below will be used for my procedure and that the anesthetic technique to be used is determined by many factors including my physical condition, the type of procedure my doctor is to do, his or her preference, as well as my own desire. It has been explained to me that sometimes an anesthesia technique which involves the use of local anesthetics, with or without sedation, may not succeed completely and therefore another technique may have to be used including general anesthesia.

☐ General Anesthesia	Expected Result	Total unconscious state, possible placement of a tube into the windpipe.
	Technique	Drug injected into the bloodstream, breathed into the lungs, or by other routes.
	Risks	Mouth or throat pain, hoarseness, injury to mouth or teeth, awareness under anesthesia, injury to blood vessels, aspiration, pneumonia.
☐ Spinal or Epidural Analgesia/ Anesthesia ☐ With sedation ☐ Without sedation	Expected Result	Temporary decreased or loss of feeling and/or movement to lower part of the body.
	Technique	Drug injected through a needle/catheter placed either directly into the spinal canal or immediately outside the spinal canal.
	Risks	Headache, backache, buzzing in the ears, convulsions, infection, persistent weakness, numbness, residual pain, injury to blood vessels, "total spinal".
☐ Major / Minor Nerve Block ☐ With sedation ☐ Without sedation	Expected Result	Temporary loss of feeling and/or movement of a specific limb or area.
	Technique	Drug injected near nerves providing loss of sensation to the area of the operation.
	Risks	Infection, convulsions, weakness, persistent numbness, residual pain, injury to blood vessels.
☐ Intravenous Regional Anesthesia ☐ With sedation ☐ Without sedation	Expected Result	Temporary loss of feeling and/or movement of a limb.
	Technique	Drug injected into veins of arm or leg while using a tourniquet.
	Risks	Infection, convulsions, persistent numbness, residual pain, injury to blood vessels.
☐ Monitored Anesthesia Care (with sedation)	Expected Result	Reduced anxiety and pain, partial or total amnesia.
	Technique	Drug injected into the bloodstream, breathed into the lungs, or by other routes producing a semi-conscious state.
	Risks	An unconscious state, depressed breathing, injury to blood vessels.
☐ Monitored Anesthesia Care (without sedation)	Expected Result	Measurement of vital signs, availability of anesthesia provider for further intervention.
	Technique	None.
	Risks	Increased awareness, anxiety and/or discomfort.

I hereby consent to the anesthesia service checked above and authorize that it be administered by ____________________ or his/her associates, all of whom are credentialed to provide anesthesia services at this health facility. I also consent to an alternative type of anesthesia, if necessary, as deemed appropriate by them. I expressly desire the following considerations be observed (or write "none"):

____

BLOOD TRANSFUSIONS

The likelihood of needing a blood transfusion for this procedure is: ☐ highly unlikely, ☐ possible, ☐ probable.

I understand that there are potential risks from blood transfusions, though rare, and that some of these include transfusion reaction, hepatitis, and AIDS (Acquired Immune Deficiency Syndrome). *Initial in appropriate box:*

☐ I give consent to receive blood or blood products as determined by my anesthetist and doctor to be necessary for my well-being.
☐ I give consent to receive blood or blood products only as an emergency life-saving measure.
☐ I do not want to receive blood or blood products under any circumstance.

I certify and acknowledge that I have read this form or had it read to me, that I understand the risks, alternatives and expected results of the anesthesia service and that I had ample time to ask questions and to consider my decision.

PATIENT IDENTIFICATION

Patient's Signature *Date and Time*

Substitute's Signature *Relationship to Patient*

Witness

Developed by the American Association of Nurse Anesthetists - 1991

B

P91-5

Figure 14–2—continued.

probe. *All the above actions must be noted on the intraoperative record.*

The preinduction period is also the time when laboratory values are reviewed to assess fluid and electrolyte status and nulla per os (nothing by mouth; NPO) status. Allergies are reviewed and the airway reexamined for potential difficulty during induction. This information, as well as time and dosage of preoperative medication, which should include steroids or antibiotics (if any) and availability of blood for transfusion, must be documented in the appropriate location of the anesthesia record for quick reference. Other pertinent documentation that should be written on the record concerns pads or other devices employed to ensure patient safety placed prior to induction. Any antibiotic or other drug therapy instituted prior to beginning anesthesia administration must be documented. In summary, everything that is done to the patient before induction should be documented concisely, accurately, and completely.

Equipment Malfunction Checklist

Among those pieces of information that require written notation on the anesthesia record or other permanent record of the patient chart is the equipment checklist. Essential to any anesthetic is the proper function of equipment because "the majority of incidents involving anesthesia equipment are a result of failure to check the equipment prior to use."[8,9] The Joint Committee on Accreditation of Health Care Organizations (JCAHO) believes so strongly about the issue of safe anesthesia equipment that it states "prior to administering anesthesia, the anesthetist shall check readiness and working condition of all equipment used in the administration of an anesthetic."[10] Additionally, the Food and Drug Administration (FDA) developed a "checkout procedure" that was endorsed by the AANA in 1986 (Fig. 14–3).

Strict protocol for evaluation of anesthetic equipment prior to the anesthetic must be in place in every anesthesia department. Proper checkout procedure for gas machines and other equipment provides some evidence and security that the equipment was functioning at the beginning of the anesthetic. Methods by which anesthesia personnel adhere to this standard of care vary from a check mark or indicator on the anesthesia record to a separate record with a descriptive checklist. Should a check mark be used as the method of documentation, protocol for equipment malfunction checkout needs to be incorporated into the department policy and procedure manual, and personnel education of such procedure should be ongoing.

INTRAOPERATIVE DOCUMENTATION

The intraoperative record, commonly called the "anesthesia record," is a surveyable monograph of the entire course of actual anesthesia administration. Documentation stimulates continuous observation of the patient and affords the user the capability of tracking trends of the patient's response to surgery, anesthesia, and any anesthetic interventions. Documentation arranged in a logical, sequential manner also facilitates review or extraction of data.

The intraoperative anesthesia record is usually a two-sided sheet or a document with carbon paper attached which is designed with a grid on which hemodynamic measurement can be entered and tracked. A comment section for preoperative, intraoperative, and postoperative information is usually included. The best design for an anesthetic record is one that minimizes the incidence of incomplete documentation. Opinions vary regarding whether compliance to procedures is best served by a checklist format or by a section that requires detailed data or narrative entry. Regardless of format, the designer of the intraoperative anesthesia record should bear in mind that the more care delivered during actual anesthetic management, the more documentation is required; any additional need for documentation increases the chance that important data may be unintentionally omitted. A record-keeping system that accommodates ease of data entry encourages a more accurate and complete record of pertinent intra-anesthetic events. A format that more closely meets this need is one that is task-oriented, since it allows a more com-

Anesthesia Apparatus Checkout Recommendations, 1992

This checkout, or a reasonable equivalent, should be conducted before administration of anesthesia. These recommendations are only valid if the anesthesia system includes an ascending bellows ventilator and the following monitors: capnograph, pulse oximeter, oxygen analyzer, respiratory volume monitor (spirometer) and breathing system pressure monitor with high and low pressure alarms. This is a guideline which users are encouraged to modify to accommodate differences in equipment design and variations in local clinical practice. Such local modifications should have appropriate peer review. Users should refer to the operator's manual for specific procedures and precautions.

Emergency Ventilation Equipment

1. Emergency Equipment is Available and Functioning

High Pressure System

2. Check Oxygen Cylinder Supply
   a. Open O_2 cylinder and verify at least half full (about 1000 psi).
   b. Close cylinder.

3. Check Central Pipeline Supplies
   a. Hoses are properly connected, and pipeline gauges read 45-55 psi.

Low Pressure System

4. Check Initial Status of Low Pressure System
   a. Flow control valves and vaporizers' are off.
   b. Check fill level and tighten vaporizers' filler caps.
   c. Remove O_2 monitor sensor from circuit.

5. Perform Machine Low Pressure Leak Check
   a. Verify that the machine master switch and flow control valves are OFF.
   b. Attach "Suction Bulb" to common (fresh) gas outlet.
   c. Repeatedly pump until fully collapsed.
   d. Verify bulb stays *fully* collapsed for at least 5 seconds.
   e. Open one vaporizer at a time and repeat 'b' and 'c' as above.
   f. Remove suction bulb, and reconnect fresh gas hose.

6. Turn On Machine Master Switch
   and all other necessary electrical equipment.

7. Test Flowmeters
   a. Adjust flow of all gases through their full range, checking for smooth operation of floats and undamaged flowtubes.
   b. Attempt to create a hypoxic O_2/N_2O mixture and verify correct changes in flow and/or alarm.

Breathing System

8. Check Initial Status of Breathing System
   a. Selector switch is in "Bag" mode.
   b. Breathing circuit is complete, undamaged, and unobstructed.
   c. CO_2 absorbent is adequate.

9. Install Accessory Equipment
   to be used during the case.

10. Calibrate O_2 Monitor
   a. Calibrate to read 21% in room air.
   b. Reinstall sensor in circuit and flush breathing system with O_2.
   c. Monitor should now read greater than 90%.

11. Perform Breathing System Leak Check
   a. Set all gas flows to zero (or minimum).
   b. Close APL valve and occlude Y-piece.
   c. Pressurize breathing system to 30 cm H_2O with O_2 flush.
   d. Gauge value should not noticeably drop in 10 seconds.

Figure 14–3. Anesthesia apparatus checkout recommendations. Documentation that this checklist has been performed is required on every anesthesia record of every case. (From the Department of Health and Human Services, Food and Drug Administration, Rockville, MD, 1992.)

Continued

Scavenger System

12. Check APL Valve and Scavenger System

a. Pressurize breathing system to 50 cm H_2O and insure it remains intact.
b. Open APL valve and insure that a pressure decrease occurs as the valve is opened.
c. Insure proper scavenging connections and adjust waste gas vacuum.
d. Fully open APL valve, and occlude Y-piece.
e. With minimum O_2 flow, insure negligible negative pressure at the absorber pressure gauge.
f. With O_2 flush activated, insure negligible positive pressure at the absorber pressure gauge.

Ventilator

13. Functional Test of Ventilator and Undirectional Valves

a. Place reservoir bag on Y-piece.
b. Set appropriate ventilator parameters for next patient.
c. Set O_2 flow to minimum, other gas flows to zero.
d. Turn ventilator ON and pressurize system with O_2 flush.
e. Insure cycling of ventilator and free movement of bellows.
f. *Check for proper action of unidirectional valves.*
g. Exercise breathing circuit accessories to assure appropriate function.
h. Turn ventilator OFF, and return bag to bag mount.

Monitors

14. Check, Calibrate, and Set Alarm Limits of all Monitors

Capnograph — Pulse Oximeter
Oxygen Analyzer — Respiratory Volume Monitor (Spirometer)
Pressure Monitor with High and Low Airway Pressure Alarms

Final Position

15. Check Final Status of Machine

a. All flow meters to zero (or minimum).
b. Vaporizers off.
c. Selector switch to "Bag" mode.
d. APL valve open.
e. Patient suction level appropriate.
f. Patient breathing system ready to use.

Figure 14–3—continued.

prehensive detailed documentation over a shorter period of time (Fig. 14–4).

It should again be stressed that adequate, accurate records substantiate quality of care. Evidence that quality care has been provided is supported by documentation that current practice standards were employed during anesthetic management. It is important for documentation to indicate the rationale for particular actions and the justification for clinical judgments made in selecting anesthetic techniques and drugs used during anesthetic management. Accurate charting is mandatory, regardless of the format of the actual record. The following points are often helpful in evaluating the quality of intraoperative documentation.

1 Data should be recorded at regular time intervals.
2 The time of event(s) should match the time of intervention(s).
3 Only relevant data should be recorded.
4 Only commonly accepted abbreviations should be used.
5 Trade or generic names of drugs should be used for consistency, not a mixture of the two.
6 When recording drugs, use mg or mcq, not cc or ml.
7 List only devices that are actually used.
8 Designate changes in equipment setting if and when they are made.
9 Note equipment malfunction if it occurs.

The intraoperative phase of anesthesia care begins with the induction of anesthesia and ends with report in the postanesthesia care unit (PACU). The busiest and most critical times during this period are induction and emergence; literature demonstrates that regular notation on the anesthesia record declines significantly during these two events when the patient requires strict vigilance and attention. These virtues do not, however, negate the importance of concurrent record-keeping. Trial and error has demonstrated many times that concurrent record-keeping is more accurate than reconstructing events. Although this task may be impossible at times, attempts should be made to be as concurrent as possible.[2] In the event of an urgent or emergency situation, the best approach is to have one individual assigned to document events.

Induction of Anesthesia

The technique used for induction (i.e., asleep, sedated, awake) of anesthesia and the time induction began should be noted accurately. Induction maneuvers and administration of drugs must be indicated in such a manner that they demonstrate accuracy in sequence, dose, and method of administration.

Since intubation is such an important part of the induction of anesthesia and a critical time for complications, this part of the procedure should be carefully and accurately documented. Documentation should include special procedures such as rapid-sequence induction or other unusual intubation techniques. The type and size of laryngoscope blade, size of endotracheal tube, use of an inflated endotracheal tube cuff, position of the endotracheal tube after placement, and presence and correctness of breath sounds must be documented. The importance of documenting events related to the management of a difficult airway during induction cannot be overstated.

Documentation of anatomic airway abnormalities is important, not only for the time at hand, but for future reference if the patient should need further anesthesia services. If airway difficulties are encountered, the patient and/or family need to be made aware of this information postoperatively, and any problems should be made a part of the permanent medical record. If regional anesthesia is administered, the technique, agents used, safety maneuvers, and level of block achieved must be completely documented. Some anesthesia providers chart the manufacturer's lot number and expiration date of the regional equipment if prepackaged supplies are used. Any difficulties with administration should be charted as well as complications that result.

Monitoring during induction and all phases of anesthesia must be documented in a timely, accurate fashion, as monitoring is the most valuable means of communication between the patient and caregiver during the anesthetic procedure. The increasing

Developed by the American Association of Nurse Anesthetists - 1991

ANESTHESIA RECORD

Date	OR No.	Page of	Procedure / Surgeon(s)

	START	STOP
Anesthesia		
Procedure		

PRE-PROCEDURE

Identified: ID Band Questioning
Chart Reviewed Permit Signed
NPO Since ____
Pre-anesthetic State: Calm
Awake Asleep
Apprehensive Confused
Uncooperative Unresponsive

PATIENT SAFETY

Anes. Machine # ____ Checked
Safety Belt On Axillary Roll
Armboard Restraints Arms Tucked
Pressure points checked and padded
Eye Care: Ointment Saline
Taped Pads Goggles

MONITORS AND EQUIPMENT

Steth: Precord Esoph Other
Non-Invasive B/P: Left Right
Continuous EKG V Lead EKG
Pulse Oximeter Oxygen Sensor
End Tidal CO_2 Gas Analyzer
Temp. ____ Nerve Stimulator
Warming Blanket EEG Doppler
Airway Humidifier Fluid Warmer
NG / OG Tube Foley Catheter
Art.Line ____
CVP ____
PA Line ____
IV(s) ____

ANESTHETIC TECHNIQUE

General: Pre-Oxygenation L.T.A.
Rapid Sequence Cricoid Pressure
Intravenous Inhalation
Intramuscular Rectal
Regional: Spinal Epidural
Axillary Bier Block Ankle Block
Position ____
Prep ____ Local ____
Needle ____
Drug(s) ____
Dose ____ Attempts x ____
Site ____ Level ____
Catheter ____ See Remarks
Other: M.A.C.

AIRWAY MANAGEMENT

Intubation: Oral Tube size ____
Stylet used Nasal Regular
Magill's Direct RAE
Fiber optic Blind Armored
Blade ____ Laser
Secured at ____ cm Endobronch.
Attempts x ____ ET CO_2 present
Breath sounds ____
Uncuffed, leaks at ____ cm H_2O
Cuffed Min. occ. pres. Air NS
Airway: Oral Nasal Difficult,
Circuit: Circle NRB see Remarks
Mask Case Nasal Cannula
Via Tracheostomy Simple O_2 mask

RECOVERY

Location		Time
B/P		O_2 Sat
P	R	T
Awake	Stable	Nasal Oxygen
Drowsy	Unstable	Mask Oxygen
Somnolent	Intubated	T-piece Oxygen
Unarousable	Ventilator	Oral/nasal airway

CONTROLLED DRUGS

Drug	Used	Destroyed	Returned
Provider		Witness	

TIME:

Oxygen (L/min)
N_2O Air (L/min)
(%)

AGENTS

FLUIDS

Urine (ml)
EBL (ml)

MONITORS
EKG
% O_2 Inspired (FIO_2)
O_2 Saturation (SaO_2)
End Tidal CO_2
Temp: C F

VITAL SIGNS
Baseline Values
B/P
P
R
200 180 160 140 120 100 80 60 40 20

VENT
Tidal Volume
Resp. Rate
Peak Pressure
PEEP

Symbols for Remarks

Position

TOTALS

SYMBOLS
X ANESTHESIA
⊙ OPERATION
V Λ B. P. CUFF PRESSURE
⊥ T ARTERIAL LINE PRESSURE
▲ MEAN ARTERIAL PRESSURE
● PULSE
○ SPONTANEOUS RESP
Ø ASSISTED RESP
⊠ CONTROLLED RESP
T TOURNIQUET

Anesthesia Provider

PATIENT IDENTIFICATION

REMARKS

A

P91-2

Figure 14–4 (A and B). The intraoperative anesthesia record. Two examples are provided. Either can be used depending on provider preference. (From the American Association of Nurse Anesthetists, Park Ridge, IL, with permission).

Developed by the American Association of Nurse Anesthetists - 1991

ANESTHESIA RECORD

Procedure

Date | OR No. | Page of | Surgeon(s)

	START	STOP
Anesthesia		
Procedure		

PRE-PROCEDURE

Identified: ID Band Questioning
Chart Reviewed Permit Signed
NPO Since ____
Pre-anesthetic State: Calm
Awake Asleep
Apprehensive Confused
Uncooperative Unresponsive

PATIENT SAFETY

Anes. Machine # ____ Checked
Safety Belt On Axillary Roll
Armboard Restraints Arms Tucked
Pressure points checked and padded
Eye Care: Ointment Saline
Taped Pads Goggles

MONITORS AND EQUIPMENT

Steth: Precord Esoph Other
Non-Invasive B/P: Left Right
Continuous EKG V Lead EKG
Pulse Oximeter Oxygen Sensor
End Tidal CO_2 Gas Analyzer
Temp. ____ Nerve Stimulator
Warming Blanket EEG Doppler
Airway Humidifier Fluid Warmer
NG / OG Tube Foley Catheter
Art.Line ____
CVP ____
PA Line ____
IV(s) ____

ANESTHETIC TECHNIQUE

General: Pre-Oxygenation L.T.A.
Rapid Sequence Cricoid Pressure
Intravenous Inhalation
Intramuscular Rectal
Regional: Spinal Epidural
Axillary Bier Block Ankle Block
____ Position ____
Prep ____ Local ____
Needle ____
Drug(s) ____
Dose ____ Attempts x ____
Site ____ Level ____
Catheter ____ See Remarks
Other: M.A.C.

AIRWAY MANAGEMENT

Intubation: Oral Tube size ____
Stylet used Nasal Regular
Magill's Direct RAE
Fiber optic Blind Armored
Blade ____ Laser
Secured at ____ cm Endobronch.
Attempts x ____ ET CO_2 present
Breath sounds ____
Uncuffed, leaks at ____ cm H_2O
Cuffed Min. occ. pres. Air NS
Airway: Oral Nasal Difficult,
Circuit: Circle NRB see Remarks
Mask Case Nasal Cannula
Via Tracheostomy Simple O_2 mask

RECOVERY

Location		Time
B/P		O_2 Sat
P	R	T
Awake	Stable	Nasal Oxygen
Drowsy	Unstable	Mask Oxygen
Somnolent	Intubated	T-piece Oxygen
Unarousable	Ventilator	Oral/nasal airway

Recovery Notes

FLUID TOTALS

Crystalloid ____ EBL ____
Blood ____ Urine ____

REMARKS

TIME:

FLUIDS / AGENTS

Oxygen (L/min)
N_2O Air (L/min)
(%)

TOTALS

Urine (ml)
EBL (ml)

MONITORS

EKG
% O_2 Inspired
O_2 Saturation
End Tidal CO_2
Temp.: C F

VITAL SIGNS

Baseline Values

B/P

P

R

200, 180, 160, 140, 120, 100, 80, 60, 40, 20

VENT

Tidal Volume
Resp. Rate
Peak Pressure
PEEP

Symbols for Remarks

Position

SYMBOLS

× ANESTHESIA
⊙ OPERATION
∨ ∧ B.P. CUFF PRESSURE
⊥ T ARTERIAL LINE PRESSURE
▲ MEAN ARTERIAL PRESSURE
• PULSE
○ SPONT RESP
Ø ASSISTED RESP
⊠ CONTROLLED RESP
T TOURNIQUET

PATIENT IDENTIFICATION

Anesthesia Provider

CONTROLLED DRUGS

Drug	Issued	Used	Destroyed	Returned

Provider

Witness

B

P91-1

Figure 14–4—continued.

importance of documenting data accessed through monitors during anesthesia is supported by the strong emphasis given to it in risk management, quality assurance, and medicolegal activities. Compliance with the AANA monitoring standards should be strictly observed (see Chapter 7).

Data made available through monitors is traditionally recorded every 5 minutes with the exception of temperature. Temperature values can be recorded at 30-minute intervals unless abnormal values are noted when the monitor is placed, or patient history of untoward events such as malignant hypertension are known. Additional monitors, other than those considered standard, may be required for special or more complex surgical procedures; it is the responsibility of the provider to know which monitoring techniques are considered standards of care for these procedures.

It is difficult to defend lack of documentation once a monitor has been instituted as part of a patient's care. An integrated monitoring system may lend itself to redundancy in documenting care information, but it is a valuable method of documentation, especially in the event one system fails.

Maintenance

Maintenance is the time during which an anesthetic level that provides the patient with a pain-free, relaxed, and unconscious state is reached. It is the goal of the anesthetist to maintain a documentable, homeostatic state to the extent possible, given the patient's preexisting health status and the type of surgical procedure being undertaken. All activities are directed toward optimizing patient outcomes postoperatively.

The time leading to and including the maintenance period often require frequent adjustments in delivery of anesthetic agents. These adjustments must be entered on the anesthesia record and justified by correlating the modifications to an altered physiologic state; this is usually accomplished by documented vital signs or other monitored parameter changes. Hemodynamic values continue to be charted at 5-minute intervals throughout the maintenance phase of anesthesia. If changes in physiologic status occur more frequently, recording these changes may become tedious, because most records are not designed for minute-to-minute notations of events. The anesthetist is responsible for being as accurate as possible in detailing the patient's response to surgery and anesthesia even if additional anesthesia records are required.

If the maintenance period of an anesthetic is so lengthy that relief of the anesthetist is necessary, the time and name of the individual providing relief should be entered on the record. Relief should never be accepted during induction or emergence or when a patient is unstable. A summary of the events charted during maintenance are listed in Box 14–1.

Notations concerning directions/orders from the surgeon should be made as well as notations concerning lengthy delays in intervention (i.e., delay for surgeon, radiologic reports, consultations, tissue analysis). In the event of an unexpected response or a complication, a detailed, accurate description of the occurrence plus any means of intervention should be noted. Documentation of exact times of such events may be critical for the protection of the anesthetist in a legal consequence. Language or abbreviations used in notations must be accurate. In a word, defensive charting is necessary in today's medicolegal climate.

Emergence

Decreasing the depth of anesthesia elicits several anticipated physiologic responses.

BOX 14–1
EVENTS CHARTED DURING THE MAINTENANCE PERIOD

- Hemodynamic values
- Adequacy of ventilation
- Fluid and/or blood loss
- Fluid and/or blood replacement
- Neuromuscular function
- Drug therapy
- Anesthesia drugs/doses or percentages of agents
- Patient position
- Protective devices employed
- Unusual surgical and/or anesthesia events

As the patient's awareness is increased, response to stimuli is heightened and is usually evidenced by increases in blood pressure and heart rate. These and any other responses of emergence should be noted as part of the anesthesia record.

The adequacy of muscle strength is an important assessment to make during emergence. The use of muscle relaxant reversal agents is frequently indicated, and use and doses of drugs should be documented. The anesthetist should note recovery from muscle relaxants by recording recovery of twitch response with a peripheral nerve stimulator. Notation that the patient has met the criteria for extubation and has been extubated needs to be entered on the record. The patient's physical condition and degree of awareness are important assessments that are recorded prior to arrival in the PACU. It is extremely important to note that anesthetic agents are being discontinued, and a notation should be made if the patient is transported to his or her postoperative destination with oxygen or any monitoring device.

Emergence is a busy time for the anesthetist and charting is often delayed to attend to the patient. Many times charting of important events for this period are left until after the patient has been safely transported to the PACU, again setting the stage for incomplete recording of events, particularly if pressure is exerted on the caregiver to begin the next anesthetic. Regardless, the anesthetist must continually chart vital signs and be sensitive to the fact that the entire anesthesia record should be reviewed for completeness.

POSTANESTHESIA RECOVERY UNIT DOCUMENTATION

Transport of the patient to the PACU is not without risk, and emergence from anesthesia continues en route making possible the occurrence of unexpected events. The safe practitioner should anticipate the needs for transport and not leave the operating room until all safety precautions are complete and the patient would not be jeopardized by transfer. All monitoring devices that would ensure safe transport to the PACU should be noted on the anesthesia record.

The responsibility to the patient does not end when the patient arrives in the PACU. The competent provider assures stabilization of hemodynamic values and ventilation before transferring care to the PACU personnel. The process of relinquishing care duties involves a report to include the type of anesthetic given, anesthetic events that have occurred, expectations during recovery, and orders to be initiated. It is not enough to verbally report information; documentation of a report should be made a part of the anesthesia record or the PACU record, according to protocols of the institution. Hemodynamic data on admission to PACU are the values last recorded on the anesthesia record; these entries should include, but not be limited to, blood pressure, heart rate, respiratory rate, oxygen saturation, temperature, patient color, and state of awareness. In all cases the CRNA should note on the record that the PACU nurse has accepted care for the patient.

Postoperative Documentation

Notation of a postanesthesia evaluation is considered a standard of care for anesthesia. The postoperative visit serves to assess the patient's response to anesthesia postoperatively and should include adequacy of pain management and/or control of nausea and vomiting. Time spent on such a visit can be used to disclose any unusual or unexpected responses to the anesthetic and to assess the patient's perspective of the anesthesia experience. It is a time for the patient to discuss any misunderstanding or dissatisfaction. Allowing the patient to discuss these matters will likely decrease the patient's disposition to seek legal recourse. The nature of the interaction, pertinent discussion, assessment, and notation of any postoperative complications is documented. If complications are noted, other notations of follow-up visits and/or treatment are necessary to demonstrate continuation of appropriate care.

LEGAL ASPECTS OF ANESTHESIA CHARTING

Although good documentation does not prevent anesthesia complications, it does decrease the likelihood of litigation by providing strong evidence of quality care.

Unfortunately, even though the above statement is true, expert witnesses declare poor documentation to be the most common weak link in defending malpractice suits. In cases involving anesthesia mishap, such witnesses find anesthesia documents to be incomplete and illegible. It behooves all anesthesia providers to know the legal ramifications of their record-keeping and to realize that the present legal climate allows the introduction of records without explanatory testimony from the anesthesia provider.

Introduction of a Record as Evidence

Historically, medical records introduced as evidence in a court of law without supportive testimony from the record keeper were considered hearsay. Today there are two rules, which have been successfully applied to medical records, that allow records documenting services performed to be introduced as evidence without supporting testimony from the actual record keeper. One of these rules is the Uniform Business Records Evidence Act and the other is the Shopkeepers Rule. Although the Shopkeepers Rule has no mandated mechanism for supporting testimony from a person familiar with medical records, part of the Uniform Records Evidence Act does allow a record custodian to testify as to the mode of preparation and the compliance of the record with previously documented criteria. In the case of anesthesia documentation, this custodian would be a medical records librarian. Needless to say, a poorly constructed anesthesia record would not be an asset to anyone except the plaintiff.[3]

Other methods for introducing the anesthesia record into evidence are more traditional than the two acts described above and give the anesthetist more opportunity for explanation. One of these methods is the declaration of the medical record as an official public document and another is a stipulation by the parties to the litigation that the record may be admitted into evidence.

Privileged Information

If a record is introduced as a matter of public record, it becomes important for the anesthetist to understand how this changes the commonly understood definition of privileged information or patient confidentiality. Generally any communication between a patient and health care provider is considered confidential and, therefore, privileged information. Once a lawsuit has been filed alleging that a patient has been harmed because of a medical act, the medical record, including the anesthesia record, is no longer considered privileged for the purposes of litigation. However, there is violation of confidentiality if there is disclosure of information that goes beyond that required for the lawsuit.

Common Problems Associated with Anesthesia Care Documentation

Because the medical record is often the first evidence of standards of practice and the first source of information reviewed during litigation, it has become necessary to practice what is known as "defensive charting." *Defensive charting* is the practice of documenting in a manner that will lead to a more accurate portrayal of the quality of care given. Defensive anesthesia documentation should begin with a departmental policy that specifies charting guidelines and describes a standardized record format. All department members responsible for documentation should be familiar with this policy and apprised of any changes in its content.

Most anesthesia records require documentation of data pertinent to the anesthetic management of the patient. Much of this data relate to the patient's history, present physical condition, and diagnostic test results. It is imperative that all aspects of the anesthesia records be complete or that explanations be made to clarify their deletion. Blank spaces in anesthesia documents should be avoided. If the anesthetist must rely on data not charted on specific anesthesia forms, it is the responsibility of the anesthetist to validate that such data are available elsewhere in the chart and that these data were reviewed prior to the administration of the anesthetic. To proceed with an anesthetic with only a notation that the surgeon's history and physical has been "dictated" is not acceptable.

One of the pitfalls found in medicolegal chart review is failure to confirm that records have been reviewed and considered in the planning of an anesthetic. This lack of documentation is frequently noted when the anesthetist or anesthesiologist doing the preoperative assessment has not implemented and managed the anesthetic. The assurance of quality care in these situations is best accomplished when the anesthetist actually providing the anesthesia services reassesses the patient and documents verification of important data. This documentation should also include consideration of pertinent patient information in the development of the anesthetic plan. If patient assessment is not possible, a notation should be made confirming that the record was reviewed and considered in the planning of the anesthetic.

Emergency situations may demand that the anesthetist proceed prior to adequate documentation of pertinent patient information. In these circumstances it is important to have the surgeon note that the emergent nature of the case precludes waiting for such documentation. If the surgeon refuses to provide a notation, consideration should be given to delaying the case, particularly in states when nursing standards require nurses to protect patients from harm. In these instances, following a physician's order without considering the consequences of such action may not be enough protection in a court of law or at a disciplinary hearing.[2]

Most anesthetists accurately chart names and amount of agents as well as drugs employed during anesthetic management. However, charting why these agents or drugs are given is often forgotten. For example, the amount of labetalol used prior to induction to control hypertension and tachycardia is usually charted but the rationale for its use is not. If a medication is given or action is taken as a directive or order from a physician, the physician's name should be included in the documentation. Clear explanations are important for defensive charting to adequately demonstrate quality anesthesia management and to support compliance with current standards of care. Charting also helps the anesthetist recall events during surgery and anesthesia if a lawsuit is filed.

Current standards of care require blood pressure and pulse rate to be charted at 5-minute intervals. In addition, charting frequency and depth of ventilation are considered as important as documenting pulse and blood pressure. Standards of care also require documentation of blood pressure and temperature on pediatric patients.[2]

It is illegal to delete entries from any document considered a part of a medical record. Incorrect notations may be corrected by drawing a line through the incorrect data yet leaving it legible, inserting the correct data, and initialing the change. Corrections should never be made with "Whiteout." Events may be added to a document at a later time, but these data must be dated and timed to indicate exactly when it was placed in the chart. A reason for the late entry should also be included. It is considered fraud to predate any entry on a record in an attempt to make the entry appear to have been made at an earlier time.[3]

Another illegal act that relates to destruction or lost records is *spoliation*. This term refers to any alteration, destruction, or loss of a record pertinent to ongoing litigation. Spoliation relates to whether a person altered a record as an attempt to avoid responsibility and lends to the belief that the missing or altered records would have supported the cause of the party who does not have custody of the record (in most cases this would be the patient).[3]

Completeness, legibility, and accuracy of anesthesia records is a vital part of verifying quality care in any legal issue surrounding patient care. Because this is such an important aspect of anesthesia care, any time circumstances interrupt the anesthetist's ability to chart data in a timely fashion (i.e., cardiac arrest during anesthesia), a scribe should be appointed. If this is not possible, the anesthetist should include any notations made during circumstances as part of the record even if notations are used later to reconstruct the chart.[3]

The end of anesthetic management is as important as the beginning; therefore, records should reflect that anesthetic agents were discontinued, drug and fluid replacement summarized, postanesthesia recovery score awarded, and report given to the appropriate personnel in the postanesthesia recovery area. Too many times the anesthesia record is found with no evidence of discontinuation of anesthesia and no evidence of placing the patient safely in the capable hands of the PACU nurse. One of the more common errors found in anesthesia documentation is failure to chart postoperative anesthesia follow-up. Documentation is not considered complete unless this important notation is made. The legal system takes a dim view of what it perceives to be a lack in continuity of care.

Records hold the anesthetist accountable for care that was delivered, but there is nothing to fear as long as records are accurate, complete and readable, and reveal that current standards of anesthesia care have been followed. It is important to remember that regardless of the quality of care actually given, records of that care are the windows through which others evaluate that care.

FUTURE TRENDS IN ANESTHESIA DOCUMENTATION

Anesthesia providers are very much aware of the difficulties involved in generating accurate and timely anesthesia documentation, particularly in emergency situations. Manually prepared records are often inaccurate, time-consuming, and have a limited format. Charting often becomes episodic whenever the anesthetist's full attention is directed toward the patient. Studies have shown the most inaccurate data that are manually charted are vital signs because these are often recorded after the fact and "smoothing" is inevitable.[9,11–14]

Manual charting is, indeed, time-consuming. As anesthesia becomes more technical, more data will be produced and more time will be dedicated to charting rather than to patient care. To complicate matters further, records used today in anesthesia are designed to be used by many different people. Information must be recorded by the anesthetist to satisfy other hospital personnel including the billing clerk, the researcher, and the quality assurance officer. The anesthetist, however, should not be constantly occupied filling in information not pertinent to immediate patient care since data not used or needed by anesthesia can prove to be distracting enough to jeopardize patient safety.[9]

The above-mentioned reasons are just a few of those that lead many to believe that computerized patient records would generate more accuracy in record keeping as well as free the anesthesia provider. Computerized records not only could improve accuracy of documentation but could also provide the following additional advantages.

1 Instantaneous data retrieval
2 Transmission of laboratory tests results and progress notes directly into the operating room
3 Transference of intraoperative data to the PACU at the completion of anesthesia
4 Timely, uniform, and legible documentation
5 Rapid calculation of data derived from monitors
6 Reminders built into the system that alert the anesthetist of incomplete or inaccurate information, overdose, and allergies
7 Functions that calculate drug dose and infusion rates
8 Incorporation of a central alarm system
9 Statistical analysis of large amounts of anesthesia data for evaluation of outcomes[9]

Computerized records would allow selected data to be generated. For example, all anesthesia-related data for a patient can be generated on one page. If more pages are needed due to length of case, each page generated still contains only information pertinent to anesthesia. This produces less waste because the information now found on records for other departments is not reproduced unnecessarily. Additionally, data can be visualized in more than one way. For example, if needed, vital signs may be viewed in less than 5-minute intervals. Many sophisticated computers can record and generate data from any monitor having an output port. Infrequently needed information is not visible unless specifically retrieved. Even though information in computers may be selectively viewed, computers used for patient data documentation must be capable of generating all information in a format that can become a part of the permanent record.[9]

The three major criticisms of computerized records are incorporation of artifacts as part of the record, removing the anesthetist from the information loop, and system failure. Computers cannot recognize and filter artifacts, as can the anesthetist, so that artifacts can become a part of the record. The documentation of artifacts by a computer may be edited at the time of occurrence by the anesthetist if he or she notices, or the computer may be programmed to record more frequently, making artifacts more obvious when the entire record is printed and reviewed.[9]

Although editing of computerized records is possible to rid the record of such artifacts, editing of records may lead to the question during a lawsuit of how much of the record could and was changed. Consequently, the question arises as to whether or not a jury can really be convinced, when computer-generated records are presented into evidence, that a record was indeed unaltered or was altered only for removal of artifacts.

The computer can remove the anesthesia provider from the information being recorded, thus moving him or her out of the information loop. Unlike manual record-keeping, which requires information charted to first be transferred through the anesthetist's mind, information documented by computer is done automatically without the involvement of the anesthesia provider. This raises concern that the computer could decrease the provider's awareness of the patient's status.[9]

The third disadvantage of computerized medical records is the possibility of system failure. System failure can result in the loss of an entire anesthesia record. A backup hand-documented record may not be available, which would mean total loss of all events during the anesthetic.[9]

SUMMARY

Accurate, complete, and legible record-keeping is imperative during the perioperative anesthetic course. Documentation is vital to ensure all that review the data that quality patient care was provided by a qualified anesthetist who was cognizant of adopted standards of care. All aspects of care, from the initial meeting between the anesthesia provider and the patient to the final postoperative interview, must be documented in detail. The documenter(s) must always be aware of the importance of anesthesia documentation as a part of the permanent medical record and that the future safety of the patient may depend on documentation that is accurate and beneficial to subsequent providers.

REFERENCES

1. Beecher, HK: The first anesthesia records. Surg Gynecol Obstet 71:689, 1940.
2. Storey, BM: The anesthesia record: Documenting the standard of care. CRNA Forum 5:1, 1989.
3. Markarian, CJ: The anesthesia record. In Dornette, WHL (ed): Legal Issues in Anesthesia Practice. Philadelphia: FA Davis, 1991, p. 93.
4. Jackson, SH: Humanism and anesthesia safety. Current Reviews for Nurse Anesthetists 8(11).
5. Markarian, CJ: The anesthesia record. In Dornette, WHL (ed): Legal Issues in Anesthesia. Philadelphia: FA Davis, 1991, p. 93.
6. *Sauro v. Shea*. 390 2d Pa. Superior Ct. (1978).
7. Mannino, MJ: The Nurse Anesthetist and the Law. Grune & Stratton, New York, 1982.
8. Cooper, JB, Newbower, RS, and Kitz, RJ: An analysis of major errors and equipment failures in anesthesia management: Considerations for prevention and detection. Anesthesiology 60:34, 1984.
9. Fiedler, MA: New technologies in anesthesia: Update for nurse anesthetists—the computer-generated anesthesia record. AANA Journal 58:49, 1990.
10. Accreditation Manual for Hospitals. Joint Commission for Accreditation of Hospitals and Organizations, Oakbrook Terrace, IL, 1990.
11. Zollinger, RM, Kreul, JF, and Schneider, AJL: Man-made versus computer-generated anesthesia records. J Surg Res 22:419, 1977.
12. Dirksen, R, et al: The clinical use of the Ohmeda automated anesthesia record keeper integrated in the Modulus II anesthesia system. Int J Clin Monit Comput 4:135, 1987.
13. Gravenstein, JS, et al: The electronic clipboard: A semiautomatic anesthesia record. Int J Clin Monit Comput. 4:153, 1987.
14. Logas, WG, et al: Analysis of the accuracy of the anesthetic record (abstr). Anesth Analg 66:S107, 1987.

SIX

Assessing Quality in Practice

15

Establishing Measures of Competence

Linda Callahan

OUTLINE

OBJECTIVES

On completing this chapter, the reader will be able to:

1. Define the term "competence" as it relates to clinical practice and other domains of professional endeavor.
2. Identify professional groups or agencies that impact on definitions of competence.
3. List traditional measures of competence and understand problems with each as they relate to validity.
4. Gain verbal facility in relating the theory of concept analysis and its relation to developing competence models.
5. Describe the AANA practice model and the method of defining role-specific competencies.

Anesthesia as a practice discipline requires a high level of specialized knowledge, judgment, and ability. For more than 100 years, nurse anesthetists have demonstrated an ability to translate the clinical requirements of this specialty into safe, quality care that suits patient needs. As a professional, each certified registered nurse anesthetist (CRNA) is responsible and accountable for the maintenance of an acceptable level of clinical competence. As social concerns about access to quality care continue to escalate, it is imperative that all health care professionals develop and effectively evaluate their own professional competence in practice. The ability to document competence enhances societal recognition, understanding, and trust in the professions. These activities also enhance collegiality, which practitioners must develop to fully experience the culture of the profession (see Chapter 2). Above all, the CRNA must pay requisite attention to clinical competence, as professional health care providers remain accountable solely to the public for cost-effective, quality care; and for that, we must be able to justify and document our competence in its delivery.

Before embarking on a narrative that discusses competence from a theoretic standpoint, it might be advantageous to understand what "competence" is considered to be, some domains of professional activity for which a level of competence must be determined, who determines competence, and some of the more common yardsticks of measurement. From that vantage point, this chapter addresses efforts of the American Association of Nurse Anesthetists (AANA) to develop a competence model for CRNAs to use in determining their competence profile.

WHAT DO WE KNOW ABOUT COMPETENCE?

Broadly defined, *competence* is the ability to demonstrate knowledge, skills, and abilities that underlie effective job performance. Although akin to a job description, a comprehensive competency profile is much more global in nature. It speaks to capabilities and potentials of the provider rather than specific tasks or technical maneuvers to be completed. The characteristics of any determination of competence usually include the following. First, a written description of competence should be based on measures of outcome; for instance, one measure could be continuous quality improvement data, which documents patient outcome. It should include easily identifiable and measurable behaviors that the provider can visibly demonstrate. These activities may not necessarily be limited to behaviors inherent to clinical performance alone, as we will discuss below. Finally, the process of measuring competence is dynamic and ongoing; measurement should not be limited to the classification of skills on a criteria basis beyond which there is no room for improvement. Finally, measures of competence always will and should vary from practitioner to practitioner, because each competence profile must reflect the individual CRNA's educational preparation, employment arrangement, and practice setting.

Most researchers in this area agree that there are four levels of competence. The first level includes attention to tasks or skills required for clinical practice. Examples of these would be the ability to start an intravenous line (IV), insert an invasive monitor, or intubate a patient. Next, a competence profile should address the practitioner's ability to make quality judgments or decisions that relate to practice problems. This level establishes that judgments and decisions made by the CRNA are pertinent to the problems at hand, that the practitioner has the ability to construct a "cognitive" or thinking approach to problem solving and critical thinking, and that the CRNA is able to formulate hypotheses and test potential solutions.

Third, the practitioner must demonstrate advanced knowledge and skills beyond what is considered to be minimum competence to practice. An example of this would be the need for the practitioner to manage patients with multisystem disease or some syndrome involving complex medical problems. At this stage, these competencies should be able to withstand the scrutiny of peer review, comment, and analysis. As one can readily see, the nature of competence measures is truly dynamic and ongoing. There is always something left for the practitioner to achieve in terms of improving competence, thus modifying their competence profile in an upward direction.

The fourth level of competence involves clinical activities that introduce the concept of "totality in care." That is, clinical maneuvers should now incorporate a system of problem solving and clinical decision making that accommodates the application of values from both the patient's and provider's perspective. These clinical actions or decisions should be integrated with dimensions of personal philosophies, attention to ethical standards, motivations, and intent.

DOMAINS OF COMPETENCE

Measures of competence should not be restricted only to clinical practice. There are other domains of competence that the CRNA should consider in developing a comprehensive competence profile. Again, acknowledging the fact that profiles vary between practitioners, there are selected areas of nonclinical, professional practice in which some CRNAs must be able to demonstrate competence according to their unique employment arrangement or circumstance.

For instance, one domain to which all CRNAs need to attend is the area of continuing education. Every recertified CRNA must demonstrate competence in acquiring continuing education and applying its principles in clinical practice. CRNAs must also demonstrate their understanding of professional standards and codes. That is, every anesthetist should be able to demonstrate solid skills in interpreting clinical practice standards, local and community practice standards, and ethical codes of behavior. Selected CRNAs who are teachers, scientists, or administrator/managers must be able to demonstrate competence in instructional skills, hypothesis formulation and testing, and/or personnel management and policy formulation. It is hoped that these examples provide a clearer understanding of the notion that competence profiles of CRNAs will necessarily be different, depending on practice settings. The reader should bear in mind that just because competence profiles differ, this does not indicate that one CRNA is more or less competent than another, relative to basic standards or minimum competence standards required to practice. It only indicates that each profile reflects the unique practice configuration of the individual CRNA.

WHO DETERMINES COMPETENCE?

The responsibility for determining what constitutes clinical competence should remain with the provider, as this is a basic right and responsibility inherent to the CRNA's claim of professionalism. Often competency measures are well defined by the professional association to which the provider belongs, such as the AANA. However, there are others external to the field of nurse anesthesia who would, *and sometimes do,* assume the responsibilities of defining competence.

The list of groups that seek to define the practice and competence of CRNAs is long. Among them are state boards of nursing, which are largely responsible for regulating (licensing, certifying, or designating) the nurse anesthetist. For instance, the National Council of State Boards of Nursing states that the public has a right to expect an individual board of nursing to monitor competence of nurses throughout their career. The National Council of State Boards of Nursing proposes that competence is measurable, definable, and can be monitored to reasonably assure the public health, safety, and welfare. In most states, however, local boards of registered nursing (BRNs) defer to the professional organization, such as the AANA, to define competence.

In addition to the BRNs, some medical specialty groups and federal and state governmental agencies such as the Health Care Financing Administration (HCFA) have attempted to become active players in promulgating definitions. Individual hospital policy-making bodies and medical malpractice insurance carriers have begun to define clinical practice standards, which in essence address the issue of competence. Another example might be the Joint Commission on the Accreditation of Hospitals and Organizations, which now states that there must be a process to ensure competence of providers with explicit specifications rather than implicit assumptions.

TRADITIONAL COMPETENCE MEASURES

One could justifiably ask, "How is competence really measured?" given the fact that it is claimed by some to be a rather abstract notion, not easily given to understandable jargon or practical criteria. Although some answers are forthcoming, it is clear that the study of competence is in its infancy and has yet to reveal concrete answers that have proven to be consistent, valid, and reliable.

Traditionally, competence has been measured by an initial certification examination, although most agree that this mechanism tests competence only at a discrete point in time, that is, when an individual first enters the profession. It does not speak to competence beyond that point. For that, we have devised a system of mandated continuing education (CE) every 2 years, as have many other disciplines. The problem here, however, is that the results of research are disappointing regarding the question of whether or not accumulation of CE credits in actuality assures competence. Research does tell us that any enhanced patient outcome derived from the application of learned principles from CE is rarely demonstrated unless application is introduced into clinical practice almost immediately after it is learned.

Some state regulatory agencies (for medical and nursing groups) and professional organizations have devised other means of measuring competence in clinical practice, among them the requirements to undergo peer review and audits of records, resubmitting to a competency examination at periodic intervals, requiring minimum practice hours, or attaining a certain academic degree. All proposals have their problems, and none have yet emerged as a clear indicator of competence.

Among the most promising new proposals are attempts by some professional organizations to implement competence models. These schemata have the potential to offer a conceptual framework of competence from which specific competency statements can be derived. It is from these models that some propose competence measures can be more clearly elucidated.

The next section addresses the theory behind competence as a concept and provides a background to a model proposed specifically for the nurse anesthetist.

ANALYSIS OF COMPETENCE IN TERMS OF A CONCEPT

In the educational and professional arena, a functional differentiation is made between the words "competence" and "competency," which are used interchangeably, in the broadest sense. In order to analyze the terms "competence" and "competency," one must first attempt to clarify the terminology as it is often used in the medical and nursing professions.

A *concept* can be defined as "a notion or idea that signifies what is common to a number of specific things or states of affairs."[1] Competence defines a concept because it tells us what is unique about a variety of facts, thoughts, and achievements that makes them competent. Further, "to analyze" means to take something apart, thereby revealing functional components and the relationship of those components to each other, as well as to the whole.

The previous definitions are somewhat helpful for understanding, but they do not answer the question of why we should make the effort to analyze concepts at all. Kneller[1] states that concepts are crucial because they act to filter our experience of the world. Our professional world comes to us perceptually unorganized, and we must categorize our experiences of it, so that knowledge can be gained that gives us the sense of the whole event. This process allows us to establish an identity within our world.

If we accept this premise, the first step in analyzing the concept of competence is the examination of the word in the context of common usage. In doing so, we are not seeking just the simple meaning of the word, but are looking for precisely the things or components that the word includes or excludes. It is also necessary to grasp what the analyzed term implies and under what conditions its use is appropriate.

A dictionary provides us with the meanings of words, while analysis of the words, which represent concepts, provides a rationale for meanings expressed in the dictionary. In essence, analysis allows us to define the *necessary and sufficient conditions* for the application of a concept. Concepts are often complex, with multiple layers of functional meaning. As we "unpack" the strata of subconcepts inherent to the definition, we discover individual components, or role-specific competencies. The dictionary definition of competence includes such terms as "adequate" or "sufficient to the task." Certainly, such terms are value laden and open to wide interpretation. The subconcept of a competency, for example, a single, observable, or definable skill, functions with other subconcepts to assist in identification of the necessary and sufficient conditions for comprehension of competence.

An example of the use of this particular subconcept is the definition of role-specific competencies. *Role-specific competencies* are groups of related skills and abilities specific to a given situation. Role-specific competencies that help define the overall concept of competence may be further classified as consisting of knowledge, skills, aptitudes, attitudes, and intellectual strategies, such as problem solving or the ability to deal with ambiguity.

It is tempting to look at competence as simply a process for which there are differing methodologies. Examination of subconcepts, such as role-specific competencies, allows the recognition of competence not only as a process but also as a *product* of the process. By such examination we therefore gain and increase our understanding of another portion of the necessary and sufficient conditions of the larger concept.

In attempting to "unpack" the concept of competence for learning purposes, it must be recognized that education is a practical endeavor difficult to place within abstract symbolic schema. Therefore, educational philosophers perform "linguistic analysis" or ordinary language analysis rather than analysis by symbolic logic. Symbolic logic makes use of algebraic symbols, while linguistic analysis allows one to analyze concepts in terms of useful analogies from other, prior analyses.

Ludwig Wittgenstein (1889–1951) believed that the "language game" was a key concept necessary to understanding the philosophy of language.[1] The "game" is the manner in which words are used in communal and related activities. His basic tenet for understanding was "don't ask for the meaning, ask for the use." Wittgenstein saw language as a collection of games, each with its own rules. An act of speech or writing becomes an act within the language game. To understand the act, one must know not only the game, but also the rules by which it is played. The meaning of any word then becomes equal to what it stands for in the context of the game. In other words, when one knows how the word is used, one knows what it means.[1]

Using Wittgenstein's approach, the first step in analysis is to consider the words used to help define the concept. In our current discussion, the concept is named "competence." We begin by asking what "things" would ordinarily be called by that name. In making a list of related words, one must consider when these words may be used in lieu of the concept word itself. We might include such words as knowledge, ability, application, judgment, goodness, responsibility, and capability. These words begin to define the concept and lead to the next question. Does the concept apply to a single thing, such as an activity, achievement, or underpinning, or does it represent a range of things?

Competence appears to cover a variety of terms that are used to represent processes, products, or even professions within varying contexts. It is also useful to distinguish between central and marginal corollary words of the concept. *Central corollary words* exemplify more intrinsic understandings of a concept. Knowledge, ability, and judgment are intrinsic to any understanding of competence, for they are always present in any definitional form of competence. Competence could not exist without them. For instance, goodness and responsibility are certainly descriptive of some competence parameters, but without them, competence as a concept could still be defined. These terms are not representative of words that help to identify "necessary and sufficient conditions" for the application of the concept. *Marginal corollary words* function as different language forms that communicate data that is different in nuance and cultural perspective. For example, responsibility language often deals with generalization of events associated with duty and guilt, while goodness language often deals with the individual's perception of the experience of specific acts or phenomena.[1]

The use of marginal corollary words, such as responsibility and goodness, helps define the use of the concept of competence in a descriptive fashion. This allows development of rules that guide us toward conceptual understanding via differing epistomologies, or ways of knowing. A final examination of all necessary and sufficient conditions for application of the concept of competence is complex, with many overlapping and contextually dependent speech acts in the language game.

Identification of the necessary and sufficient conditions for application of the concept of competence can be further aided by a consideration of hermeneutics, the study of understanding. The 19th century German philosopher Wilhelm Dilthy[1] argued that interpretation itself is central to understanding. Although the hermeneutical approach is built on text analysis, an observed act is deemed meaningful, hence understanding it is like reading a text. Implicit in such understanding is the presence of a number of speech acts that verbally and nonverbally inform us or others. Whether assessing text or an observed act, we seek to find out what the authors are trying to accomplish. To do this we must take their place, assume their prejudices, look through their eyes, and fully identify with them. The ability to do these things allows "empathetic understanding" or *Verstehen*. Empathetic understanding includes interpretation because it involves the recognition of a meaning that is not immediately obvious. Such recognition is *analyzed or evaluated* to be identical with the author's intention. Heidegger[1] noted that to understand something is to grasp its meaning and significance (evaluation function), whereas to interpret something is to comprehend what is signifies from a certain standpoint or situation (analysis function). We each understand events in light of our own purposes and hence from standpoints or situations defined by those purposes. Understanding is, therefore, interpretive. The term "understanding," which represents interpretation for knowledge acquisition, can be said to function as another central corollary word, which is useful for defining the necessary and sufficient condition for the application of the concept of competence.

The explicit definition of words that must accurately substitute for the original concept word would be desirable, but has proven to be impossible even in the world of pure science.[2] Simple definitions or complex analyses of concepts reflect the development of science or our understanding of the world at that time. As models for reality mature and change, definitions and analyses change.

The terms "entry level competence" and "continuing competence" are based on interpretation of a specific model of professional competence formulated at a specific point along the developmental continuum. Continuing competence builds on entry-level competence as appreciation of our professional world, expressed by a known competence model, matures. Processes and theories change and develop as perspectives mature and knowledge grows, but competence as a concept remains constant and meaningful.

Following the process of this theoretic discussion, a definition for competence in professional practice may be gleaned, examined, refined, and perhaps gradually accepted. The National Council of State Boards of Nursing has developed a definition: "Continued competence for nurses encompasses the ongoing ability to render safe, direct nursing care or the ongoing ability to make sound judgments upon which that nursing care is based."[3]

While useful in its broadness, a full understanding of the whole concept of competence, defined in the previous statement, remains dependent on the identification and culturally shared understanding of subconcepts, or specific competencies that make up the whole. Defining subconcepts, essential to the whole concept, provides one with the "pieces" that may be transmitted in a pragmatic and observable fashion to others. The concept of competence is far too complex to be understood by most people in a single exposure, but it may be refined gradually by the assumption and practice of subconcepts that change over time, yet remain the "necessary and sufficient" parts of the whole.

THE PRACTICAL APPLICATION OF A COMPETENCE MODEL

Before moving into study of the actual competence model to discern how it works, it might be helpful to review some of the basic characteristics and functions of the model.

The responsibility of a profession to define and describe the practice of its members has prompted the development and implementation of competence models by various health care organizations. In the specialty practice of anesthesia by nurses, this model can provide certifying and regulatory agencies, employers, and consumers with criteria on which to base expectations of acceptable practice by the CRNA. The model serves to replace implicit assumptions about competence with observable parameters that can be directly evaluated.

As previously stated, role-specific competencies found within the model differ from one practitioner to another. They are not designed to define optimal practice in every setting. Rather, competency statements act as guidelines for development of competency standards for individual practitioners, departments, or agencies. Each competency statement reflects the skills and abilities needed for adherence to an identified capability inherent to competent practice. The model may be used as a tool in the development of position descriptions, assessment of services provided, staff orientation, performance appraisal, and staff development. The model is descriptive and, when properly used by the individual practitioner, can provide the basis for realistic self-evaluation and/or peer review.

The practical application of the model by the practitioner requires review and selective modification of competency statements to reflect the requirements and characteristics of individual practice settings. Caution should be exercised to ensure that modifications reflect recognized standards of clinical practice, and such modifications must be broadly stated to avoid undue restrictions on scope of practice. The model design should accommodate minor modifications as practice patterns change or the practitioner assumes new professional responsibilities, such as advanced clinical services (pain management), research, teaching, or departmental management.

The use of properly modified competency statements derived from the model, when used as an individual or peer review mechanism, provides strong evidence for the practitioner's concern for autonomy and professional excellence. To maintain credible professional strength and identity, practitioners must self-monitor their practice to a greater degree than required by external agencies that are charged with monitoring practice or regulation. If this responsibility is not taken, they will likely be assumed by those agencies external to the discipline. This proactive behavior demonstrates concern for the provision of quality anesthesia care, as well as possession of requisite clinical knowledge and continuous self-evaluation.

Many feel that competency models portend the future for how health care practitioners will be monitored, assessed, and regulated. This model will allow the practitioner and employer to jointly review the document to assess practitioner compliance with desired institutional standards of care. Competence-based assessment is commonly used in personnel development and program planning offices at many institutions when employee performance is in question and remediation required. If properly used, the model can serve as a "guidepost" for activities the practitioner can follow to help correct performance deficiencies via explicit, written expectations.

THE AMERICAN ASSOCIATION OF NURSE ANESTHETISTS COMPETENCE MODEL

Recognizing the need for a mechanism of professional accountability, in 1985, the board of directors of the AANA formed an ad hoc committee charged with the development of a competence model for nurse anesthesia practice. During a 4-year period, the committee developed a conceptual framework of nurse anesthesia practice from which role specific competencies were extrapolated. To aid in development, the first step was to conduct a values clarification survey, which was sent to a representative group of practitioners. The information gained aided in the development of a preliminary philosophy statement as well as a model that addressed the knowledge, understanding, skills, values, attitudes, and interests nurse anesthesia professionals held regarding their practice. The practice model provided a basis from which competence standards and role-specific competencies could be developed.

As demonstrated in Figure 15–1 and described in Boxes 15–1 through 15–5, a nurse anesthesia practice model was developed from action words that described the philosophy of the profession. (Concepts identified in the boxes are provided to clarify the

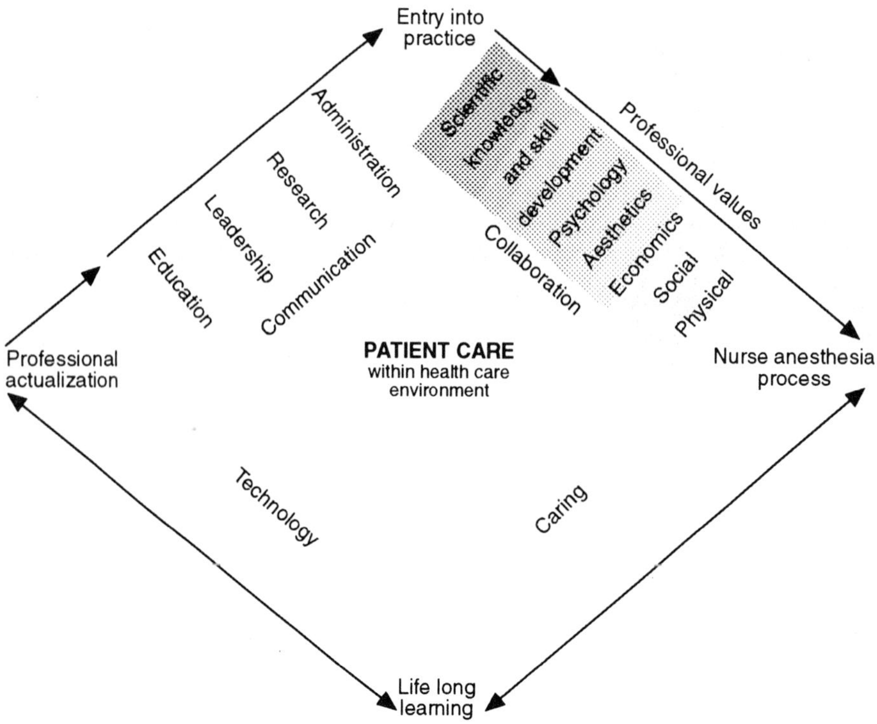

Figure 15–1. Nurse anesthesia practice model.

BOX 15–1
DEFINITION OF NURSE ANESTHESIA PRACTICE MODEL*

The advanced practice of nursing in the specialty of nurse anesthesiology has special attributes that speak to the strength and uniqueness of our role in the provision of anesthesia care in the health environment.

Caring for the patient as a holistic being is an important tenet of our professional behavior. We strive to be altruistic human beings, believing that caring is essential to one's personal development.

Collaboration between the nurse anesthetist and other members of the health care team takes place in separate and joined activities and responsibilities that are directed at attaining mutual goals of excellence in patient care.

Communication is sharing information to achieve mutual understanding. Communication skills are a cornerstone of patient interviews, imparting information to other health professionals, documentation of practice, and participation as a contributory member in meeting society's health needs.

Technology denotes an area rich in technological advances and scientific content that requires strengthening and updating through the professional life. Practitioners have the ability to apply the nursing process to complex problems at a high level of competence.

*From Munguia-Biddle and co-workers.[4]

BOX 15–2
DEFINITION OF NURSE ANESTHESIA PRACTICE MODEL*

Entry into Practice

Recognition of the attainment of a defined body of knowledge, technical skills, and professional development is essential to the beginning practitioner's entry into the anesthesia care milieu. The recognition of entry level skills attainment is confirmed by the Council on Certification of Nurse Anesthetists after the successful completion of an accredited nurse anesthesiology educational program.

*From Munguia-Biddle and co-workers.[4]

BOX 15–3
DEFINITION OF NURSE ANESTHESIA PRACTICE MODEL*

Professional Values

A profession may be defined in terms of the domains of human endeavor valued by the members of the profession. Such are the following domains within professional nurse anesthesiology practice.

Intellectual

Integral concepts within this domain are based upon advanced knowledge in the fields of anatomy, physiology, pathophysiology, technology, and pharmacology as applied to anesthetic practice. The continued development of technical expertise and competence in practice are inherent in this area of concern.

Psychological

The professional nurse anesthetist is concerned with enhancement of the patient's coping skills in a time of possible physical and emotional disruption produced by the perioperative experience. Recognition of the needs of the practitioner are expressed as concern with issues such as communication, autonomy, counseling, and impairment or incompetent practice within the workplace and the profession as a whole.

Aesthetics

Spiritual growth and religious preferences are recognized and respected as inherent to full development of human potential within the patient and the nurse anesthetist. Ethical development and involvement within the political realm encompassing the nurse anesthetist as a member of society is held to be a continual and necessary growth process.

Economics

We place great value on the historical role of the nurse anesthesiology profession in providing continuity of anesthesia care that supports an economically viable health care industry. The exploration of strategies leading to resolution of liability issues as well as mechanisms to increase feelings of potential job security are recognized as valuable to continued professional and personal growth and well-being.

Social

Valued concepts within this domain include enhancement and preservation of the professional role of nurse anesthetists in the societal health care delivery system, legal and legislative responsibility for competent patient care, constant development of improved standards of care, patient education, and continued liaison with other health care providers.

Continued

BOX 15–3
DEFINITION OF NURSE ANESTHESIA PRACTICE MODEL*—*CONTINUED*

Physical

Patient safety and the interface between technology and humankind or machines and the patient is of paramount concern. The appropriateness of physical work that considers the impact of schedules, stress, fatigue, and vigilance must be demonstrated in the clinical setting as important factors in securing the patient care environment.

*From Munguia-Biddle and co-workers.[4]

BOX 15–4
DEFINITION OF NURSE ANESTHESIA PRACTICE MODEL*

The nurse anesthesiology *process* is a problem-solving model that utilizes assessment, analysis, planning, implementation, and evaluation in the complex decision making and actions that exemplify practice within the health care environment.

Lifelong learning is a continuum of nurse anesthesiology process providing for ongoing needs assessment, analysis, planning, implementation, and evaluation. This essential process function is in concert with the rapidly changing setting of nurse anesthesiology practice in specific and the health care environment in general. It provides the vehicle for actualization of self-responsibility in meeting educational needs that are critical to patient care. Commitment to lifelong learning further demonstrates continued acceptance of accountability for the provision of quality anesthesia care for the members of society.

*From Munguia-Biddle and co-workers.[4]

BOX 15–5
DEFINITION OF NURSE ANESTHESIA PRACTICE MODEL*

Professional Actualization

Professional actualization is a dynamic, ongoing endeavor to realize maximum development of professional potential.

Education

Provides an environment that allows for exploration and application of strategies to facilitate the preparation of future practitioners, thereby assuring continuance of the profession.

Leadership

Demonstrates the ability to define reality, set goals, communicate a vision, and influence the willing participation of others in purposeful action that is directed to goal achievement.

Research

Encourages active involvement in scientific inquiry as a consumer, participant, or contributor. It is the driving force of actualization that validates our role in the provision of anesthesia services, enhances growth for the nurse anesthetist and the profession, and leads to new knowledge and improved safety in patient care.

Administration

Provides the interface between people, groups, departments, organizations, professions, and society that enhance individual and collective professional growth.

*From Munguia-Biddle and co-workers.[4]

model set forth in Fig. 15–1.) Basic tenets of the model incorporated the following philosophic notions.

Demonstrate our respect for the worth and dignity of the individual that enters the health care system;

Reaffirm our commitment to equal and quality patient care;

Value integrity and accountability as inherent to our role in the health care system;

Promote a concept of responsibility for lifelong learning as a means of maintaining competence;

Encourage the continuing growth and development of the individual and the profession;

Recognize, initiate, and adapt to society's demands for change in the health care system;

Nurture the potential for and development of advanced nurse anesthesiology practice, education, leadership, administration and research;

Educate the patient and the public in wellness attitudes that contribute to life and health enhancement.[4]

Following initial development of the practice model, a growth model (Fig. 15–2) was developed to demonstrate the need to describe the necessary relationship between our specific practice model and the social structure within which it must function. This growth model clearly indicates movement, change, and interrelationships among elements of the initial model (see Fig. 15–1) and the health care system at large, as well as society. Circular, interlocking gears were chosen to demonstrate the dependence and mutual effects these three subsets had on one another. The equality in size of the gears indicates that each component may be the driving force or may be driven by each of the others. Whichever gear supplies the impetus, all must move together in response. This model is dynamic and applicable to all CRNAs regardless of their chosen professional role. Specific examples of these relationships are found in Table 15–1.

A final model for nurse anesthesiology practice accountability was developed (Fig. 15–3). To enhance understanding, the design of this final model was similar to that of the nurse anesthesiology growth model. In this model, the practice setting should reflect the analysis by the CRNA of individual qualities and performance that reflect agency or employer goals. Included may be items such as administrative skills, organization, promptness, scheduling, call coverage, or cost containment. The interlocking gears of competence contain statements regarding role-specific competencies that are based within the cognitive, psychomotor, and affective domains of practitioner behavior and learning. It is important to note that role-specific competencies should reflect the need to accommodate needs of the employer or practice setting and that competence levels demonstrated will necessarily "drive" the gears of the practice setting.

Boxes 15–6 and 15–7 provide examples of role-specific competencies in the area of patient assessment. The reader should appreciate the fact that this is only a single area of professional endeavor within which the CRNA should maintain competency. This example is provided as the skill of assessment is generic to all CRNAs. It is at this point, however, that the individual CRNA must devise his or her own specific competence statements as they reflect their professional role, practice setting, employment configuration, education, and individual capacities within the model provided and the prevailing standards of care.

SUMMARY

The concept of competence readily lends itself to definition within a conceptual model. However, the more pragmatic concerns of clinical practice deal with overt, behavioral activity. As such, the evaluation of anesthesia services requires observable or demonstrable evidence. Therefore, criteria that are accepted as evidence of competence should be presented as a list of competencies that may be assessed by observation in the practice setting. This allows separate evaluation of component parts of the concept of competence. Appropriately developed, nurse anesthesiology competence statements should reflect the broad range of abilities that link generic knowledge to the essential activities and skills that are descriptive of clinical practice.

An understanding of the process of con-

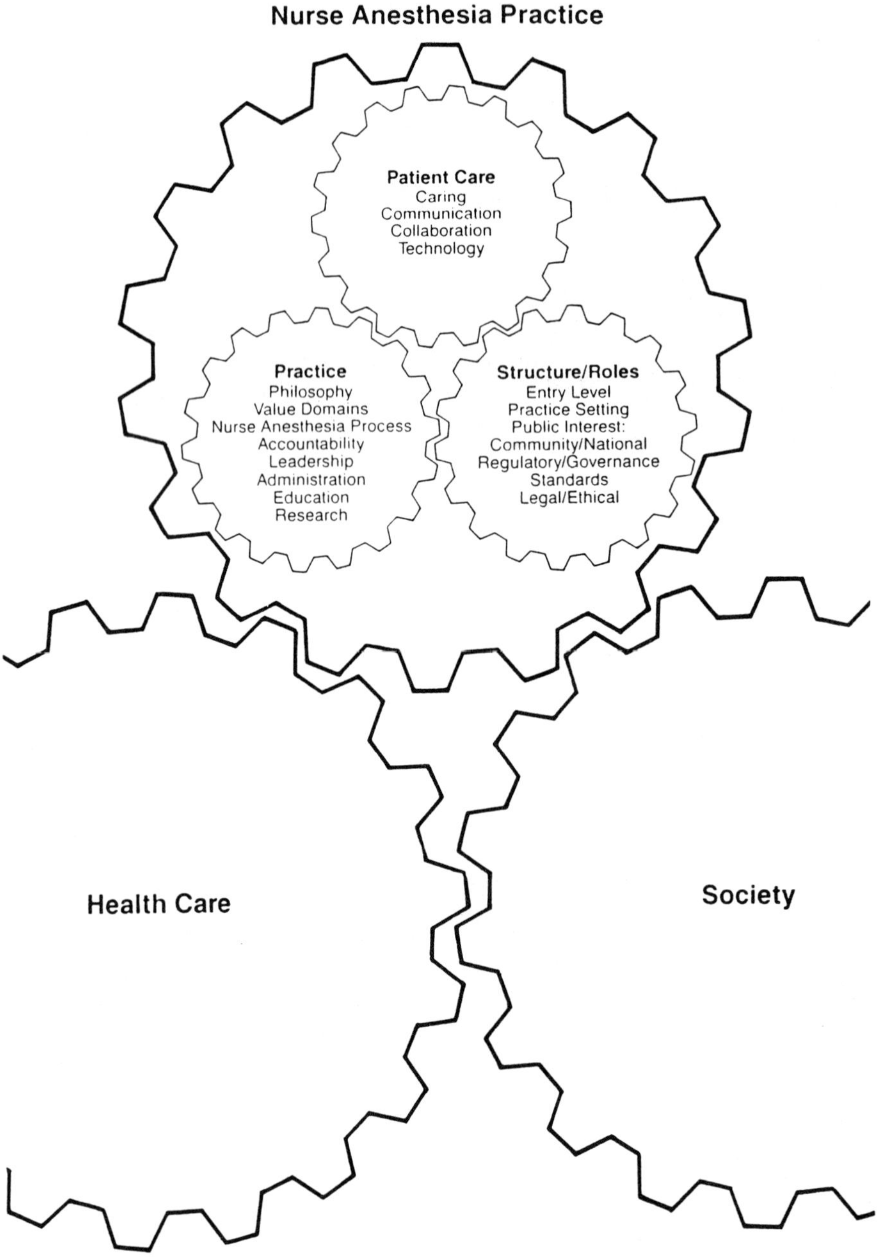

Figure 15–2. The growth model.

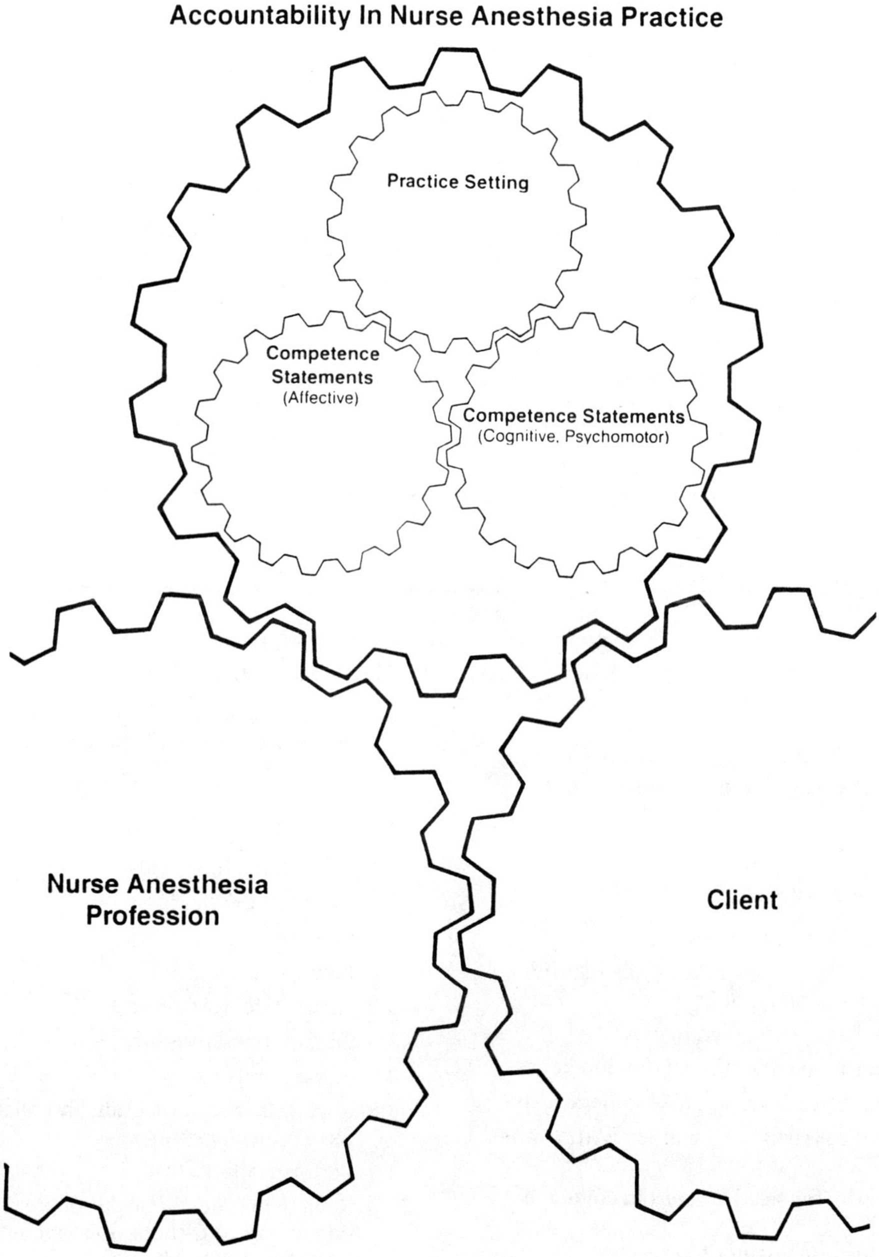

Figure 15–3. The final model.

TABLE 15-1

GROWTH MODEL OF NURSE ANESTHESIA PRACTICE APPLICATION IN VARIOUS PROFESSIONAL ROLES*

Role	*Client*	*Caring Manifested by*
Clinical practice	Patient	Providing pain relief and protecting physical and psychological integrity
	Surgeon	Providing optimal patient conditions for a medical intervention
Education	Nurse anesthesia student/CRNA	Education for entry and/or excellence/or additional role function in specialty
	Public or other health care providers	Professional writing or speaking
Research	Scientific community/CRNA practitioner/other	Participating in research as an investigator, collaborator, data collector, communicator, and disseminator of research findings through professional writing and speaking
Administration	Organization/personnel	Effective efficient planning, allocation, direction, and evaluation of organization or unit; human, fiscal, or material resources
Consultation	Clients (individual) Institutions (organizations)	Assisting in development/ implementation of various programs or problem solving
Leadership	The profession/professional colleagues/society	Maximizing potential Effecting change to 1. Better serve society 2. Maintain vitality and relevance

*From Munguia-Biddle and co-workers.[4]

BOX 15–6
ROLE-SPECIFIC COMPETENCIES BASED WITHIN THE COGNITIVE AND PSYCHOSOCIAL DOMAINS*

Assessment

The CRNA should be able to establish a patient database of verifiable information.

Measurable Criteria

1.0 Patient History

1.1 Obtain patient history
1.2 Obtain previous anesthesia history of patient and family
1.3 Assess exercise tolerance
1.4 Determine patient's last oral intake
1.5 Initiate appropriate preanesthetic tests
1.6 Identify risks associated with transmission of infectious disease
1.7 Identify the need for steroid coverage

2.0 Physical Assessment

2.1 Assess general appearance of patient
2.2 Palpate and inspect anatomic landmarks for regional anesthesia
2.3 Inspect patient for signs of venous distention, jaundice, hepatomagaly, ascites

3.0 Organ System Review

3.1 Auscultate lung fields
3.2 Percuss lung fields
3.3 Palpate trachea
3.4 Inspect upper airway
3.5 Auscultate heart sounds
3.6 Obtain blood pressure
3.7 Palpate pulse
3.8 Review electrocardiogram and related cardiovascular studies
3.9 Perform Allen's test
3.10 Review preanesthetic parameters for impact on anesthetic management, including the following
- Nervous system
- Cardiovascular system
- Renal system

*From Munguia-Biddle and co-workers.[4]

BOX 15–7
ROLE-SPECIFIC COMPETENCIES BASED WITHIN THE AFFECTIVE DOMAIN*

The CRNA has the ability to demonstrate caring, committed concern for the welfare of others.

Measurable Criteria

1.0 Gives full attention to the patient and his or her needs during the entire anesthetic process
2.0 Assists other personnel in providing needed care as appropriate
3.0 Expresses active concern about social trends/issues
4.0 Advocates formal and informal liaisons with other health care professionals

The CRNA has the ability to accept and respect all individuals as possessing equal human rights, privileges, and/or status.

Measurable Criteria

1.0 Provides anesthesia care based on the needs of the individual, irrespective of personal characteristics
2.0 Communicates and collaborates with other providers in a nondiscriminating fashion
3.0 Verbalizes ideas regarding individual access to appropriate anesthesia health care
4.0 etc.

*From Munguia-Biddle and co-workers.[4]

cept analysis, recognition of the importance of conceptual modeling to the understanding of both individual and global professional concepts, and thoughtful identification and definition of role-specific competencies demonstrate the ability of practitioners to measure accountability and define the professional culture unique to those nurses educated and certified to administer anesthesia.

REFERENCES

1. Kneller, GF: Movements of Thought in Modern Education. John Wiley & Sons, New York, 1984.
2. Jaeger, RM (ed): Complementary Methods for Research in Education. American Educational Research Association, Washington, DC, 1988.
3. National Council of State Boards of Nursing, Inc.: Position Paper On Continued Competence. Chicago, 1984.
4. Munguia-Biddle, FP, et al: Nurse Anesthesiology Competence Evaluation: Mechanism for Accountability, unpublished document. American Association of Nurse Anesthetists, Park Ridge, IL, 1990.

BIBLIOGRAPHY

American College of Nurse-Midwives: Report of the Education Committee, and Decker, C: Core Competencies. Washington, DC, 1985.

American College of Nurse-Midwives: ACNM Statement on Practice Setting. Washington, DC, 1983.

American College of Nurse-Midwives: Core Competencies in Nurse Midwifery. Washington, DC, undated.

Andrusyszyn, MA: Clinical evaluation of the affective domain. Nurse Education Today 9(2):75, 1989.

Association of Operating Room Nurses: A model for perioperative nursing practice. In AORN Standards and Recommended Practices for Perioperative Nursing. Denver, CO, 1986.

Bara, M and O'Toole, M: Competency based education. RNABC News 22(4):17, 1990.

Becker, J and Ellson, SK: How to develop a competency-based head nurse orientation program. Journal of Healthcare Education and Training 4(3):32, 1989.

DiMauro, K and Mack, LB: A competency-based orientation program for the clinical nurse specialist. Journal of Continuing Education in Nursing 20(2):74, 1989.

Dirschell, KM: A mandate for standards of care. Nursing Health Care Journal, 8:27, 1987.

Fawcett, J: A framework for analysis and evaluation of conceptual models of nursing. Nurse Educator, 5:195–200, 1980.

Gosnell, D: A conceptual model, evaluating continuing education in nursing. Journal of Continuing Education in Nursing 15(1):9, 1984.

Hercules, P, Kneedler, J, and Roth, R: Perioperative nursing competencies. AORN Journal 43(1):259, 1986.

Hickey, M, et al: Competence statements for differentiated nursing practice in critical care. Focus on Critical Care 18(4):286, 1991.

Rethans, JJ, et al: Competence and performance: Two different concepts in the assessment of quality medical care. Fam Pract 7(3):168, 1990.

Rew, L, et al: Intuitive skills in crisis management. Nursing Connections 4(2):3, 1991.

Sams, L, Baxter, K, and Palmer-Smith, P: A competency based model for nurse internships. Journal of Nursing Staff Development 6(2):93, 1990.

Wolf, RM: Evaluation in Education: Foundations of Competency Assessment and Program Review. Frazier Publishers, New York, 1984.

16

Quality Assessment and Improvement for the 1990s

Jonathan T. Lord
Gary P. Kraus

OUTLINE

OBJECTIVES

On completing this chapter, the reader will be able to:

1. Recount the brief history of quality assurance and measurement in health care.
2. Describe the difference between structure, process, and outcome measurements as they relate to quality assessment.
3. Describe an overview of traditional quality assessment programs.
4. Describe the JCAHO 10-step model of evaluation and measurement.

The focus on quality in health care continues to occupy the attention of the public, regulators, and leadership of health care organizations. "Quality" has been an elusive target, often defined divergently by the different constituent groups of users, payers, and providers. Traditionally, the public views the emphasis on quality as a shroud around medical "mistakes," which yields information that too often is not released to the public as useful data for the improvement of patient care. Payers view quality measures as largely irrelevant because of the lack of aggregate data and the absence of linkages between clinical outcome data and cost information. Physicians and other providers view quality assessment (QA) activities as a paperwork exercise focused on ill-defined care problems, and health care administrators see it as a regulatory burden. Still, the concept of QA remains an emerging discipline that many feel will guide the way in which health care services are practiced and delivered.

HISTORY

Formalized quality review dates back to the beginning of this country with the writings of Codman and the American College of Surgeons. These early efforts were directed at structures of professional staff, case reviews, medical record documentation, and support services. These issues were incorporated into the American College of Surgeons Hospital Standardization Program in 1917 (Box 16–1). By 1951, the core elements of this program were more formally coordinated through a hospital accreditation program that was developed by a newly formed organization that included the American Medical Association, the Canadian Medical Association, the American College of Surgeons, and the American College of Physicians, called the Joint Commission on Accreditation of Hospitals (JCAHO). In the intervening period from 1951 through 1992, JCAHO has undergone membership and functional changes, emerging as the premier nongovernmental organization in the world concerned with the quality of health care.

During the 1960s, two watershed events effecting the concept of quality measurement occurred. First, the passage of federal Medicare and Medicaid legislation, and second, the landmark work of Dr. Avedis Donabedian on the structure-process-outcome theory of health care quality. This federal legislation adopted formal requirements for measuring the quality and appropriateness of care and sanctioned the processes for this measurement, embodied in JCAHO standards, as a qualification and approval for Medicare payments.

Dr. Donabedian's work drew 60 years' worth of peer review together with industrial concepts of quality into a comprehensive theory that has been the basis for traditional quality assurance from 1970 through the early 1990s. His theory introduced several new concepts including structure measurements, process measurements, and outcome measurements. *Structure measures* referred to the various traits, features, or resources within a particular health care environment that would enable a provider to deliver quality health care. Examples could include requisite equipment and facilities, specialty services, or accreditation status of the institution. *Process measurement* referred to what is done to and for the patient by individuals, teams, or systems. In other words, process measurements sought information from the organization that could be evaluated against professional standards of quality care relative to how care was provided. *Outcome measurements* determined the health or wellness of patients after care was delivered. These statistical data could then be used to compare the desired results of care given between one institution or provider group and another group, or against some predetermined care goal. Succinctly, structure and process measurements are aimed at causes, whereas outcomes measure the effects of care.

Initial QA efforts in the 1970s focused on the appropriateness or utilization of services by a health care organization and was implemented by "structure-process" based audits. By the end of the 1970s, assessment activities shifted from the unidimensional character of retrospective audits to the identification of actual problems. The problem-focused approach, albeit an improved methodology, suffered from the fact that the

BOX 16–1
THE MINIMUM STANDARD

1 That physicians and surgeons privileged to practice in the hospital be organized as a definite group or staff. Such organization has nothing to do with the question as to whether the hospital is "open" or "closed," nor need it affect the various existing types of staff organization. The word "staff" is here defined as the group of doctors who practice in the hospital inclusive of all groups such as the "regular staff," the "visiting staff," and the "associate staff."

2 That membership on the staff be restricted to physicians and surgeons who are (a) full graduates of medicine in good standing and legally licensed to practice in their respective states or provinces, (b) competent in their respective fields, and (c) worthy in character and matters of professional ethics; that in this latter connection the practice of the division of fees, under any guise whatever, be prohibited.

3 That the staff initiate and, with the approval of the governing board of the hospital, adopt rules, regulations and policies governing the professional work of the hospital; that these rules, regulations, and policies specifically provide:
a. That staff meetings be held at least once each month. (In large hospitals the departments may choose to meet separately.)
b. That the staff review and analyze at regular intervals their clinical experience in the various departments of the hospital, such as medicine, surgery, obstetrics, and the other specialties; the clinical records of patients, free and pay, to be the basis for such review and analysis.

4 That accurate and complete records be written for all patients and filed in an accessible manner in the hospital—a complete case record being one that includes identification data, complaint, personal and family history, history of present illness's physical examination, special examinations, such as consultations, clinical laboratory, x-ray and other examinations, provisional or working diagnosis, medical or surgical treatment, gross and microscopic pathologic findings, progress notes, final diagnosis, condition on discharge, follow-up, and, in case of death, autopsy findings.

5 That diagnostic and therapeutic facilities under competent supervision be available for the study, diagnosis, and treatment of patients, these to include, at least (a) a clinical laboratory providing chemical, bacteriologic, serologic, and pathologic services; and (b) an x-ray department providing radiographic and fluoroscopic services.

From the Minimum Standard of the American College of Surgeon's Hospital Standardization Program, 1913.

single "problem" was too static and did not comprehensively assess an institution's responsibility for a continuous, system-linked assessment. These approaches eventually gave way to more systematic monitoring and evaluation procedures to assess continuous quality of care. However, most of the assessment efforts described had a common focus: to find the negative outcome, event, or failure of the process and fix it. The approach did not look at "systems" causes of events, rather it focused on the individual in a rather punitive manner.

This approach to quality management had a predictable affect on various groups within the health care industry. Practitioners generally considered it demeaning and an intrusion into traditional professional prerogatives such as practice autonomy. Health facility administrators treated it as another aspect of an ever-increasing industry bound by bureaucratic red tape, complicating the management of the institution and contributing significantly to costs.

One positive effect of these efforts, however, was that they spawned the development of a new occupational group in health care whose primary role was quality information management. Quality assurance professionals come from many occupations but most often from nursing and medical records administration. Like other professionals, they have organized their own societies to advance the discipline of quality improvement, the largest of which is the National Association for Healthcare Quality located in the Chicago suburb of Skokie, Illinois.

AN OVERVIEW OF QUALITY ASSURANCE

Contemporary quality assurance activities are generally derivatives of the implicit review process that draw on components of Donabedian's structure-process-outcome theories. These activities have been organized along organizational structural lines of health care institutions, including their major components, medical staff, hospital, and governance.

Within these major components, traditional quality assessment mechanisms or implicit review activities have been segregated by professional discipline and subspecialty and have focused on events or problems in a retrospective fashion. Unfortunately, quality assurance has been and is generally performed in isolation from other activities in the organization, with a primary emphasis on meeting minimum regulatory expectations and requirements.

The typical quality assurance function in organizations today is outlined in a quality assurance plan for the institution that is written to meet the requirements of the JCAHO. In addition to a hospitalwide plan, some organizations have developed department- or section-specific plans for quality assessment. Unfortunately, many of these institutionally generated documents have usually been read by few in the organization. Consequently, their universal application has been sporadic and not wholly successful.

The organizational plans for assessing quality within an institution usually contain the following major sections.

- General description of the QA plan with clear goals and objectives
- Outline or scope of activities to be assessed
- Assigning responsibilities for activity assessment
- Methodology for data collection
- Mechanisms for reporting and oversight
- Process for assessment of effectiveness

THE 10-STEP MODEL OF MONITORING AND EVALUATION

Beginning in 1984, the primary methodology employed for QA has been described as a planned and systematic process to monitor and evaluate the quality and appropriateness of care. Many organizations have adopted the JCAHO's 10-Step Model of Monitoring and Evaluation. This systems approach propagated by the JCAH is basically a variation of the management concept of the closed loop. The purpose of the closed management loop and its incorporation into the 10-step model described below is to require within a managed unit (such as a hospital department) a mechanism by which all aspects of the management processes can be documented.

Within the closed loop paradigm, all evaluative processes are linked together cyclically rather than being disjointed and disconnected. Consequently, when decisions or goals are made, tasks and activities necessary to implement them are assigned and implemented, resulting in conclusions being reached and recommendations being made. Results are then compared to the original decision and corrections made if needed. The process is then repeated.

This process offered a solution to many of the causes of quality-related problems that the JCAH frequently found during years of conducting accreditation surveys. When an institution studies quality problems, the underlying cause is usually due to lack of effective communication and coordination between operational departments and subunits. The 10-step model was designed to ensure greater interaction among caregivers and ensure that every step of the process was complete and incorporated by components of the system. Figure 16–1 is a diagram of the process that incorporates the equivalent steps of the 10-step model that is discussed in the following section.

The tasks and activities of the 10-step model are

1. Assign responsibility.
2. Delineate scope of services.
3. Identify important aspects of care.
4. Identify indicators.

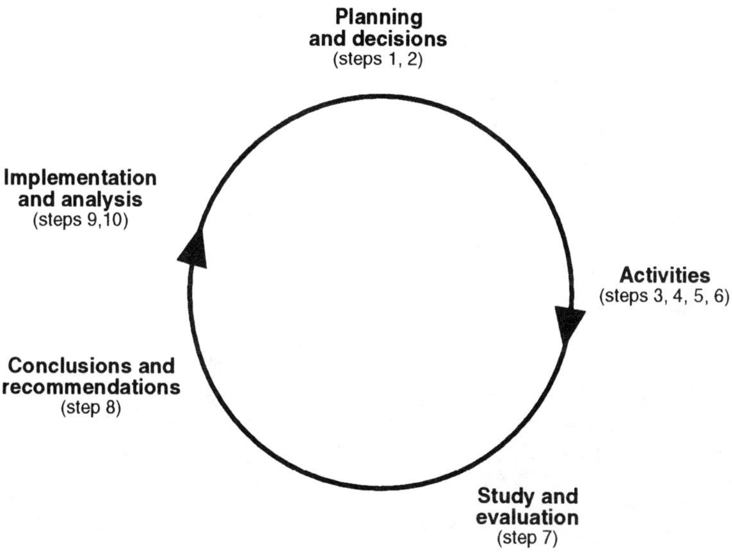

Figure 16–1. Modification of the closed-management loop.

5 Establish thresholds for evaluation.
6 Collect data.
7 Analyze data.
8 Take actions to improve services.
9 Assess the impact of actions taken.
10 Communicate the results to relevant components of the organization.

Indicators in Step 4 and *thresholds* in Step 5 are key features that describe the system linkages found within the historical implicit review process. *Indicators* are defined by the JCAHO as a measurement tool used to monitor and evaluate the quality of important governance, management, clinical, and support functions. Common types or categories of indicators are the desirable indicator, outcome indicator, process indicator, rate-based indicator, sentinel event indicator, structural indicator, and undesirable indicator. Typical indicators employed in most hospitals are derived from an analysis of cases, including such indicators as patient death, medical complications, unexpected event, complaints about services, and other failed outcomes.

A *threshold,* for the purposes of the model above, is the level at which a trigger point is reached that signals the need for the management to begin the process of evaluation and determine why the threshold was crossed. For instance, if the institution has set the acceptable nosocomial infection rate at 4 percent, and institutional data demonstrates that the rate has increased to 5 percent, a systematic process of focused evaluation of cause and remediation is triggered. The following text outlines the 10-Step JCAHO model of evaluation and monitoring.

Step 1. Assign Responsibility

Organizational leaders are responsible for the overall design of a quality improvement system and for obtaining an organization-wide commitment to CQI (see Chapter 17 for a more in-depth discussion of continuous quality improvement [CQI] and its relationship to QA). They are also responsible for assigning responsibility for the various phases of the plan, setting priorities, and making sure the plan is carried out. Leadership commitment and involvement are crucial to the success of any QA or CQI plan.

The responsibility for quality management in the anesthesia department usually rests with the director of that department. However, it is important to remember that the provision of anesthesia is only one part of the total process of patient care. To influence quality care, it is incumbent on all anesthesia providers to be familiar with the facility's patient care and service activities from the time of admission to discharge and know who is responsible for various aspects of patient care.

For example, it is usually the admission department's responsibility to communicate to patients how they should prepare for a given procedure at the time it is scheduled. Since the information needed by the patient originates with the anesthesia department, it is important that there be clear communication and coordination between the anesthesia department and admissions. Another example of information that must be communicated to the patient from the anesthesia department is the requirement that the patient abstain from food or liquids for a certain number of hours prior to the commencement of general anesthesia. This type of necessary communication is often put in the form of an information brochure drafted by the anesthesia department and supplied to the admission department and other providers. It is often up to the admission office to provide patients with this information and advise them to read it carefully. The anesthesia provider must, of course, check with the patient to make sure that the information was understood and followed. Follow-up with the admission department is necessary to correct problems that may ensue or when changes in protocols are made.

By reviewing the total patient care process, the head of the anesthesia department is in a much better position to design the approach necessary for effective anesthesia CQI, identify the responsible persons with whom the anesthesia providers must interact on an ongoing basis to maintain CQI, and establish the necessary priorities for assessment and improvement. The person responsible for the anesthesia department's CQI should, at a minimum, discuss the nature and scope of anesthesia CQI with admissions, nursing (both inpatient and outpatient), recovery, surgery, laboratory and radiology, pharmacy, and the discharge planning staff.

In addition, CQI design and implementation should be discussed with the key facility employees responsible for risk management and quality assurance. Arrangements should be made for the anesthesia department to be appropriately involved in any quality assurance or risk management planning and review activities, and specific linkages should be set up to properly coordinate activities and communication within the facility. Also, mechanisms must be set up for the interface of the anesthesia service with medical staff and hospitalwide monitoring functions (Fig. 16–2). These functions typically include

- Surgical case/invasive procedure review
- Blood usage review
- Drug usage evaluation
- Pharmacy and therapeutics
- Medical record review
- Infection control
- Utilization review
- Safety

Responsibility for performing the various steps in the process can, of course, be delegated to other members of the department. In fact, it is critical that the entire staff feel they have a role in CQI. It should also be a major component of each anesthesia provider's job description and performance evaluation.

Step 2. Delineate the Scope of Care and Service

This step involves taking an inventory of all care and services provided in an organization or department. The purpose of this step is to ensure that consideration has been given to every individual in the organization and to every essential activity or function performed. In an organizationwide CQI program, this might include leadership, information management, patient satisfaction, human resources management, and others.

From this list of services provided, the most important functions should be identified for monitoring and evaluation. Important functions are those that have the greatest effect on the quality of care the patient receives, including clinical, support, managerial, and governance activities. In addition, essential elements for consideration should include

- Types of patients served
- Conditions and diagnoses treated
- Treatments and activities performed

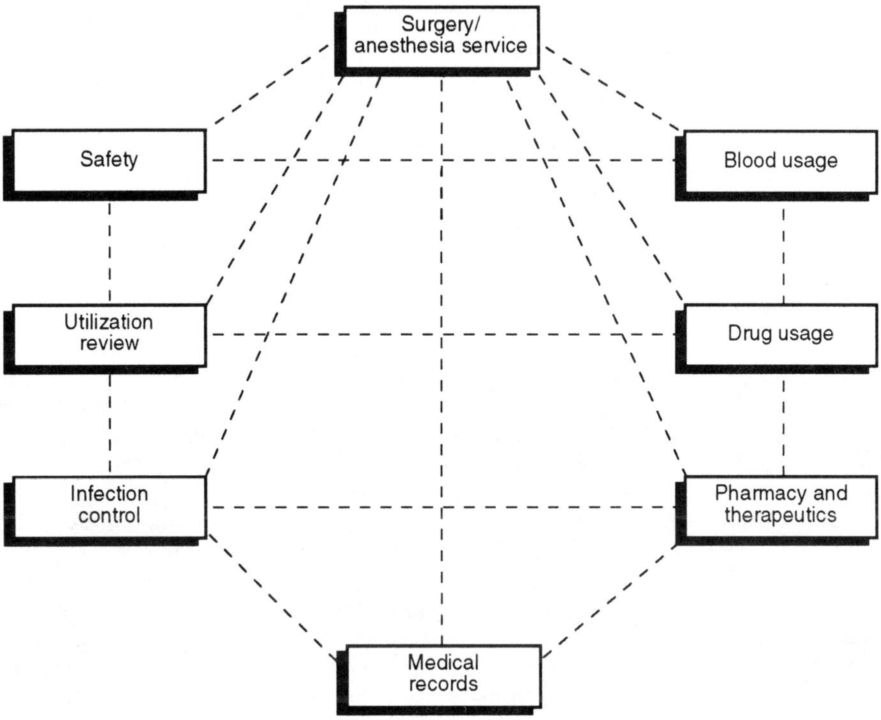

Figure 16–2. Interface with hospitalwide functions.

- Types of practitioners providing care
- Sites where care is provided
- Times when care is provided

Types of Patients Served

Consider the various age groups treated and the setting of their care. For example, inpatient, outpatient, observation status.

Conditions and Diagnoses Treated

Consider the general categories of conditions and diagnoses treated. If at all possible, include statistics to assist in identifying the categories that are high-volume for the particular organization.

Treatment and Activities Performed

Consider the full range of treatments providers render and activities performed both on a daily basis and during crisis situations. An obvious example would be physiologic monitoring. Less obvious examples would be equipment maintenance and inventory control, but these activities can be critical to the efficiency with which the job is performed.

Types of Practitioners Providing Care

Consider the entire team involved in serving the patient. Include technicians, "float" and/or agency personnel, as well as employed professional staff. It is obvious from the exercise addressed in step 1 that the people over whom one has the least control can often be key to successful quality review activities. Thus, it is important that they be identified and their advice and consultation sought during the planning stages of CQI as an aid to determining priorities for review activities.

Sites Where Care Is Provided

Consider every possible site where care or services may be offered. Include both the primary service site and other ancillary service areas, especially those areas where conditions are less than optimal. Again, the areas where there is least control, such as those that require the use of portable equipment, and/or are assisted by staff unfamiliar with provider needs, may be the very areas where the focus of monitoring activities should be maintained. At the very least, these variables will be critical elements to consider when analyzing the data collected and determining possible actions to take in correcting problems or improving care.

Times When Care Is Provided

Consider whether care is provided every day, at all hours, or on a more limited basis. Again, remember that examining service activities only during normal business hours may result in missed opportunities for providing optimal care to patients who, for instance, receive emergency care at night.

Step 3. Identify Important Aspects of Care and Service

In this step, the subjects for ongoing monitoring and evaluation are selected and prioritized. Using the scope of care and service as a basis, select those aspects of care and service important enough to warrant ongoing monitoring and evaluation. These aspects of care may be important functions, procedures, treatments, processes, or other activities that affect patient care. In keeping with a CQI philosophy, this step should be done by an interdepartmental team covering the gamut of patient care from beginning to end. Remember that the goal of CQI is to find ways to do the right thing, do it well, and continually improve the quality of care and service.

One should not focus solely on the treatment or procedure but the point in the process that is most important. One way to assign the designation of "most important" is to determine whether such activity or treatment is high-volume, high-risk, problem-prone, or any combination of the three.

High-volume activities or treatments can be defined as those that occur frequently or affect a large number of patients. If statistics are available, this determination proves to be a relatively simple task. Examples of high-volume aspects of care in an anesthesia department might be preanesthesia evaluation, patient monitoring and anesthesia induction, maintenance, and emergence.

High-risk activities or treatments can be defined as those that place patients and/or staff at risk if they are performed incorrectly, inappropriately, or are omitted. Examples of high-risk aspects of care in an anesthesia department might be intubation or reintubation of an anesthetized patient.

Problem-prone activities or treatments can be defined as those that are low-volume but high-risk, involve a new procedure or technology, involve new and complex equipment, are dependent on interdepartmental cooperation or assistance, are dependent on a degree of compliance or understanding, involve resource personnel external to the department or organization, incur high cost, or occur when staffing is at a minimum or technical support is unavailable.

Examples of problem-prone aspects of care in the anesthesia department might be anesthesia induction and emergence. Once aspects of care are prioritized, the team evaluates those with the higher priority and selects the aspects of care they consider to be the most important to improving quality of services provided in the facility.

Step 4. Identify Indicators

Before proceeding to the identification of indicators, it is important to understand what an indicator is and, possibly more importantly, what it is not. At this point, one should review the definition of indicators found in previous portions of narrative within this chapter. *Indicators* are the tools used to monitor important processes and outcomes. An indicator is not an indication of good or poor quality in and of itself. Indicators merely serve to point the provider in the direction of possible issues to be evaluated further. Indicator selection is a way of examining discrete aspects of care and identifying how, and at what point, evaluation or assessment of this care aspect needs to occur. The JCAHO has developed 13 anesthesia indicators for monitoring and evaluation. All 13 of these indicators are contained in the AQ+ risk and quality management collection form found in Chapter 17.

There are several types of indicators: outcome indicators (all of the JCAHO indicators are of this kind), process indicators, rate-based indicators, and sentinel event indicators. *Outcome* indicators relate to expected results of treatments or care (what happens to the patient). Outcome indicators can be used to assess an event that is either desirable or undesirable. Examples of desirable outcomes include 0 percent induction delays during a certain time period and no unplanned admissions to the intensive care unit (ICU). Examples of undesirable outcomes include adverse or unexplained anesthesia reactions, unplanned respiratory arrest, and unexpected return to surgery. It is important to recall, at this time, that indicators do not definitively measure quality. Instead, they provide a tool for prioritizing a review of activities and focus for further investigation.

Process indicators are used to measure a series of events, actions, or steps performed during the course of patient care, either direct care (e.g., the documentation of preexisting conditions) or to support patient care. The best process indicators identify processes closely linked to patient outcomes. For example, carrying out preanesthesia evaluations should result in better patient outcomes.

Rate-based indicators either provide information about the rate at which events occur within a defined period of time or draw attention to individual occurrences of events *(sentinel event indicators).*

An indicator must possess two important attributes that together determine its usefulness as a performance measure. These are reliability and validity and they must exist in measurable degrees. *Indicator reliability* is the degree to which the indicator accurately and completely identifies all indicator occurrences from among all cases at risk of being indicator occurrences. *Indicator validity* is the degree to which indicators correctly identify events that merit further review.

When an indicator is not complete, clear, and measurable, it is necessary to develop criteria that will make it so. For example, delays in induction must be quantified so that everyone understands what constitutes a delay in induction. Each organization should establish its own criteria for what it considers appropriate. For example, delays in induction greater than 30 minutes are recorded and monitored. Through data collection, one is able to determine if the indicator has been met. By analyzing the information, along with a related outcome indicator, it may be possible to determine potential cause and effect. By tracking indicators for several months, other process indicators may become apparent which, in turn, may deserve or require further analysis.

Step 5. Establish a Means to Trigger Evaluation

In this step, using data and other sources of feedback, a mechanism is established for each indicator to determine when further evaluation will be triggered. A wide range of acceptable variables can significantly impact on the provision of care and services, such as lack of patient compliance, the necessity of triage for emergent cases, and others. Establishing a means to trigger evaluation at a level beyond what is considered acceptable or controllable is the step in the process that allows for such variables.

These mechanisms are set according to the significance of the indicator being measured, clinical experience, past performance of the provider, and patient needs. Indicators considered "sentinel," or critical clinical events, are set at 0 or 100 percent, depending on whether they are worded as positive or negative events. For example, any occurrence of myocardial infarction following administration of an anesthetic agent would trigger individual case review. Rate-based indicators, on the other hand, would be triggered by an accepted norm or benchmark that has been established either through experience or because it is a national norm.

The setting of a triggering mechanism is critical to the process and should not be done arbitrarily. Clinical literature and historical data should be researched and referenced to provide legitimacy and meaning to the selection of this value.

Step 6. Collect and Organize Data

There are a myriad of departmentally generated forms on which data pertaining to QA can be gathered. As JCAHO mandates this data collection activity, there are few hospitals without at least a passing acquaintance of these forms. Chapter 17 will introduce the AQ+ collection form, designed for the flexible and ongoing collection and organization of data to fulfill the requirements of this phase of CQI. The AQ+ data collection system is designed to be either a standalone system or an integrated data collection system within an existing department or hospital CQI program.

In addition to the data collection form, other quality-related feedback mechanisms, such as surveys from patients and families, employees, and others who use the organization's services, should be developed and used in the effort to improve patient care and service.

Collection of data is ideally performed on a concurrent, ongoing basis; that is, consequent with the time patient care is delivered. Although it is possible to perform this activity retrospectively, its value decreases, since it is dependent on accurate and thorough documentation from the medical record. It is also a time-consuming task for the staff and makes ongoing and systematic participation difficult to maintain. Using the data collection sheet concurrently proves valuable because it is timely, the elements collected are fresh in the minds of the participants, the task is shared equally among the staff, and it can be assimilated quickly into the routine process of rendering and documenting care.

Data collection is more than simply the accurate and timely collection of information, although that is clearly important. The data collection process must be managed in the same way as any other aspect of service delivery. This requires planning to ensure that all of the persons affected understand the purpose of the data collection effort and how it is to be done. It also requires directing and monitoring to determine whether or not the data collection functions are being carried out as planned, such that data will be useful.

Step 7. Initiate Evaluation

After reviewing the data, both from ongoing monitoring and other quality-related feedback, such as patient satisfaction surveys, or comments from staff or patient's families, a decision must be made to initiate evaluation. Those individuals who can best evaluate all facets of the particular aspect(s) of care and service should be brought together to form a team to make these decisions. When necessary, these teams should be composed of members from different departments and services.

Certainly, one component of improving quality must be to help find and solve the chronic problems, whether those problems are systems, equipment, or personnel. But the greatest opportunities to improve the quality of care and service lie in improving the overall performance of the systems, equipment, and personnel. Opportunities for such improvement are most often found in ongoing processes rather than in isolated individuals. Determining the patterns of care that triggered evaluation may often be more valuable in improving overall care than will the findings of peer reviewers looking at individual cases. However, when intensive review of occurrences related to a particular practitioner must be undertaken, a peer review should be conducted.

The importance of implementing statistical quality control cannot be emphasized enough. Some of the charts and graphs used as tools in statistical quality control are discussed below.

Control Charts

A *control chart* shows performance data over a period of time to illustrate trends along with the average performance, the upper control limit, and the lower control limit. The control chart shows variation in a process and whether that variation requires action. Performance moving toward a limit and performance outside the limit require action.

Cause-and-Effect Diagrams

A *cause-and-effect diagram* illustrates a process as a set of causal factors and their consequences.

Flowcharts

Flowcharts are often used to illustrate a decision-making process. Flowcharts present a series of steps and their sequels depending on whether the preceding step takes place or not. In quality improvement, a flowchart can be used to understand a process and find problematic steps.

Pareto Charts

Pareto charts are used to determine priorities. If, for example, a cause-and-effect diagram showed 10 possible causes of delayed surgeries, data would be collected to determine how frequently each cause comes into play. The most frequent cause would be the place to focus problem-solving actions.

Run Charts

A *run chart* displays performance over time to illustrate trends. A run chart could be useful to show the number of delayed anesthesia inductions over a designated period of time.

Histograms

Histograms measure the rate and frequency of an occurrence. They can be used to measure productivity. A histogram could, for example, show the frequency at which medical records are completed within a given number of days after discharge. A histogram is used to examine common events and could be useful in formulating reasonable expectations for just how frequently the event occurs.

Scatter Diagrams

Scatter diagrams show the relationship between two variables. Like the Pareto chart, a scatter diagram provides data with which to evaluate cause-and-effect relationships. For instance, an evaluation could be made to determine the relationship between delays in anesthesia induction and cancellation of surgery. Data collected could show what appeared to be an increase in the number of cancellations of surgery or delays of more than 30 minutes in induction. A run chart (Fig. 16–3) was prepared using the raw data. This would confirm the fact that the trend was toward increasingly delayed or cancelled cases.

The flowchart example in Figure 16–4 was designed to show the process from the time surgery was scheduled until the patient was given anesthesia. This showed that there could be many reasons for the delays and cancellations and many different departments might be contributing to the overall problem. A cause-and-effect diagram in Figure 16–5 illustrates the process as a set of causal factors and their consequences.

The task is to look at various factors that

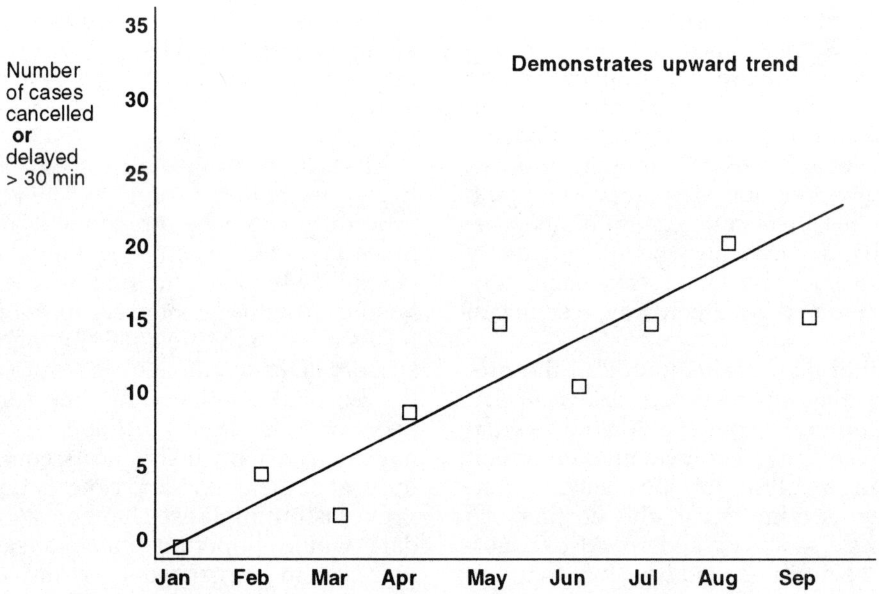

Figure 16–3. A run chart depicting surgery delays and cancellations.

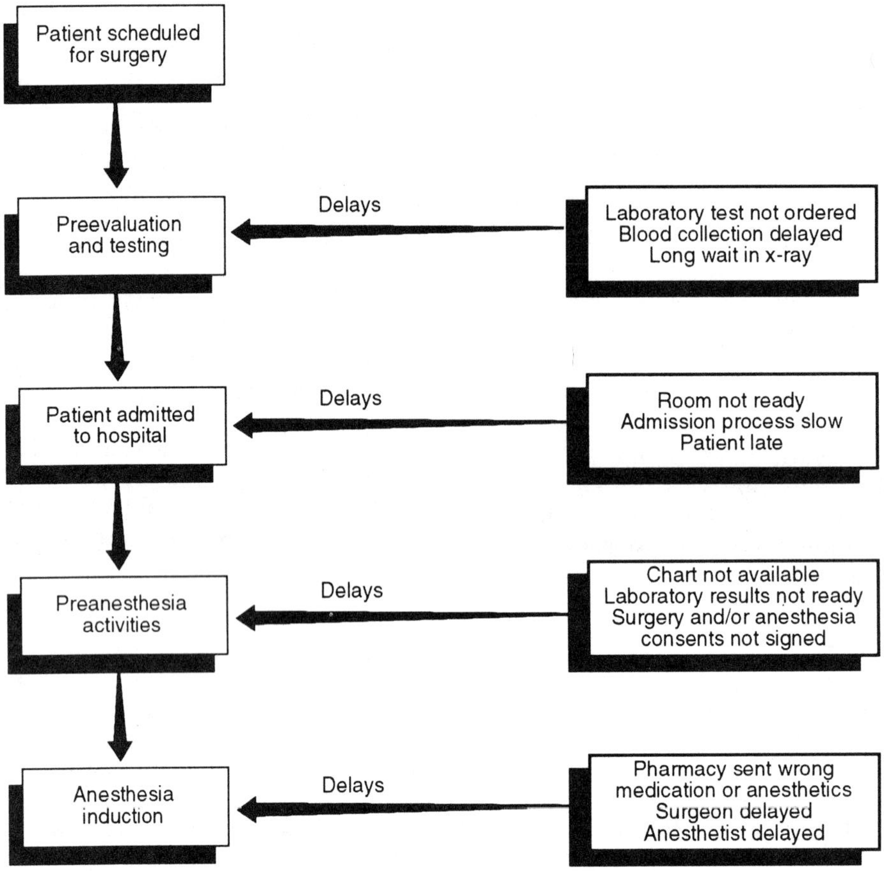

Figure 16–4. Flow chart describing the relationship between scheduled surgery time and anesthesia induction.

may be contributing to the problem and work out a plan of action. The first step might be to assemble a team from each of the departments involved: admissions, laboratory, housekeeping, surgery, and any others. The team would look at the entire process, noting any opportunities for improvement. It could be that there is no communication between the department scheduling surgery and the laboratory, so that preevaluation testing is not ordered in a timely way, resulting in delays.

After thorough evaluation of all the processes leading up to delays and cancellations in surgery, it could be determined that the problem was a cumbersome admission procedure, resulting in long delays in getting patients admitted to the hospital, so everything else was backed up. Also surgeries were being scheduled too close together so that it was almost impossible for preevaluations to be done and consent forms obtained before the next scheduled surgery. It might also be found that outpatients were arriving late on the day of admission to the hospital.

After discovering the problem, it is relatively easy to find a solution. The admission procedure could be streamlined and more time allotted between surgeries. Also, outpatients who lived a long way from the hospital might be housed in motels and hotels close to the hospital the night before surgery. This would allow them to arrive at the hospital in plenty of time for all the necessary presurgical activities. The cost of housing is usually insignificant compared to the cost of the delays and cancellations.

On instituting these changes, subsequent data would hopefully show a significant decrease in surgery delays and cancellations. This information should be communi-

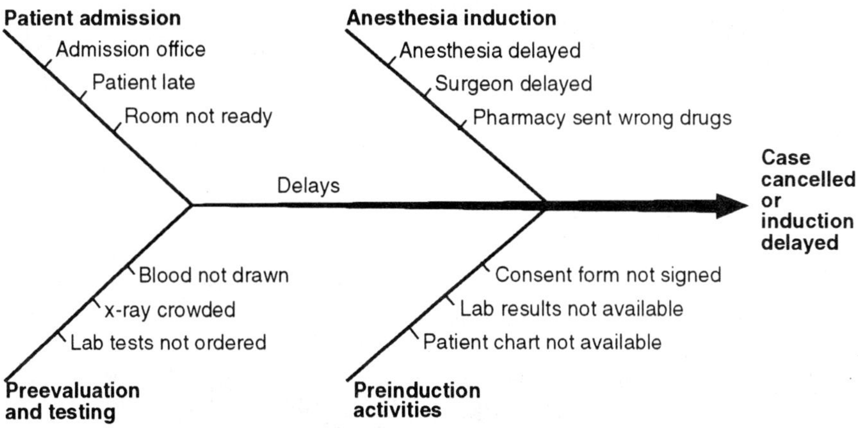

Figure 16–5. Cause-and-effect diagram.

cated to all of the original team members and to the hospital administration. Some system of charting the evaluation and follow-up of those processes or outcomes that require it must be developed, similar to those worksheets found in Chapter 17.

Step 8. Take Actions to Improve Care

This step includes determining the actions to take, assigning responsibility for these actions, and setting a time frame for completion and expected improvement. In organizationwide CQI, this step should be done by a team of experts from all of the involved departments.

If the anesthesia department is doing its own CQI, people from other departments or those with special expertise should be consulted. It is important at this stage to be as precise as possible about the specific person or persons responsible for implementing the recommendations, the timeframe within which the action will take place, and the improvement or change expected. The expected change should be measurable.

Actions may take one of three general forms: organizational/systems actions, knowledge/ability actions, or behavior/motivational actions. Organizational/systems actions are those requiring changes in the way services are designed, structured, and/or documented. Remember that approximately 85 percent of quality issues are system-driven rather than practitioner-driven. That is, rather than changing modes of practice, most problems are addressed through changes in the way the service delivery system operates within the facility. Possible actions include

- Changing or improving channels of communication
- Revising policies, procedures, and protocols
- Adjusting staff complements
- Updating or changing equipment
- Redesigning charts or charting processes

Knowledge or ability problems relate to an individual's intellectual and physical capacities to perform the required work at an acceptable level. Actions addressing problems in this area include

- Providing education programs (in-service, continuing)
- Improving report availability, accessibility, and data collection
- Circulating needed information to staff
- Job performance coaching (on-the-job training)

Problems falling in the area of behavior/motivation are usually related to an individual's volition (i.e., willingness and responsiveness) to perform as expected or required. Problems in this area result not from individuals' inability to perform, but from their choosing not to, for whatever reasons. This is an especially difficult area to address, and actions usually take the form of

- Counseling
- Changing assignments or level of responsibilities
- Disciplinary action (suspension, reduction, termination of privileges for independent providers)
- Suspension or termination of employment

After deciding what needs to be done, who will do it, and how and when the actions will be accomplished, documentation is required.

Step 9. Assess Effectiveness of Actions and Ensure that Improvement is Maintained

As the CQI process becomes operational, ongoing monitoring occurs. The results of continued data collection and monitoring and evaluation activities should be documented to provide a record of the efficacy of actions taken. If the quality of care in a specific area does not improve, then the deficiency, its cause, and the action taken to improve it should be reassessed and new action taken and the effectiveness of this action assessed. Also, important aspects of care, indicators, and triggering mechanisms should be reviewed and assessed on a regular basis for possible revision.

At a minimum, the documentation required by this section should describe how often follow-up should occur, who is responsible, and how this responsibility is carried out. The follow-up should then be monitored carefully and often to ensure that the actions taken have been effective. It will be helpful to format findings in a manner that will allow the QA manager to readily ascertain not only whether a threshold has been met, but also whether there has been any improvement or decline in results.

Step 10. Communicate Results to Appropriate Individuals and Groups

This final step is meant to "close the loop." It provides for the communication of findings, recommendations, actions, and the forwarding of results to staff, management, and administrative personnel. It provides a mechanism for raising the awareness of key people to the issues considered important in the delivery of care and services. It also allows managers an avenue for demonstrating where barriers exist and gives them opportunity to remove them.

The information provided assists the facility in setting budgetary priorities and developing an organizationwide strategic plan. It may be a golden opportunity for focusing the attention of the organization on a critical need specific to a department, such as anesthesia. When compiling reports and formatting data, be sure important ideas are readily understandable to those who may not be familiar with a particular clinical area.

Establish strong working relationships with the institution's quality management director. This individual should prove to be an excellent resource person and an invaluable ally in efforts to bring issues and problems to the attention of key personnel. Remember that a quality management director's primary role is to facilitate individual, departmental, and institutional efforts, and to coordinate information and findings from all areas.

QUALITY ASSESSMENT AND IMPROVEMENT FOR ANESTHESIA: THE FUTURE

Applying these principles to an anesthesia department or service has a profound impact on how quality assessment is performed. Ideally, anesthesia of the future will not be functioning as a separate department but instead will be functioning in an organizational matrix with surgical, obstetric, postanesthesia care unit (PACU), and pain management services. These organizational matrices would include physicians, nurses, support staff, physician office staff, key management personnel, and members from key customer groups such as patients and third-party payers. Within each matrix, data would be assessed to identify important services currently being performed and strategically important services for the future. Once identified, teams would be formed that would include anesthesia providers to assess current activities and design methods for the optimal provision of service, and develop indicators that would relate to clinical outcomes, customer perception of service, and cost of production. Within this spectrum of activities, examples of anesthesia-related indicators include

1. Factors associated with preparation of patients and clearance for anesthesia
   a. Patient education, medical protocols of complicated patients (e.g., diabetic patients), the process for preanesthetic evaluation
   b. Measures related to patient perception of services, the rate of canceled or delayed procedures due to inadequate preparation or evaluation, and the costs of preanesthetic evaluation/testing
2. Factors associated with the performance of the anesthetic procedure
   a. Procedure selection (general, regional, conscious sedation), agent selection, use of fluid and blood replacement therapies
   b. Measures to assess variations in approach and techniques compared with the way the process was "designed," perception of "customers" including surgeons, nursing, and pathology in the way procedures are performed and cost analysis including procedure times and room turnover times
3. Factors associated with outcome
   a. Clinical outcome at the time of the end of surgery, release from recovery rooms, patient discharge, and long-term outcome analyzed in the context of the above factors

SUMMARY

This chapter is designed to give the reader a historical perspective on the development of quality measures in health care. In addition, it serves as an introduction to Chapter 17 on the emergence of CQI and a specific application of its principles in a discussion of the American Association of Nurse Anesthetists (AANA) Anesthesia Quality Plus Program. As changes in health care financing and the political and social climate of the 1990s unfold, and the systems approach and transition to CQI theories develop, those fundamental organizational structures and functions become the new "tradition" for health care organizations. These challenges create many opportunities to deliver better health care and anesthesia services in the future.

BIBLIOGRAPHY

Berwick, DM: Curing Health Care, New Strategies for Quality Improvement. Jossey-Bass Publishers, San Francisco, 1990.

Deming, WE: Out of Crisis. Massachusetts Institute of Technology, Cambridge, MA, 1986.

An Introduction to Quality Improvement in Health Care. Joint Commission on Accreditation of Healthcare Organizations, Oak Brook Terrace, IL, 1992.

Lohr, KA (ed): Medicare: A Strategy for Quality Assurance, Vol. 1. Institute of Medicine, National Academy Press, Washington, DC, 1990.

17

The AANA Quality Assurance and Risk Management Program and Member Services

Gary P. Kraus

OUTLINE

OBJECTIVES

On completing this chapter, the reader will be able to:

1. Provide definitions and conceptual comparisons of quality assurance and CQI.
2. Describe the objectives and features of the AANA AQ+ Program.
3. Describe the advantages to a clinical CRNA of participating in a CQI program.
4. Describe the role of patient satisfaction surveys as a component of CQI.
5. Describe the relationship between CQI and provider reimbursement.

The past two decades have seen the nation's health care providers engaged in a crisis of medical liability. These crises have had a serious impact, not only on hospitals and physicians but also on nursing, particularly on nurses involved in a specialty, high-risk practice, such as anesthesia. Anesthesia misadventures generally do not happen often, but when they do they tend to produce devastating damages and large monetary awards. As a result, insurance companies experience millions of dollars in claims. During the height of the insurance crises of the 1970s, some insurance companies decided to suspend writing malpractice insurance for anesthesia providers and other high-risk specialties such as obstetrics, neurosurgery, and orthopedics. Other insurance companies cancelled professional liability insurance altogether and completely withdrew from some states, such as Florida. The principal effects of the first malpractice crisis were dramatic increases in insurance premiums and a lack of availability of insurance in some locations. The primary impact of the second crisis, in the 1980s, was to increase the premiums that certified registered nurse anesthetists (CRNAs) had to pay; however, access to insurance continued to be available throughout the country.

Since anesthesia is classified as a low-frequency, high-severity risk, the impact of the insurance crises was substantially more serious for CRNAs than for many other nursing specialties. It was not unusual for a CRNA to spend $17,000 a year for malpractice insurance in some high-risk jurisdictions: however, premium rates have declined substantially since those years.

In response to requests from its members, the American Association of Nurse Anesthetists (AANA) assisted CRNAs in obtaining insurance policies from agencies and their underwriting companies. The AANA's primary role was facilitator for contracting with an agency and assisting it to market insurance to AANA members. In 1986, the AANA decided to take a more active role in the malpractice insurance service arena and discuss the possibility of forming its own insurance subsidiary. At the same time, the Association sought to provide its members with services pertaining to quality assurance (QA) and risk management, programs that would emphasize prevention, safety and proactive assessments, and documentation of the quality of care provided to patients by CRNAs.

In 1989, the AANA board of directors established a for-profit insurance corporation subsidiary, for which the Association would serve as a holding company and sole stockholder. This action resulted in the establishment of Anesthesia Professional Liability Services, Inc. Within this AANA-owned subsidiary, there were formulated two separate departments, Anesthesia Quality Plus (AQ+), to deal with issues of quality assurance and risk management services to members, and Anesthesia Plus (A-Plus), which deals exclusively with providing liability insurance to CRNAs.

Although not the focus of discussion for this chapter, A-Plus today serves over 2500 CRNA subscribers. A-Plus provides a unique service to AANA members in terms of detailed information about CRNA professional liability insurance. It offers lecturers to national and state association meetings about a range of professional issues, from those concerning insurance acquisition and transfer to more timely issues that might be affecting the insurance market. Representatives are available to members at all times for questions, even without the requirement to purchase insurance.

To complement this new member service, in 1990, the AANA established a Department of Quality Assurance and Risk Management to provide CRNAs with a range of quality assurance and risk management activities that would assist them in assessing, documenting, and improving the quality of care provided to patients. This department was charged with the responsibility of developing and managing the AQ+ program, which will be explained in greater detail in later sections of this chapter. With the advent of AQ+ programming, the AANA became the first health care organization in the nation to demonstrate its commitment to the public for the provision of quality anesthesia care. These efforts would eventually culminate in a variety of benefits to Association members and in turn, the public.

1 Within the emerging discipline of continuous quality improvement (CQI; formerly termed QA) the AANA became

known as a national leader and trend setter in the field of quality improvement in the health care disciplines.

2 For the first time, CRNAs could provide evidence of the quality of care provided to patients via comprehensive data collection on patient outcomes. These data would be important for those CRNAs in practice settings where no mechanism existed previously to document patient events, such as those in private practice or small rural settings.

3 Through this documentation, the CRNA could provide evidence to regulatory boards, liability carriers, third-party reimbursers, and governmental decision makers of the quality of care provided.

4 Finally, and most importantly, the AQ+ program provided to CRNA subscribers an innovative mechanism to assess their own personal clinical practice profile and determine areas that, if improved, would greatly enhance the care (and outcome) of patients.

To the AANA, the evidence appeared clear: the future viability of any type of health care provider would come to depend in large part on the ability of the provider to demonstrate his or her record of clinical performance in meeting practice standards of the discipline. The Association believed that benefits afforded by the AQ+ Program could potentially become mandatory in future years in order for the CRNA to maintain registration, certification, liability insurance, reimbursement rights, and the trust of the public.

THE TRANSITION FROM QUALITY ASSURANCE TO CONTINUOUS QUALITY IMPROVEMENT

Before embarking on a detailed description of the AQ+ program, it may be beneficial to acquaint the reader with some pertinent terminology. For most, the notion of quality assessment activities has been synonomous with the term "quality assurance." However, in recent years, terminology has changed to the term "continuous quality improvement" (CQI). As the reader will soon come to realize, the concept of CQI is much more comprehensive than mere data collection and interpretation. Also, the AQ+ program incorporates a comprehensive approach to total quality management and evaluation.

The historical background provides a clearer understanding of the renewed emphasis given to quality management in the health care industry. In recent years it has become obvious to America's business and industrial leaders that, in order for American products to compete with those of the rest of the world, particularly Germany and Japan, quality must improve. The improvement of quality in a product or service requires more than a statement from the administration or leadership of a particular corporation; it requires a firm commitment, resources, and training necessary to achieve the goal.

With the collapse of many businesses during the Great Depression, writers and professors published and lectured on methods for improving the quality of business in this country. Several theories were advanced. One that centered on the quality of the product or services produced stated that production of a good-quality product should be a primary concern of a business organization. This theory stated that, with quality as a primary objective, profits will flow and the product will maintain its competitive edge and increase its market share. This "quality" philosophy was advanced by W. Edward Deming, Joseph M. Juran, and Phillip B. Crosby.

The opposite approach was the "bottom line" or profit approach taught by the Harvard Business School and others. This viewpoint has been espoused by American business leaders for the past four decades. Its premise is that the foremost objective of an organization is to make profits and to do whatever is necessary to achieve that end. As a result, as American industries attempted to show profitable balance sheets, the quality of their products diminished.

In recent years it became apparent to business leaders that the bottom line approach was failing, and in fact was the cause of many of America's economic problems. Business leaders began to realize that the quality approach should have been their focus from the onset. As a result, there was a major shift to quality improvement in this country, a shift that spread to the health care industry as well.

The difference between QA and CQI is too substantial to be dealt with here in detail (see Chapter 16); however, it is important to explain the difference between quality assessment, QA, and quality improvement. *Quality assessment* pertains to the measurement of the technical and interpersonal aspects of care and outcomes. Actually, the term "quality assessment" has long been the correct one for describing what heretofore has been called quality assurance.

Quality assurance refers to the full cycle of activities involved in maintaining quality of care by stressing individual performance rather than other factors. *Quality improvement* is a combination of principles that creates both a quality- and customer-focused environment and the ability to identify, assess, and constantly enhance the efficiency and effectiveness of those processes that determine important organizational outcomes.

There are many functional differences between quality assurance and CQI, or total quality management, as some refer to it. One difference lies in the reason for doing it and the factors that motivate it. Quality assurance is externally driven, that is, it is required by accrediting and governmental agencies and others, whereas quality improvement is internally driven by an institution's desire to improve quality. Quality assurance follows the organizational structure; it is compartmentalized within each department, whereas quality improvement follows a patient from before he or she enters the institution until he or she returns home or achieves wellness. It is basically a patient-focused effort that must be carried out by all individuals within an institution.

Quality assurance is usually assigned to a few persons within an organization to implement and monitor, whereas quality improvement is based on the theory that the people who are best able to improve the quality of a product or service are those who produce that product or perform that service every day. The focus of QA is on the individual, and the outcomes of care are of primary concern. When things do not go well, they are blamed on an individual rather than on the institution.

In quality improvement, the focus is on process and structure; structural characteristics deal with measuring the resources in the delivery system. The process deals with what is done to and for the patient by those who run the system. Structure and process identify causes, whereas outcomes identify effects.

While QA implies perfection, that is, assurance of quality, CQI is based on the idea that, regardless of how things are done, there is always room for improvement. In QA, quality is not linked to efficient outcomes. In CQI, outcomes, efficiency, and effectiveness are integrated.

There are several shortcomings associated with the QA approach to quality management. Notwithstanding the fact that it is focused on individuals and does not adequately deal with efficiency and effectiveness as well as outcomes, the most serious problem with QA is that it impairs professional motivation. It has a negative effect on performance. Frequently, QA uses no external benchmarks, because it is department- and discipline-specific. Unfortunately, QA focuses only on clinical activities.

Quality improvement, on the other hand, focuses on process indicators as well as outcomes. Part of the philosophy of CQI is that outcomes are affected not so much by individual incompetence as by problems in the structure and process of the organization. In essence, a bad process creates an environment for poor performance. Therefore, by making a concentrated effort to look at structures as well as outcomes, through CQI improvement, the causes of poor performance can be determined.

The tools and methods of QA and quality improvement differ as well. In QA, data is collected on high-volume, high-risk activities, whereas in CQI, variations and customer feedback are examined. Quality assurance traditionally carried out in individual clinical departments, but CQI must be carried out throughout the hospital.

In QA, evaluation of care is based on inspection and documentation, whereas CQI evaluation is based substantially on customer satisfaction. Here, QA follows the traditional organizational structure; CQI follows the patient flow throughout the enterprise. In QA, the focus is on special and common causes. It is focused on peer review, whereas in CQI, the focus is on systems improvement. Finally, QA focuses on actions directed toward people, whereas in CQI the action is directed toward the process environment.

In order to carry out CQI, a substantial amount of information must be available throughout the institution to allow the performance of the detailed analysis necessary to identify causes of quality problems in both process structures and outcomes. In QA, a few indicators of poor quality are identified, and data is collected only on those cases where a critical indicator has occurred. As a result, information in the QA program reveals only that an indicator was violated. Statistically, this could represent only a small fraction of the total number of cases performed within an anesthesia department at any given time.

In CQI, it is necessary to track information on all cases, regardless of whether one of the indicators occurred. By collecting information on demographics, types of procedures, agents used, preexisting conditions, patient positioning, and other information called for on the AQ+ risk and quality management collection form, all aspects of patient care can be examined, not only those cases where indicators occurred. The use of common statistical tools is a hallmark of CQI. In order to do good statistical analysis and concentrate efforts on areas where statistics indicate there should be more attention, a large amount of in-depth information must be collected over a period of time. This is one of the problems faced by anesthesia providers. Traditionally, health care providers reported information only when outcomes fell below a particular standard. However, in CQI, data must be collected on every case to provide a pool of information that is sufficiently large to conduct good statistical analysis.

It is common in risk and quality management for a bad outcome to be preceded not simply by one particular event but by a cascading series of events. Experience has shown that, when analyzing a catastrophic event, many small things that ordinarily would be overlooked are seen to have contributed to the mistake that caused the bad outcome. With CQI, attention can be focused on problems dealing with the organizational structure and the process that makes it easy for employees to make errors. Subsequently, by focusing attention on both process and structure as well as on outcomes, quality of care can be improved on a continuing basis.

OBJECTIVES OF THE AQ+ PROGRAM

The primary mission of the AQ+ program is to reduce or prevent risks associated with anesthesia services by improving patient safety and quality of care. Specific objectives of AQ+ encompass three major areas: education, research, and member services. Each area contains several ancillary goals that speak to the broader subject. The objectives of the AQ+ program were designed to be congruent with the overall strategic plan of the AANA developed in 1990. Recent trends in health care in general will soon mandate explicit documentation of care activities. The underlying philosophy of the program is based on the commitment that chief among the responsibilities of the professional CRNA is the need to continuously monitor, evaluate, and improve patient care.

Prior to the establishment of AQ+, AANA offered to its membership only limited QA and risk management resources. During the 1980s, surveys of AANA members indicated that many CRNAs performed the anesthesia department QA activities mandated by the Joint Commission on Healthcare Organizations (JCAHO). Many members requested more information from AANA, prompting it to publish a monograph, *Implementing a Quality Assurance Program in Anesthesia Departments and Action Plan,* in 1982. Members also asked that anesthesia QA and risk management sessions be scheduled as part of AANA-sponsored programs. Accordingly, education became one of the primary missions of AQ+.

Since the inception of the AQ+ program, the AANA has sponsored numerous regional workshops to acquaint CRNAs with the concepts of CQI, risk management, and of course implementation of the AQ+ program. The program also provides a bimonthly newsletter in combination with the *AANA NewsBulletin* which highlights trends in CQI, problem solving case reports, anesthesia safety, pertinent legislative actions, and articles about upcoming AQ+ workshops or meetings.

The most comprehensive and detailed publication produced by AQ+ is the *Anesthesia Providers Guide for Continuous Quality Improvement* which accompanies the purchase of the AQ+ software program. This 3-inch-thick looseleaf manual contains over 250 pages of original work to acquaint the user with the theoretical precepts of CQI, an overview of the JCAHO quality improvement model, a self-assessment guide to document the quality of anesthesia departments and services, recent monographs and classic works in the area of CQI, a patient satisfaction survey system, and finally a detailed and systematic explanation of the AANA computer-based system for QA data collection and evaluation.

Another primary objective of AQ+ was to promote research in the area of CQI. The ability to conduct research in this area would provide AANA members with several distinct benefits. First, such a program would establish a mechanism to collect consistent, comprehensive, and verifiable data that could be tested and used to establish and refine quality standards in anesthesia practice, thus improving patient care. Second, by studying the characteristics of nurse anesthesia practice across various practice settings, it would be possible to influence governmental decision makers as to what should rightly constitute cost-effective, comprehensive, and safe practice patterns within the discipline of anesthesia at large. Policy decisions, such as reimbursement or supervision levels, are too often based on specious and undocumentable assumptions about what constitutes competent care. This information would facilitate more justifiable decisions. Most importantly, the computer-generated database of QA information would allow ongoing closed-claim studies on anesthesia occurrences.

A third objective of AQ+ was to provide specific technical services to the membership, services that would help CRNAs become better able to manage CQI efforts within their particular institutions and practice settings. These activities have come to include a speaker's bureau, consultation services, usually in preparation for JCAHO visitation, and a plaintiff and defendent expert witness referral service.

FEATURES OF THE AQ+ SYSTEM

The AANA approach to the issue of CQI improvement is broad ranging and comprehensive in its approach. Although there is a natural tendency to highlight and even promote the actual automated management information system, there are other essential components necessary for an all-encompassing system of continuous evaluation and improvement.

The system provides a quality and risk management profile self-assessment checklist and departmental quality management plan and instructions. These programs help to facilitate a thorough self-assessment of an anesthesia department or service. The guide may also be useful in creating a quality and risk management profile. The primary target users of this instrument are anesthesia providers. It may also be of value to other health care professionals such as administrators, medical directors, educators, risk and quality managers, accreditation personnel, and practice and management consultants.

The departmental profile not only identifies strengths and weaknesses related to the provision of anesthesia services, but also establishes a framework for CQI. The assessment tool addresses quality management, quality assessment, risk management, clinical privileges, environmental safety, anesthesia equipment, drugs and supplies, and types of documentation. Recommendations drawn from these analyses can then be utilized by department leadership to develop goals and objectives for improving the overall quality of the anesthesia service. The use of this instrument on an annual basis provides a quality management tool that can assist in maintaining effectively administered anesthesia services.

Guidance is also provided to the user in other important areas. It includes work forms for conducting the JCAHO 10-step model of monitoring and evaluation of departmental services, including traditional and expanded anesthesia quality indicator definitions. Model anesthesia records as well as informed consent model forms are included with instructions.

The important complement to CQI activities are those involving risk management. To guide the CRNA in avoiding undue risk, the system provides documents including clinical guidelines for nurse anesthesia practice, infection control guidelines for anesthesia, a risk management guide, and numerous documents delineating professional and legal issues pertinent to nurse anesthesia practice.

For the future, AQ+ has proposed establishing a quality and risk management profile service clearinghouse. This service is a computerized database system designed to perform information processing necessary to support the provider with "performance-based credentialing" of his or her quality and risk management activities. By participating in the program, CRNAs can have their professional performance maintained in a confidential file and made available to any person or organization they designate. The material can be used to support one's role within an institution's QA program, for future employers, and for additional uses mandated by the JCAHO and other regulators. The CRNA's performance can also be matched against national or regional standards as evidence of competent practice in the event privileges are challenged.

The same service is also proposed to serve identical activities of the department or group practice, just as the provider profile service is designed to serve the individual. This system would be of value to providers needing assistance for JCAHO accreditation, insurance renewals, Medicare quality evaluations, and other third-party reviews.

THE AUTOMATED SYSTEM FOR CONTINUOUS QUALITY IMPROVEMENT

The centerpiece of the AANA's quality management program is the AQ+ system for CQI in anesthesia. In 1990, the Quality Assurance and Risk Management Task Force was established to develop a variety of evaluation tools members could use to perform QA within their own practice settings which would not only comply with JCAHO critical indicators, but would also go beyond to specify in more detailed accounts the quality of care provided by CRNAs throughout the perioperative course. Specifically the program was designed to provide the following.

1 Document quality patient care
2 Comply with JCAHO requirements
3 Monitor competence of anesthesia care providers
4 Provide data for recredentialing
5 Analyze practice trends
6 Assist in budgetary planning
7 Identify equipment problems
8 Demonstrate the efficacy of monitoring interventions
9 Provide data for clinical research studies

Predominant among those evaluation tools was the development of a computer-based information system designed to assist in the collection and processing of QA data. Via this mechanism, a variety of hard copy reports could be produced that itemized specific provider performance or patient outcome data. These reports could then be used by the CRNA to measure personal or departmental performance against predetermined criteria or site-specific critical indicators.

With establishment of an automated information system which provided a consistent reporting format for QA information, it was then possible to establish a national pool of anesthesia data on patient outcomes. Such a pool would provide not only verifiable, personal CRNA performance records, but also data required to document to external agencies, including congressional, governmental, and regulatory groups, the quality of care provided by CRNAs. It should be noted that data collected by a specific provider or institution is strictly confidential. A decision to release any provider or institutional specific data is reserved to the provider or institution alone.

The automated data collection system was tested in both alpha and beta phases by CRNAs from across the country. Approximately 25 institutions and 10,000 forms were analyzed. The system was refined on the basis of those testing phases and is managed by the Department of Health Services Management at the University of Missouri at Columbia, which provided computer and consultation support.

AQ+

Anesthesia Quality Plus

RISK AND QUALITY MANAGEMENT COLLECTION FORM

PLEASE READ THE *AQ PLUS* INSTRUCTION MANUAL BEFORE COMPLETING THIS FORM.
SPECIAL NOTE: Refer to the manual for explanation of items with an asterisk*

* ENTER SUBSCRIBER NUMBER or Place Label Here ___ ___ ___ - ___ ___ - ___ ___ ___ ___

* LOCATION CODE ___ ___ ___ ___ ___ (zip code) ___ ___ ___ ___ (+ four) ___ ___ (dept.)
Case # (optional) ________________

PATIENT INFORMATION

Date of Anesthesia Administration ___/___/___

Patient's age: ____ years ____ months ____ days

Sex: ____ Male ____ Female

Weight: ____ lbs. ____ kg. ____ gm.

Payment Source (Check one)
___ Medicare
___ Medicaid
___ HMO
___ PPO
___ Commercial Ins.
___ Self Pay No Ins.
___ Workers Comp.
___ Unknown

***ASA CLASS**
____ I
____ II
____ III
____ IV
____ V
____ E

Race
_____ American Indian/ Alaskan Native
_____ Asian/ Pacific Islander
_____ Black
_____ Caucasian
_____ Hispanic
_____ Other ____________

*** Primary Provider Information:**
Social Security Number: ___ ___ ___ - ___ ___ - ___ ___ ___ ___
____ CRNA
____ ANESTHESIOLOGIST
____ SRNA
____ ANESTHESIOLOGY RESIDENT
____ OTHER PHYSICIAN*
____ OTHER RN*
____ OTHER (specify) ____________

*** Secondary Provider Information:**
Social Security Number: ___ ___ ___ - ___ ___ - ___ ___ ___ ___
____ CRNA
____ ANESTHESIOLOGIST
____ SRNA
____ ANESTHESIOLOGY RESIDENT
____ OTHER PHYSICIAN*
____ OTHER RN*
____ OTHER (specify) ____________

Site of Anesthesia Administration:

Hospital
____ Surgery Suite
____ L & D Suite
____ Birthing Room
____ Emergency Room
____ Radiology
____ ICU
____ Catheterization
____ Clinic/Procedure Room
____ Other In-Hospital Location

Nonhospital Facilities
____ Ambulatory Surgery Center
____ Dr. Office
____ Other ____________

Admission Status
____ Inpatient
____ Outpatient - Planned Admit
____ Outpatient

Write Principal Surgical Procedure here OR enter CPT Code Below

___ ___ ___ ___ ___
CPT Code

Figure 17–1. Data collection form on which is checked pertinent patient data. The form normally takes about 2 minutes to complete per patient and may be inputted into a hand-held computer in the operating room or other clinical environment. (From the American Association of Nurse Anesthetists, Park Ridge, IL with permisssion.)

Software was designed to produce approximately 10 styles of reports, as well as a method to permit users to design their own special reports. The AQ+ standard reports meet 90 percent of all institutional QA requirements, including those of the JCAHO and other regulatory agencies.

The automated form (Fig. 17–1) was designed to be used as a manual checkoff list or could be completed via data input into a palmtop computer (Hewlett-Packard [HP] 95LX) in the operating room (Fig. 17–2). The AQ+ system was further designed to accommodate a range of users. A subscriber could use the paper and pencil method of data collection and forward the hard copy to

WERE BLOOD/BLOOD PRODUCTS GIVEN? ___Yes ___No

PREINDUCTION ACTIVITIES

Were there circumstances/conditions that interfered with the completion of ALL Preinduction Activities? _____ Yes _____ No If yes, please check those activities not completed (or substantially affected) by the conditions/circumstances.

- ___ Anesthesia assessment reviewed
- ___ Anesthesia care plan documented
- ___ Institution approved preop equipment check
- ___ Reviewed chart
- ___ Reviewed EKG
- ___ Reviewed lab tests
- ___ Reviewed other tests
- ___ Surgery & anesthesia consent signed

Agent (s) Used By Any Provider

I = INDUCTION M = MAINTENANCE E = EMERGENCE

I	M	E	INHALANTS
___	___	___	Air
___	___	___	
___	___	___	Enflurane
___	___	___	Halothane
___	___	___	Helium
___	___	___	Isoflurane
___	___	___	Nitrous oxide
___	___	___	Oxygen

I	M	E	INTRAVENOUS AGENTS
___	___	___	Etomidate
___	___	___	Ketamine
___	___	___	Methohexital
___	___	___	Propofol
___	___	___	Thiopental

I	M	E	ANALGESICS
___	___	___	Alfentanil
___	___	___	Fentanyl
___	___	___	Meperidine
___	___	___	Morphine
___	___	___	Sufentanil
___	___	___	Toradol
___	___	___	Other ________

I	M	E	ADJUNCTS
___	___	___	Anticholinergics
___	___	___	Antiemetics
___	___	___	Cardiotonic
___	___	___	H_2/antacids
___	___	___	Relaxant antagonist

I	M	E	MUSCLE RELAXANTS
___	___	___	racurium
___	___	___	Curare
___	___	___	Doxicurium
___	___	___	Mivacurium
___	___	___	Pancuronium
___	___	___	Pipecuronium
___	___	___	Succinylcholine
___	___	___	Vecuronium
___	___	___	Other ________

I	M	E	SEDATIVES/ HYPNOTICS
___	___	___	Diazepam
___	___	___	Droperidol
___	___	___	Lorazepam
___	___	___	Midazolam

I	M	E	LOCAL ANESTHETICS
___	___	___	Bupivacaine
___	___	___	Cocaine
___	___	___	Chloroprocaine
___	___	___	Epinephrine added
___	___	___	Etidocaine
___	___	___	Mepivacaine
___	___	___	Procaine
___	___	___	Tetracaine
___	___	___	Xylocaine
___	___	___	Other ________

Planned Anesthesia Technique

- ___ Epidural
- ___ General-endotracheal
- ___ General-mask
- ___ IV regional
- ___ Local anesthetic infiltration
- ___ Monitored anesthesia care
- ___ Nerve block
- ___ Spinal
- ___ Other ______________

Primary Patient Position During Anesthesia Administration

- ___ Jackknife
- ___ Kneeling
- ___ Lateral
- ___ Lithotomy
- ___ Prone
- ___ Sitting
- ___ Supine
- ___ Other ________

PATIENT MONITORING

- ___ Arterial pressure
- ___ Blood pressure cuff
- ___ Capnography*
- ___ Central venous pressure
- ___ EKG
- ___ End-tidal gas analysis*
- ___ Fetal heart tone (FHT)
- ___ Intracranial pressure
- ___ PA catheter
- ___ Peripheral nerve stimulator
- ___ Precordial Doppler
- ___ Pulse oximetry
- ___ Stethoscope
- ___ Transeso. echo (TEE)
- ___ Temperature
- ___ Other ____________________

TIME	SURGERY	ANESTH
30 min. or less	___	___
31 min. to 60 min.	___	___
61 min. to 90 min.	___	___
91 min. to 120 min.	___	___
121 min. to 150 min.	___	___
151 min. to 180 min.	___	___
3+ hrs.	___	___
4+ hrs.	___	___
5+ hrs.	___	___
6+ hrs.	___	___
7+ hrs.	___	___
8+ hrs.	___	___
9+ hrs.	___	___
10+ hrs.	___	___
11+ hrs.	___	___

Figure 17–1—continued.

Continued

the AANA for processing. Other participants indicated that they would be willing to download the information into the computer after which the AANA would produce standard and special reports. Still others could obtain the entire program on computer disk, collect data, and generate their own reports.

The information system was designed to produce reports that include the total of all categories (1) by location, (2) by provider, (3) by location and provider, and (4) by subscriber. The subscriber is the entity that usually owns the system. Subscribers can be hospitals, group practices, or individuals. Each owner receives a subscriber number

PREEXISTING CONDITIONS

RESPIRATORY
___ Abnormal airway anatomy*
___ Airway foreign body
___ Airway tumor
___ Chest tubes
___ Hypoxemia*
___ Laryngeal fracture
___ Limited neck ROM
___ Obstructive disease
___ Pneumonia/atelectasis
___ Restrictive disease
___ Smoker
___ Tracheostomy
___ URI*
___ Ventilator support
___ Other ______________

CARDIOVASCULAR
___ Aneurysm
___ Angina
___ CAD
___ Cardiac shunt
___ Cardiomegaly
___ CHF
___ Dysrhythmia
___ Embolus
___ Hypertension
___ MI-6 mos. or more
___ MI-less than 6 mos.
___ Pacemaker
___ Peripheral vasc. insufficiency
___ Shock*
___ Valvular disease
___ Other ______________

CENTRAL NERVOUS SYSTEM
___ Comatose
___ Convulsive disorder
___ Cord injury
___ CVA
___ Dystrophies/dystonia
___ Epi/subdural hematoma
___ Parkinson's disease
___ Peripheral neuropathies
___ Psychiatric disorder
___ Tumor/aneurysm
___ Visual/auditory disorders
___ VP/VA shunt
___ Other ______________

GASTROINTESTINAL
___ Ascites
___ Esophageal abnormalities
___ Foreign body
___ Full stomach/NPO less than 6 hrs.
___ Hiatal hernia
___ Motion sickness/NV
___ Nausea & vomiting (NV)
___ Obesity
___ Obstruction/distention
___ Past history of postoperative NV
___ Peritonitis
___ Other ______________

ENDOCRINE/RENAL
___ Adrenal disease
___ Diabetes (on medication)
___ Hyperthyroid
___ Hypothyroid
___ Liver disease/hepatitis
___ Pancreatic disease
___ Parathyroid disease
___ Pituitary disorder
___ Renal dysfunction
___ Other ______________

SPECIAL
___ Abnormal lab tests*
___ Acid base/elect. disorder
___ Acute/chronic alcoholism
___ Aids/immuno disorders
___ Arthritis
___ Blood dyscrasias*
___ Cancer
___ Chemotherapy
___ Chronic drug therapy*
___ Connect. tissue disorder*
___ Enzyme deficiency*
___ Glaucoma
___ Hyperthermia > 101 F
___ Hypothermia < 96 F
___ Malignant hyperthermia
___ Metabolic disease
___ Myasthenia gravis
___ Neuromuscular disorder
___ Poor dentition*
___ Pregnancy -- abnormal*
___ Pregnancy -- normal
___ Sepsis
___ Substance abuse
___ Thermal injury
___ Trauma
___ Other ______________

If you had an anesthetic/patient event, then continue, otherwise stop here.

ANESTHETIC/PATIENT EVENTS

I = Induction
M = Maintenance
E = Emergence
R = Recovery

1. Equipment Failures:	I	M	E	R
Anesthesia machine	___	___	___	___
Breathing circuit	___	___	___	___
Laryngoscope	___	___	___	___
Monitor	___	___	___	___
Tourniquet	___	___	___	___
Ventilator	___	___	___	___
Other ______________	___	___	___	___

2. Airway Incidents:	I	M	E	R
Dental injury	___	___	___	___
Difficult intubation	___	___	___	___
Obstructed endotracheal tube	___	___	___	___
Postintubation croup	___	___	___	___
Soft tissue/naso/oropharyngeal injury	___	___	___	___
Unplanned bronchial intubation	___	___	___	___
Unplanned extubation	___	___	___	___
Unplanned reintubation	___	___	___	___
Unrecognized esophageal intubation	___	___	___	___
Unsuccessful intubation	___	___	___	___
Other ______________	___	___	___	___

Figure 17–1—continued.

that is assigned by AQ+. This number is applied to the form using labels that are given to each subscriber at the time he or she purchases the system and periodically as more are needed. By using a subscriber number, along with location and provider numbers, users who are in a group practice and serve multiple institutions have separate data from each location so that data belonging to hospital A or physician B would not be comingled with data belonging to hospital C or physician D.

A second standard report includes all patient events with preexisting conditions, age, and American Society of Anesthesiologists (ASA) class. A third report includes critical events and incorporates all of the JCAHO's required indicators as well as oth-

ANESTHETIC/PATIENT EVENTS (CONTINUED)

3. Respiratory Problems:	I	M	E	R
Abnormal breath sounds				
ARDS				
Bronchospasm				
Hyperventilation-Pa CO_2<25				
Hypoventilation-Pa CO_2>50				
Hypoxemia-SaO_2<90% or PaO_2<55				
Laryngospasm				
Obstruction				
Pneumo/hemo/chylothorax				
Pulmonary aspiration				
Pulmonary edema				
Unplanned postoperative ventilation				
Unplanned respiratory arrest				
Other ______				

4. Cardiovascular Problems:	I	M	E	R
Acute MI				
Air or other emboli				
Asystole				
Atrial fib/flutter				
CHF				
Coagulopathy				
Hypertension - > 110 diastolic				
Hypotension - < 80 systolic				
New PVCs - > 5/minute				
New ST segment changes				
Sinus bradycardia < 40				
Sinus tachycardia > 120 (child > 180)				
Unplanned intra-art. inject.				
Ventricular fibrillation				
Ventricular tachycardia				
Other ______				

5. Central Nervous System Problems:	I	M	E	R
Anticholinergic crisis				
CVA				
Delayed arousal period > 4 hrs PO				
Extrapyramidal symptoms				
Failure to return to preanesthesia LOC				
Hyperthermia temp. > 101 F CORE				
Hypothermia temp. < 96 F CORE				
Seizure				
Unplanned patient awareness				
Other ______				

6. Endocrine/Renal Problems:	I	M	E	R
Adrenal suppression - CV collapse				
Anuria				
Hyperglycemia > 400				
Hypoglycemia < 50				
Hyperkalemia > 6.0				
Hypokalemia < 3.0				
Oliguria < 0.5 cc/kg/hr				
Thyroid storm				
Other ______				

7. Integumentary Problems:	I	M	E	R
Burn				
Corneal abrasion				
Ecchymosis				
Infiltrated IV				
Laceration				
Pressure/nerve injury				
Tourniquet injury				
Other ______				

8. Regional: I M E R

Block Performed by:
☐ Primary Provider ☐ Secondary Provider

8. Regional:	I	M	E	R
Brain stem anesthesia*				
Epidural wet tap*				
Failed block				
Greater than 3 attempts at insertion				
Hematoma				
High sub/epidural block with CV or resp. insufficiency				
IV injection of local anesthesia*				
Persistent paresthesia				
S/S local anesthesia toxicity*				
Spinal headache (postural puncture)				
Sustained hypotension > 15 min				
Other ______				

9. Medical Problems:	I	M	E	R
Adverse/unexplained anesthesia reaction				
Allergic/anaphylactoid reaction				
Drug administration error				
Inadequate reversal of relaxants				
Narcotic excess requiring naloxone				
Postop delirium requiring tranquilizer				
Transfusion reaction				
Other ______				

10. Miscellaneous	I	M	E	R
Alternative anesthesia plan required				
Arterial/central line complication				
Case canceled preinduction				
Case canceled postinduction				
Death				
Induction delayed > 30 min				
Patient/family dissatisfaction				
Protracted vomiting				
Pruritis				
Surgical complication*				
Unexpected return to surgery				
Unplanned admission to ICU				
Unplanned outpatient surgical admission				
Unplanned PACU over 2 hours				
Other ______				

Figure 17–1—continued.

Continued

ers. It cross-references five characteristic extremes of age, weight in excess of 100 kg, ASA Classes II or over, emergency cases, anesthesia time of more than 5 hours, and preexisting conditions. The critical indicator and patient event reports are also produced by subscriber, location, provider, and by location/provider. Reports detailing patient events with preexisting conditions and the AQ+ critical indicator report are the most common ones hospitals request from a clinical department for the JCAHO's survey process. Users who send this data to AQ+ for processing receive standard reports in 2 weeks. These standard reports are produced every month, as well as quarterly and annually. Additionally, those subscribers who produced their own reports are encouraged

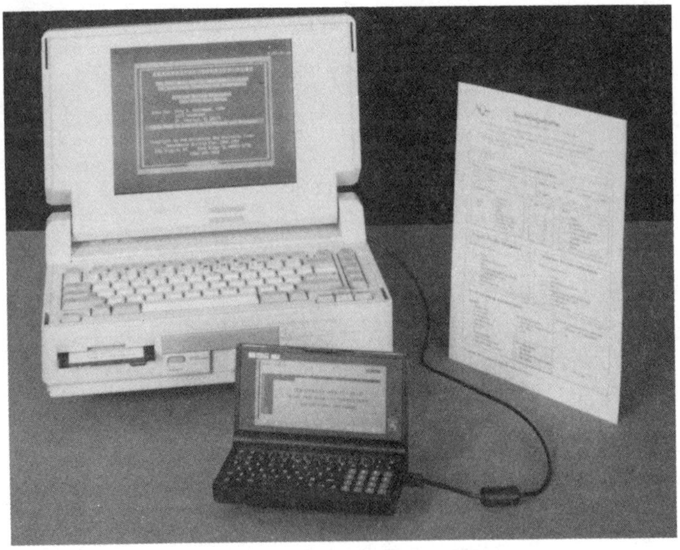

Figure 17–2. Hardware accommodation of the AQ+ computer program and the hand-held computer to facilitate data entry. (From the American Association of Nurse Anesthetists, Park Ridge, IL, with permission.)

to provide their data to the larger, centralized database, called the National Anesthesia Data Pool.

Subsequent to collection and collation of the data is the necessary and vital task of interpretation, evaluation, and remediation, if required. This is accomplished by carefully examining preexisting critical indicators to determine if threshold has been reached; that is, a critical level of performance beyond which remediation or change in practice habits are required. Figure 17–3 provides an example of the AQ+ record-keeping mechanism that tracks this information, including the aspect of care being evaluated, the threshold indicator, the evaluation (findings, conclusions, and recommendations), and the action taken by the responsible party. Time frames for expected change to occur and follow-up plans are also addressed, as the essence of productive change to achieve quality involves the integrity to act on information that indicates change is required. Without this last, final step, the arduous task of CQI fails to yield intended results.

PATIENT SATISFACTION AS A COMPONENT OF CONTINUOUS QUALITY IMPROVEMENT

The feelings and perceptions of the patient have often been overlooked by health care providers in assessing the quality of care delivered. In recent years, JCAHO has called for a method of randomly sampling complaints from patients and their families. Anesthesia Quality Plus developed the patient satisfaction system, which is sold both as a separate program and as part of the AQ+ CQI system for anesthesia.

This patient satisfaction system contains three distinct parts: monograph, a model form, and software. The monograph explains the reason for a patient satisfaction program and why it should be used by an anesthesia department. It also explains the reasons for each question on the model satisfaction survey form. In addition, the monograph deals with the administration of the satisfaction form and mechanism for collecting and collating the data, either by using the software program or batch-processing the information. The monograph also discusses collating the data. It advises administrators regarding ways to compare questions, and explains the meaning of each question as it affects the patient's perception of anesthesia quality. It also tells how to relate the patient satisfaction data to QA or CQI information.

One of the advantages of the patient satisfaction system is that it presents the perceptions of quality from the patient's point of view. A QA or CQI system, however, produces information from the provider's point of view. By interrelating data, anesthesia management can determine whether it is collecting adequate information from a qual-

STEP VIIB: EVALUATE CARE
STEP VIII: TAKE ACTION
STEP IX: ASSESS EFFECTIVENESS OF ACTION

Page 1 of _____

Aspect of Care	**Indicator Threshold**	**Evaluation** (Findings, Conclusions, Recommendations)	**Action** (Responsible Party, Timeframe for Expected Change)	**Follow-up**
Preanesthesia Evaluation	Preinduction activities not completed/ 100%	98% (threshold not met). Of 100 cases, only 98 contained evidence of a complete anesthesia evaluation. No pattern was identified related to procedure or practitioner. However, all cases involved outpatient surgery.	The Medical Director will share results of monitoring at the next staff meeting. Emphasis will be placed on the importance of documentation on both inpatient and outpatient procedures. Improvement of 1% is expected within one quarter.	Continued monitoring

Figure 17–3. This AQ+ Data Assessment Form is to be used during the evaluation, remediation, and action phase of CQI. An example is provided of an important aspect of care, preanesthesia evaluation, and its threshold indicator. (From the American Association of Nurse Anesthetists, Park Ridge, IL, with permission.)

ity perspective and whether the patient's perception of quality is consistent with that of the providers, which helps verify the quality of the data being produced in a QA program. The patient satisfaction form is available to any interested party in both English and Spanish.

The third component of the patient satisfaction program is the computer software developed by AQ+ for the purpose of providing the user with a tool to process patient satisfaction data. The software is written in the same computer language as the AQ+ CQI system to enable it to be interfaced. Users of the AQ+ CQI program can download the patient evaluation program as a module in a total CQI system.

Although patient satisfaction is an important component of QA, it is absolutely essential that it be used in CQI. One of the principal philosophies of CQI is that it be customer-based. Consequently, patient satisfaction information is essential for any institution that plans to perform CQI rather than QA.

CONTINUOUS QUALITY IMPROVEMENT AND THE QUESTION OF REIMBURSEMENT FOR SERVICES

Recently, it has become apparent to many leaders in quality management that, in the future, provider reimbursement may well be tied to quality assessment. The Physicians Payment Review Commission (PPRC) has held a series of meetings to share data for use by governmental organizations in carrying out quality management activities, including practitioner profiling. As recently as 1992, it was stated that if an acceptable data pool were established and practitioner profiles were created, an individual practitioner's credentials and privileges could be controlled and limited to services that he or she can demonstrate he or she can perform well and competently. In a reimbursement scheme based on the quality of performance, if physicians or other providers operated beyond their scope of privileging and credentialing, no payment would be made. This potential requires that every CRNA become a student of the political process that may lead to such decisions, since these actions would undoubtedly be controversial and would have great impact on all of anesthesia practice, regardless of provider.

SUMMARY

In the future, all CRNAs will be required to participate in CQI to sustain practice privileges, certification eligibility, acquisition of liability insurance, and reimbursement for services. Above all, it should become a mandate for the benefit of our public trust, the patient.

BIBLIOGRAPHY

American Association of Nurse Anesthetists: Anesthesia Providers Guide for Continuous Quality Improvement. American Association of Nurse Anesthetists, Park Ridge, IL, 1992.

Joint Commission on Accreditation of Healthcare Organizations: Accreditation Manual for Hospitals. Joint Commission on Accreditation of Healthcare Organizations, Oakbrook Terrace, IL, 1991.

Joint Commission on Accreditation of Healthcare Organizations: An Introduction to Quality Improvement in Health Care. Joint Commission on Accreditation of Healthcare Organizations, Oakbrook Terrace, IL, 1992.

SEVEN

Continuing Challenges in Professional Practice

18

Ethical Decision Making in Anesthesia

Ron McManus

OUTLINE

OBJECTIVES

On completing this chapter, the reader will be able to:

1. Recount the history of ethical debate as it relates to the disciplines of medicine and nursing.
2. Define pertinent terms relating to philosophy, morals, and ethical decisions.
3. Define the major ethical theories and applicable ethical principles of autonomy, nonmaleficence, beneficence, and justice.
4. Define the major issues related to advanced directives and do-not-resuscitate orders.
5. Describe the process of ethical decision making.

ESTABLISHING A CONTEXT FOR THE STUDY OF ETHICS

Socrates is said to have taught that the unexamined life is not worth living. Perhaps the same can be stated about professional life, in that the unexamined profession is not worth practicing. Health care professionals, particularly in this era, are asked and expected to examine their professional lives. During the last 400 years, the medical profession has accumulated an enormous amount of knowledge. Advances in science and technology have progressed accordingly; consequently, the health sciences make many demands on the character, education, and abilities of the practitioner.[1] Society and the professions themselves are voicing a renewed demand that the health care professional be guided by moral considerations, and the health care provider is expected to be knowledgeable of health care ethics and the process of ethical decision making.[1] In health care ethics, the responsibility is neither to discover some new moral principles on which to build a theoretic ethical system nor to evolve new approaches to ethical reasoning, but to prepare the foundation for the application of established moral rules.[2]

This chapter is concerned with the nurse anesthetist and the issue of health care ethics. Health care ethics is applied ethics; thus the issue at hand becomes how the Certified Registered Nurse Anesthetist (CRNA) can best apply ethics to clinical practice problems. Ethics falls under the domain of the discipline known as philosophy, also referred to as moral philosophy. More specifically, ethics deals with important questions concerning human conduct.

Due largely to developments in scientific thought throughout the past several centuries, the study of ethics has taken on a more quantitative rather than qualitative approach. In essence, 20th century science has separated itself from philosophic concerns (human values).[3] Unfortunately, it becomes more and more clear that science is not value-free, and attention must be paid to the study of values and their effect on human behavior.

> The scientific revolution of Newton, Galileo, Descartes, and others, which replaced Aristotelian medieval science with "modern science," was based on a value judgment, namely, that it was better or more desirable to explain the world in mathematical terms, by one set of laws at the expense of qualitative distinctions, than to persist in science that did justice to the fact that the world contained many different kinds of things, and insisted that each thing be explained according to its own kind.[3]

Judgments of value are constantly made in medicine. The way diseases are labeled is but one example. The current "definitions of alcoholism and wife-beating as sickness rather than badness shows the value basis of medicine, as does the American Medical Association's (AMA) declaring obesity a disease, not a cause thereof, and the waxing and waning of premenstrual syndrome (PMS) as a disease."[3] Ethics is clearly within the purview of science, scientists, and the health care professional.

The argument about the ideology of ethics being applicable to science has had a stormy past. The 1960s brought about a social awareness that influenced the health care profession dramatically; public disenchantment with science and technology was raised to a socially conscious level. Perhaps this attitude, along with other factors, exposed ethics as a popular topic of public discussion. These discussions have prompted many diverse opinions about what constitutes proper professional behavior. "The mass media reflects those concerns in the use of phrases such as 'quality of life,' 'heroic measures,' 'right to die,' 'right to live,' and 'the rights of people to humane and enlightened health care' "[1] (p. ix). In short, the issue can be reduced to what "is" and what "ought" to be. Perhaps the study of ethics can best be capsulized by the understanding that all health care professionals assume the responsibility of asking the "whys" of what "ought" to be.

Definitions

The nurse anesthetist, as a health care professional, is expected to make ethically "right" decisions in patient care. Albert Schweitzer observed that "good is to know pity, to help others conserve their life, and to spare their suffering . . . (it occurs when) we reach true understanding of ourselves."[4] It often seems difficult to know ourselves in this changing world. In our society, we are bombarded with information. Consciously and unconsciously, we make selections from compiled data and draw conclusions about ourselves and life. The data carry equal weight until we assign value to the information. If the information is valued enough, further investigation should follow. "For perfect knowledge, therefore, one must know the various elements of a thing one by one: its parts, its capacities, its distinctive features."[5] If the health care professional is to pursue the good and right, it becomes necessary to clarify terms associated with such a pursuit, requiring clues along the route. Definitions serve as the clues when one pursues the often elusive concept of "ethical behavior."

The health care professional faces many problems and makes many choices in clinical practice. All problems are not ethical problems, and all the choices are not moral choices, yet in the field of medicine ethical dilemmas do occur. A *dilemma* is a choice between equally undesirable alternatives. It happens when one choice is deemed better, when goods are mutually exclusive, or when there is difficulty deciding the "right" among choices. "Ethical dilemmas in medicine occur when the enforcement of law does not appear to bring about justice, when there is no obvious right or wrong behavior, when right behavior appears to have the wrong outcome or when personal sacrifice is the consequence of following ideals."[6] Answers to ethical dilemmas will have a profound and far-reaching effect on personal perceptions of fellow human beings, society, and the relationship of human beings to the world.[7] *The two essential components of an ethical dilemma are the existence of a real choice between other possible courses of action and that the decision-maker places different values on each possible action, or on the outcome of that action.*

Morality has been defined as a social enterprise, being social in its origins, sanctions, and functions. Humans are born into a society that had developed and continues to maintain morals, laws, and ethical codes.[8] A moral problem is a situation in which a person has grounds for believing that there are moral reasons or considerations to support each of two courses of action. Both cannot be chosen, and it is not known which is the more important morally.[9]

The word "morals" is derived from the Latin *moralis* meaning customs or habit. There are qualities of human beings that are called personal virtues; even in animals there are the beginnings of such traits. In subhuman social groupings there exist the rudiments of such social virtues as self-sacrifice, sympathy, and cooperation.[10] "Our morals, like our bodies and social life, are the product of long periods of development and of adaptation to changing environmental conditions."[10] Uniform ways of acting became ways of meeting human needs. These common met needs, called customs, are passed down from generation to generation. The customary actions became expected behaviors, or moral acts, which were accepted without reflection and became known as customary morality or group morality.[10] "Changes in custom come when strain appears."[10] Customs eventually develop into statutory laws. These laws provide a definition of a situation and aim at making it uniform for all members of society. Conflicts in society call for inner laws, conscience, and the voice of the community in us.[10] Morality is seen as a reflection of custom, law, and conscience.

Philosophy consists of theories and analysis about conduct, thought, knowledge, and the nature of the universe.[11] A central task of philosophy is to aid culture in clarifying its view of reality and values.[12] Philosophy concerns itself with the nature and validity of various spheres of human life. Philosophic investigation into a sphere of human life can cause humans to change the ways they behave within the sphere.[13] Philosophies attempt to offer rational answers to life's questions, the goal being to find answers that can be defined by rational argument.

The branch of philosophy called ethics (moral philosophy) deals with questions of human conduct. The word "ethics" is derived from the Greek term *ethos,* meaning customs, habitual usages, conduct, and character.[1] Ethics demands intense study, logic, and analysis, and is not an opinion or a gut reaction to a situation.[14] Today the term is used in the context of personal conduct, character, and motives of action. Ethics concerns itself with the nature of the moral dimensions of life, involving duties, responsibilities, conscience, justice, and other societal concerns and issues. Ethical investigation can make a difference in moral behavior.

Ethical theory is understood as inquiry concerning the meanings or functions of ethical terms and ethical judgments, the status of ethical judgments, the justification of ethical judgments, and the relationship of ethical judgments to nonethical factual statements.[15] The nonethical factual statement concerns the "is" of the action, while the ethical judgment concerns the "why" of the action. Morals have become the "shoulds" or the "should nots" of society, while ethics is concerned with the "why." The "why" becomes the reason for the "should" or "should not."[16] In this way, ethics and morals are often seen as synonymous.

Ethics may concern itself with theory, descriptions, or norms of behavior. Theoretical ethics evaluates the presuppositions and approaches used in examining the moral dimensions of behavior. Descriptive ethics describe what is, while normative ethics (applied ethics) prescribe what ought to be. Normative ethics explore ethical obligations and duties, what is right or wrong, what we are to be, and what we are to value. The roots of ethics were originally based on a concern for reason, at least for Socrates (c. 469–399 B.C.).

Metaethics carry us "beyond ethics" and delineate the extent to which moral judgments are reasonable or otherwise justifiable.[1] If ethics discuss the reasons for morals, then metaethics discuss the reasons for ethics. For example, questioning if a situation is an ethical issue is metaethics. It answers general logical questions about normative ethical judgments.

In health care, it is appropriate to determine if a decision is a matter of clinical judgment rather than an ethical issue.[16] If it is deemed an ethical issue, then it is important to be reminded that "unlike scientific reasoning, ethical reasoning cannot offer definitive proof as to what is the right or wrong action in a given situation."[17] However, ethics may serve as a guide to a well-traveled trail, a trail that leads to better behaviors and better actions among people.

Ethics can be applied to science and the advancements science offers. When ethics are applied to medicine, the discipline is known as bioethics. "Biomedical ethics (bioethics) is one type of applied ethics . . . the application of general ethical theories, principles, and rules to problems of therapeutic practice, health care delivery, and medical biological research."[18] The prefix "bio" means "life"; the biomedical realm addresses the span of time between conception and death. Bioethics is the marriage of ethics and science.

A History of Concerns

Years ago, a physician wrote an article for *American Weekly,* a newspaper supplement. In it he said: "If a man is good in his heart, then he is an ethical member of any group in society. If he is bad in his heart, he is an unethical member. To this author, the ethics of the medical practice are as simple as that."[19] The meaningful simplicity of this statement does have some shortcomings. Disagreements concerning actions have existed for centuries, even among people with the purest hearts. Since the time of Hippocrates, the medical profession has sought to "develop and maintain dignity, honor, honesty, and both an attitude and a reality of service to mankind among the members of their own profession."[19] A brief history of how a need for rules emerged and how principles of ethics became pertinent follows.

The history of ethics of life dates back to Biblical times and probably to the prehistoric period of human existence.[16] Ethics, as it relates to medicine, has historically received varying degrees of emphasis by practitioners. The term "medicine," derived from the Latin root word *medicus,* suggested the concept of healing or making whole again. Nursing is derived from the Latin word *nutrio,* meaning to nurture. The argument is made that the ethics of nursing and medicine fundamentally differ.[20] A historical perspective may sharpen the distinction.

Professional controls on the practice of medicine have existed since the 5th century B.C., the time of Hippocrates. Control was maintained by professional organizations, with encouragements and exhortations to follow high moral standards. Emerging professional values were classified under four headings: (1) the education of medical practitioners, (2) consultations with other practitioners, (3) transactions between physicians and patients, and (4) relationships between medical practitioners and communities.[20] All four of these categories pertained to interpersonal relationships which comprised the identifiable foci of early medicine.

Prior to the Middle Ages, the sick remained at home and were cared for by the family. When hospitals surfaced in the Middle Ages, these new institutions called for new ways of thinking and posed new problems.[1] Services of physicians and attendants to care for the sick evolved out of necessity. The problems concerning these attendants were[1]:

> How to secure nurses who would provide devoted service, and how to train them to give this service in an efficient manner. The first concern reflects a matter of ethical or religious ideals, while the latter reflects a scientific objective. These considerations, in turn, involve many questions concerning the relationship of nurses to patients, on the one hand, and the relationship of nurses to physicians, on the other hand (p. 52).

In the 1700s the British physician John Gregory (1724 to 1773) presented lectures about the qualifications and duties of physicians. His ideas involved the education of a physician and the nature of medical science.[20] The British physician Thomas Percival (1740 to 1804), a contemporary of John Gregory, drafted a code of rules to regulate and govern practitioners at Manchester Hospital. Percival wrote about public health obligations and the ethical significance of legal requirements. A unique contribution of Percival's was the recognition of the impact these laws had on professional ethics. "Jurisprudence" signified moral injunctions to Percival.[20]

As perceptions were changing concerning the physician, perceptions were also changing toward nursing. Nursing moved out of the watchful eye of the church and into a more secular mode. There was basically no training available, and nursing practice was a matter of unpleasant and difficult routine.[1] In the mid-19th century in England, Florence Nightingale instituted nursing reforms for nursing education and practice. She maintained that nursing school should teach the mind as well as form the character.[1] As a result, nursing regained a conscience.

In 1847, the AMA came into existence, and a comprehensive code of medical ethics was adopted. This was a milestone in the development of strict ethical regulation of medical practice in the United States, since before that time there was no unilateral regulation of professional behavior.[21] Part of the reason to develop such a code can be found within the context of the era. Formal medical education was characterized by low standards of education and limited apprenticeships. Consequently, the profession was not viewed favorably in the public's eyes. In an attempt to remedy some of these problems, the medical profession resorted to formulation of ethical guidelines. The code of ethics drafted by Thomas Percival in 1796 served as a model for the AMA code. Percival's concern for ethical behavior dealt with conduct in hospitals, private practice, conduct toward apothecaries, and medical jurisprudence. The AMA's code dealt with relationships of physicians to one another, to their patients, and to the public.[21] "This new code reflected the desire of the physicians to enjoy the full confidence of their patients"[21] (p. 10). The code advised doctors to modify their actions wherever possible to impress patients favorably, honor professional communications with secrecy, avoid telling the patient of impending death, regulate the frequency of visits, dispense charitable services, treat fellow physicians free of charge, and acknowledge that patients should appreciate all the conscientious services they receive.[21]

The AMA Code of Ethics went through various revisions over the years. In 1903, the new code was called Principles of Medical Ethics, and became an advisory document instead of an enforcement policy.[21] In 1957, the revised Principles of Medical Ethics consisted of only 10 short statements[21] including recommendations to

> merit confidence of patients, to improve their medical knowledge and skill, to seek consultations upon request or when they might benefit the patient, to respect professional confidences as permitted by law, to advise public health, to observe the laws of society and the profession and to expose

> practitioners who did not, to practice only under conditions which did not restrict free judgment or reduce quality of service, to avoid unnecessary association with practitioners whose method of healing lacked a scientific basis, to elicit no patients but to serve all needs in emergencies thought normally free to refuse service, and to limit professional income to fees commensurate with services rendered and ability to pay.[22]

By continually emphasizing professional conduct through the codes, the medical profession revived the idea that medicine was a dignified and honorable calling. The codes called for covenant (agreement) between the professional and patient, and today it is viewed as a social contract. Eventually, these codes became foundation statements and models for many other health care professionals.

During the early 1900s, ethics began in the nursing profession to be a more focused issue. Before that time the tactic used to promote ethical behavior appears to be shame-based. The nurse would be shamed by unethical behavior, and the profession would be blamed, criticized, and humiliated. In 1937, C.A. Aikens wrote *Studies in Ethics for Nurses* and included chapters devoted to truth in nursing report, discretion in speech, obedience, being teachable, respect for authority, discipline, and loyalty.[23] The early ethics books in nursing "delved into the private life and morality of nurses, reflecting the status of nursing students in an apprenticeship system and the stereotype of the intellectually and morally weak woman."[1] Such concerns focused on the individual's morality and the nurse's duties, obligations, and loyalties.[24]

Nursing does have its own issues, problems, and principles, and applying medical ethical theories to nursing is an argumentative issue for some. Historically, nursing has ascribed to the ideals of treating persons rather than diseases and the notion of the superiority of prevention over cure. Medicine historically has emphasized curing as a response to the presence of a disease. The contrast of the professions is often striking. Nursing is sometimes termed a health-oriented profession, while medicine is often termed a disease-combatant profession. With a different orientation of history for each profession, it is argued that nursing and medicine will have and do have different values and ethics. Perhaps nursing ethics is a distinct genre or type of ethics. If so, the term "nursing ethics" will separate itself from "medical ethics." The debate concerning this topic continues.

It is obvious, then, from the history of the health care professions, that medical ethics is not a recent invention. It is simply a newer term for ethics applied to a particular area of life. Medical ethics involves some heart-rending and difficult decisions. Complex problems caused by new technologies, new legal issues, and new economic situations offer a challenging context for ethical thinking and ethical behavior. New terms have arisen and new technical crises exist, but basic issues are as old as the first time in history when someone aided someone else who was hurt or in pain.

THE DEVELOPMENT OF ETHICAL CODES

History reveals that the health care professional has inherited a tradition of elaborate professional ethical codes. It is sometimes suggested that this heritage of codes had its beginning in sixth-century China.[7] These codes of ethics, or codes of conduct, existed to answer questions about behavior that is expected and behavior that warrants criticism. Codes, policy statements, oaths, pledges, creeds, vows, and bylaws offer professional policy regarding behavior. As such, they are usually developed and promulgated by the profession. They function as an articulation of professional values, offering important merging themes that are consistent concerns of the professional such as confidentiality, patient rights, patient dignity, professional relationship, professional responsibilities, and others. They attempt to provide an enforceable standard of minimally decent behavior.

According to *Webster's Collegiate Dictionary*, a *code* is a "system of principles or rules (moral)."[25] The professional code refers to shared values and norms, and it is designed to bring about good and minimize harm.[26] Often these codes speak to disciplinary action that might be taken if members misrepresent themselves, act negligently, become incompetent, or are engaged in professional misconduct not in keeping with the determination of a professional board. The American Association of Nurse Anesthetists (AANA) has developed such a code for its own membership (see Appendix) as well as bylaws that speak to issues of censure and revocation of professional membership.

ETHICAL PRINCIPLES

All ethical dilemmas involve moral principles. These universal principles are among the most longstanding and revered constructs of our society, having first been proposed and discussed from the times of ancient civilizations. They, together with other more contemporary principles, provide the foundation of ethical theory discussed in the following section. Principles can be generally exemplified by promoting the good (the best choices), causing no harm, and preventing harm from occurring. Principles are important because ethical decisions cannot be reached "simply by following handy formulas. No matter how carefully one issue has been resolved, the solution cannot be applied in cookbook fashion to another problem. Rather each issue . . . must be examined in the context of its particular circumstances."[27] The four important principles for the nurse anesthetist to appreciate are autonomy, nonmaleficence, beneficence, and justice.

Autonomy

The principle of autonomy, or patient self-determination, is a basic social value. An autonomous action is an act of intention; one independent of coercion by others. The American Nurses Association (ANA) Code for Nurses supports patient self-determination as a moral right.[28]

> The right to control one's body and one's treatment and the emphasis given to self-determination, privacy, freedom, autonomy, the emphasis on not being deceived, and being given complete and truthful information, all point to an important aspect of a rights-based view, namely the role of an individual patient's will in individual decision making.[29]

Autonomy must be a principle acknowledged and respected by the health care professional. It has been argued that the only permissible reason to remove a person's social or personal autonomy is to prevent harm to others. Moral principles, such as autonomy, suggest or propose certain behaviors, and they do not cause or command particular actions.[30] Autonomy in the medical setting involves a threshold element (competence), information elements (disclosure of information), and consent (voluntariness). It expresses general properties and relations rather than identifying persons or associations. It imposes an order on conflicting claims, and it offers finality, even overriding what law and custom require.

Nonmaleficence

Nonmaleficence is the concern for doing no harm or evil. As a principle, or as a governing law of conduct, harm to a patient is to be avoided. The language changes here from what "should" be done to what "ought" not be done. Harm may be defined either narrowly or broadly. The reference is mainly to physical harm, pain, disability, and death. Actions that inflict harm always require moral justification. Surgery inflicts harm but is morally justified by the premise of bringing about good or betterment. Difficult decisions are those concerned with "killing" or "letting die." Doing something or doing nothing are both actions, determined by decisions. In extreme circumstances, it is argued that mercy killing, or *euthanasia,* may be justified, but killing as a policy is certainly not justified. The extreme circumstances cited are a patient's uncontrollable pain and autonomous wishes. Allowing a patient to die also requires moral justification, but the conditions usually are not as extreme as those involving euthanasia.

Withdrawal of treatment is a nonmaleficence decision. It often means the withdrawal of medical nutrition and hydration. If withdrawal of treatment, "letting die," is seen as justifiable, then the withdrawal of medical nutrition and hydration is usually seen as justified. There is no evidence in the literature that foregoing artificial feeding and hydration is associated with increased pain or suffering, although the action may cause stress for the health care professional.

The principle of doing no harm necessitates an interpretation of values:

> One might conceptualize the progression from health to disease and, finally, death as a journey down a funnel. Beginning at the widest part, one encounters a countless variety of disease processes, injuries, and physiologic disruptions, which are caused by a comparable variety of etiologic agents. Journeying down this metaphorical funnel toward death, the slope becomes steeper, and the disease process begins to affect more and more of the organism's vital functions. As the funnel narrows, we find a gradually diminishing number of possible conditions, any and all of which will lead to a relatively limited pathophysiologic "common pathway" of death. . . . While a number of nonmedical values may compete with the goal of maximizing the longevity at the top of the funnel, decisions contrary to that goal are usually reversible, and have statistical and remote, rather than concrete and immediate, effects on the length of life. Nearing the bottom of the funnel, the consequences of nontreatment are immediate and irreversible.[31]

Consideration of risks and benefits are a part of the thoughtful and careful action dimension of nonmaleficence.[1]

Beneficence

The principle of beneficence can be understood as promoting or doing good.[8] Beneficence is action-oriented and requires positive steps. The beneficence principle requires the provision of benefits and a balancing of harms and benefits.[18]

An ethical dilemma arises for the health care professional when benefits are conflicting. Assume that the health care professional is willing to lie because it is thought the lie will benefit the patient. The principle of beneficence appears to be at odds with the principle of veracity (truthfulness). Should a nurse anesthetist lie? Several opinions are offered: Everyone has an uncompromising duty to be truthful even if the truth might be harmful[32]; some actions, such as lying, are intrinsically wrong and can be made right only if they are necessary to avoid greater evil[8]; there are times when lying is justified, but truthful alternatives should be sought[33]; lying is a temporary measure to prevent harm or death.[34] Several options are available to the health care professional, including the whole truth, partial truth, silence, lying, and decision delay.[34] Specific criteria can be used to determine whether or not a paternalistic lie is justified:

> 1. The lie benefits the person lied to; that is, the lie prevents more evil than it causes for that particular individual.
> 2. It must be possible to describe the greater good that occurs.
> 3. The individual would have wanted to be lied to; if the evil avoided by the lie were greater than the evil produced by it, the person would be irrational not to want to be lied to.
> 4. We would always be willing to allow the violation.[35]

Justice

As a guiding principle, justice involves weighing the issues and responding to the facts that are present. There is no general consensus as to what constitutes justice.[1] It is an important guiding concept when medical decisions are made. This concept could apply to medical advances and technology (deciding the recipient of a donated organ) and to the scarcity of time (deciding who needs your attention first, or most).[1] The health care professional is responsible for distributing just behavior and comparative treatment of individuals. "A fundamental need for something indicates that a person will be harmed if that thing is not obtained"[1] (p. 45). Health care needs "are things we need to prevent, maintain, restore, or compensate for departures (such as disease) from normal species functioning."[36]

Retributive justice comes into play as reparation for harm done. If a patient is harmed, there are means by which to right the wrong. The system works effectively if moral principles are followed. When they are not, the system becomes dysfunctional.

> With few exceptions, the prevailing attitude of . . . (professionals) toward disciplinary enforcement ranges from apathy to outright hostility. Disciplinary action is practically non-existent in many jurisdictions; . . . that (professionals) will not appear or cooperate in proceedings against each other . . . but

> instead will exert their influence to stymie the proceedings; . . . the members of the disciplinary agency simply will not make findings against those with whom they are professionally and socially well acquainted; . . . (I)n states with a small . . . (professional) population or in which disciplinary jurisdiction is vested in small local units, prominent (professionals) . . . guilty of misconduct received an unofficial immunity from disciplinary action because of the reluctance of the disciplinary agency to proceed against them. . . . (T)he disciplinary process is stymied, public confidence in the profession is destroyed and continued depredations upon the public are made possible.[37]

For years, the medical profession has been implicated, harassed, vilified, and degraded by charges from attorneys, the courts, and legislators of a conspiracy of silence.[37] Law students learn about medical malpractice, the practice of the medical profession of protecting its own.[38] When principles are used inappropriately by a profession, justice demands the organization be held accountable. Justice must be more than a word; it must be an active process.

THEORETICAL APPROACHES

Once the practitioner understands some of the basic ethical principles, it is possible to appreciate how some philosophers have proposed to configure these notions into a theory-based approach to ethical analysis. Ethical decision making, then, is guided by these theoretic constructs. This section discusses various theoretic approaches called *ethical theories*. Decisions need to be made on a morally justifiable basis, and knowledge of ethical theory can aid in this decision-making process. Thomas L. Beauchamp suggests that philosophy is primarily concerned with criticism and justification, and ethics is concerned with justifying some moral point of view.[39] The issue of justifying decisions and actions is addressed here.

The health care professional has many responsibilities, duties, and obligations that cause decisions to be difficult. Basic questions that are repeatedly asked are: "What is true? What is good? What is the purpose of life?" Ethical systems attempt to address these various issues. They consist of principles and theories, actions and judgments. Principles suggest what actions should be taken or what judgments should be made. Ethical theory is concerned with offering ways to balance divergent, individual opinion and social motives and conduct.

Specific theories have been proposed for helping health care professionals make bioethical decisions.[40] The theories concern themselves with how people make choices, ethical choices in particular, and aid the professional in analyzing situations and offering courses of action. Moral theories appear in three variants: the emphasis on compliance with rules, the emphasis on consequences, and the emphasis of dispositions relevant to behavior.[41] The variants fall within two broad approaches, non-normative and normative.

Non-normative approaches further divide into three major traditions: ethical emotivism, ethical skepticism, and ethical relativism. Ethical emotivism suggests that statements about right and wrong express or evoke emotions but do not state facts. The conclusion, then, is that moral judgments have no basis in fact. Ethical skepticism claims that people cannot distinguish between right and wrong. When individuals disagree about ethical issues, agreement cannot be reached. Opposing views cannot be right, therefore people cannot know right from wrong. Ethical relativism asserts that there is right and wrong, but the rightness or wrongness of an action is determined by a specific context. The context may be an individual, a culture, or a situation.

Normative ethics is the attempt to provide systematic and justifiable answers to moral questions. It presupposes there are universally applicable principles of right and wrong, good and bad.

The two traditional ways of assessing the "rightness" or "wrongness" of an act are to examine the intent of the actor or the consequences of the act.[42] The two workable approaches are deontology (duties) and teleology (results).[7]

Deontology

The Greek *deontais*, translated "duty," originally meant obedience to rules. The word is often translated as rules, principles, or binding duties. An act has specific characteristics that make it right or wrong regardless of the consequences, such as truth-telling, doing good, promise keeping, justice, and similar ideas. Promises are always kept. Truth is always disclosed. Harm is never inflicted. Acts of kindness and rules for goodness become the norm. Right is measured by actions that are considered to be right.

Deontologists believe that such principles as autonomy, beneficence, and nonmaleficence are crucial guides to moral actions. Two perspectives may be taken: focus on duty and universal rules to determine right action, or focus on the general social principle that rational persons in certain ideal situations agree on and adopt. A rule-based morality is advocated. Outcomes are not considered under this theory; the act determines the correctness of the situation. Deontologists propose that a sense of duty consists of a rational respect for the fulfillment of obligations to other human beings.[7] Any act congruent with duty is right and, conversely, any act contrary to duty is wrong. Some duties for the health professional are binding, such as the duty not to murder. The commanding duty is to respect people and their right of self-rule (autonomy).[41] The deontologic approach suggests that "rights are entitlement to protection, course of action, goods, and control over information"[41] (p. 481).

The philosopher Immanuel Kant (1724 to 1804) asserted that respect for persons is the primary test of duty.[7] There is an ultimate norm, or supreme duty (moral law), and an act is moral if it springs from good will. Kant formulated the categorical imperative: All persons have equal moral worth, and no rule can be moral unless all people can apply it autonomously to all other human beings. He stressed motive and the duty to do good things, yet offered little direction about what to do when ethical principles conflict. Most modern-day deontologists suggest that several principles can be applied at the same time to a dilemma. The health care professional who works with the individual patient often favors the deontologic approach.

Teleology

In contrast to deontology is teleology. The teleologic theory (sometimes called utilitarian) is a consequentialist approach. The terms "teleologic" and "utilitarian" are often used interchangeably, but it is suggested that the notion of teleology is the larger concept of which utilitarianism is a part.[16] The Greek term *telos* means the end of the consequences. This approach focuses on the effects of actions in deciding a dilemma. All actions are evaluated in terms of the extent to which they achieve desirable results. The "rightness" or "wrongness" is determined by the actual consequences achieved; the right action being that which leads to the best consequences.

Jeremy Bentham (1748 to 1832) and John Stuart Mills (1807 to 1873) were proponents of this approach. According to Bentham, utility is the greatest good for the greatest number. He developed "hedonistic calculus," the concept that all people are governed by two masters: pain and pleasure. Ethics functions to minimize the first and maximize the second. According to Mills, utility is the creation of happiness. His is a "goal-based ethics." The approach uses a "cost/benefit" analysis for determining the greatest happiness.[26]

Act utilitarianism is concerned with the rightness of the act, and rule utilitarianism is concerned with the rightness of the rule. Evaluation of the outcome is determined by the consequences of the act or the rule. Action is determined by examining all the available alternatives, foreseeing the consequences of performing each alternative, and evaluating the consequences in terms of which is the best.[13] A rule is determined by the amount of happiness or unhappiness produced if it is generally applied. What makes an act or rule right or wrong is its utility. Useful acts produce the greatest amount of good or the greatest amount of happiness.[7]

The best decision produces the greatest good or happiness (or the least unhappiness). This is often seen as the stance behind health care policy. The approach is the problem of defining the greatest good, deciding for whom, and assigning a weight to that goodness.[16] Thus, this approach is considered paternalistic.

Virtue

Other ethical theories expound or modify deontologic or teleologic methods; virtue ethics is often considered to be a third theoretic approach. This approach attempts to consider the issues of purpose and principle based on the goodness of the persons who select obligations and rules. It assumes that all human beings have inherent capacities that constitute the ultimate basis for all ethical claims. Actions are morally right if they are in accord with our nature as human beings. The stress is on the disposition for individuals to act morally, to be virtuous. This approach is concerned with what attributes are characteristic of persons who are considered virtuous.[43]

The theory can be traced to the time of Plato, who saw virtue as being synonymous with excellence in living a good life.[42] Such excellence could be attained by practice. "Goodness" and "virtuousness" became associated with the concept of the virtuous person doing good things, and good things were those acts that were virtuous. These are traits of human behavior that make one praiseworthy and blameworthy.[44] Aristotle wrote about everything striving to fulfill its potential. Natural law theory states that people are capable of establishing a standard of morality that is based on human nature. Acts are considered right when human potential is actualized.[7]

There is value in knowing the various theories and approaches. Each theoretic approach has strengths and weaknesses. Many of the strengths of consequentialism are the weaknesses of rule-based moralities, and rule-based moralities share similar problems with consequentialism.[13] The teleologic approach is sometimes seen as an attempt to weigh too many variables in deciding the best results. The deontologic approach is problematic because people place different values on principles. Nurse anesthetists will find the several aspects of the various ethical theories useful when pondering their own ethical dilemmas.

DECISION-MAKING MODELS

A viable decision-making model offers the health care professional self-examination and self-knowledge. Clinical decisions almost always contain a moral dimension, but the decision is rarely solely a moral decision.[45] "Clinical decisions often involve weighing moral values against political, economic, aesthetic, and prudent values."[45]

How can a moral dilemma be analyzed? The final decision may be an intuitive guess, or it may be a reasoned decision of what is best. Socrates argued that people must let reason, rather than emotion, determine ethical decisions.[8] "It is not enough to appeal to what people generally think, since they may be wrong, but we must find an answer by informed reasoning that we regard as correct"[1] (p. 3). Ethical reasoning can assist the health care professional. However, "if one's object is to discover unambiguous answers to ethical dilemmas quickly and effortlessly, then most likely he will be bewildered by the complexity of these dilemmas"[1] (p. 3). The application of principles, rules, and theories to a situation must justify the judgments that are made; knowledge of moral theory is not sufficient for improvement of moral practice. Theoretic interest is concerned with knowing and the practical interest is concerned with doing.[46] The task of knowing the good and doing the good is an ambitious one.

In an article on effective decision making for the occupational health nurse manager, Brown[47] discusses several kinds of decisions. These examples are applicable for the nurse anesthetist. Operational decisions are made in relation to day-to-day activities. Ten-second decisions require an immediate reading of the situation at hand and a response. Finally, there are decisions that tend to bring about discomfort to the parties involved.

Decisions are made within a context.

> Ethical decision making is synonymous with critical thinking. Commitment to thinking through a given clinical situation, identifying the ethical dimensions and issues, and applying moral reasoning precepts afford the best assurance that the final decision or course of action will be the "best" (morally right) one. Intelligent, sensitive, caring individuals do make mistakes; but when they use a critical reasoning process, there is less chance for mistakes based on ignorance, personal biases, or strong parentalism.[48]

Many bioethical decisions made by the health care professional carry the limitation of having incomplete knowledge of a patient's condition.[1] It is in this situation when advanced directives are extremely important and where clear communication between all involved parties is essential. The health care provider has a legal and ethical duty to provide safe, effective, and competent care and to intervene when such care is not being provided. The nursing profession has historically had a strong sense of moral obligation in upholding the welfare of the individual patient.[49] This sense of responsibility mandates that the health care professional clarify a personal value system, which in turn promotes self-knowledge.

Ethics has both an easy and a difficult aspect.[26] The easy aspect is that an ethical or moral issue emerges whenever good or harm results, and the difficult aspect is that of justifying what is determined to be good or harmful.[26] The study of ethics itself explains that there is not a single science of morals, for there are numerous alternative models emphasizing various central themes. A Kantian categorical imperative model of decision making emphasizes duty-based actions and responsibilities. An epicurean model emphasizes pleasure-centered values. A utilitarian model emphasizes actions that bring about the greatest happiness. An egoism model emphasizes self-interest. These various models call for different behaviors, so it is important that professions choose their models for behavior and decision making wisely.

A viable personal model may not be a workable professional model. Ultimately the consequences for the individual must be considered.

> In medical ethics the consequences change as technique and conditions change. One hundred and fifty years ago, before blood typing and matching, blood transfusions were almost universally fatal and so generally unethical as well. Ten years ago, the risks were small and blood transfusion generally posed no ethical problems. Today, with the spread of AIDS, there are again ethical problems with the system that supplies blood for transfusions. Sometimes our knowledge of the consequences and alternative treatments change, with the result that both the medical and ethical status of a treatment must be revalued.[39]

In medical professional life, applied ethics looks to the concrete and practical.[39] Applying knowledge differs from simply knowing. Applying ethics means making decisions, and decisions are best made if a decision-making frame of reference (decision-making model) is understood. Decision making by intuition has become an indefensible position in our time.

> All decisions, including ethical decisions, occur in a context that consists of an inner and outer environment. An inner environment consists of the sum total of one's experiences. . . . One's outer environment consists of those factors that are extrinsic to the person: the actions and reactions of others, time constraints, material resources. . . . Knowledge of one's self arises from experience gained from observation of the world and from experience gained from interaction with other living beings[7] (p. 41).

Ethical decision making is a complex process.[50] It is based on sorting out what is good, what the preferred action is and why, and what are the consequences of that action if it is taken.[51] It is suggested that there are three levels of decision making: "1.) the immediate level, in which there is no time for reflection; 2.) the intermediate level, in which there is some time for exploration and reflection; and 3.) the deliberate level, in which there is adequate time to explore, examine, and reflect in order to reach a rational, thoughtful decision"[7] (p. 40). Ethical decision making means making the decision, acting on the decision, and justifying the actions. In some situations the nurse anesthetist is a participant, and in others merely shares a point of view.

Since the 1970s, various decision-making models have been suggested for the health care professional. In 1976, Howard Brody developed an act-utilitarian ethical model and a deontologic ethical model.[52] The models involve moral reasoning, making choices from alternatives, and taking action. These two models are patterned after the major philosophic theories, utilitarianism and deontology. Rita Payton's 1979 pluralistic ethical decision-making model combined Brody's models with decision theory, "that is, problem identification, availability of alternative action, prediction of consequences of each proposed action, and selection of an ethically correct choice. The models . . . focused on 'dilemmas' as 'triggers' for ethical analysis."[53] The Thompson and Thompson Decision Model for Nursing involves a problem-solving process. It provides for "critical review of situational variables, and highlighting of the ethical issues raised by the situation."[53] The following is the Thompson and Thompson model.

1. Review the situation and identify
   a. Health problems
   b. Decision(s) needed
   c. Key individuals involved
2. Gather information that is available in order to
   a. Clarify the situation
   b. Understand the legal implications
   c. Identify the bureaucratic or loyalty issues, if any
3. Identify the ethical issues or concerns in the situation and
   a. Explore the historical roots
   b. Explore current philosophic/religious positions on each
   c. Identify current societal views on each
4. Examine personal and professional values related to each issue, including
   a. Personal constraints raised by the issues
   b. Guidance from professional codes or standards
   c. Moral obligations to individuals
5. Identify the moral positions of key individuals by
   a. Direct questioning
   b. Consideration of advance directives, if any
   c. Consideration of substituted judgments
6. Identify value conflicts, if any, including
   a. Potential sources of each
   b. Possible strategies for the resolution of each
7. Determine who should make the final decision, considering
   a. Who owns the problem
   b. Whether the patient can participate in the decision process
   c. Who can speak on behalf of the patient (substituted or best interests judgment) when patient cannot
8. Identify the range of possible actions and
   a. Describe the anticipated outcome for each action
   b. Identify the elements of moral justification for each action
   c. Note if the hierarchy of principles or utilitarianism is to be used
9. Decide on a course of action and carry it out
   a. Knowing the reasons for the choice of action
   b. Sharing the reasons with all involved
   c. Establishing a time frame for a review of the outcomes
10. Evaluate the result of the decision/action and note
    a. Whether the expected outcomes occurred
    b. If a new decision process is complete
    c. Elements of the process can be used in similar situations[53]

An analysis of the Thompson and Thompson model suggests:

Step One: Review the Situation. The first step involves identifying significant components of the situation as well as the individuals involved in making the decision. A clear understanding of the situation facilitates each subsequent action.

Step Two: Gather Additional Information. Additional information that may influence the situation is collected in this step. Demographic data, socioeconomic status, health status, prognosis, level of understanding, preferences, competence, family members, and/or significant others involved with the situation are examples of additional information that needs to be assessed.

Step Three: Identify the Ethical Issues. Understanding ethics and ethical principles is essential to identify accurately the issues of the situation. Another key to successful identification of the ethical issues is to gain a historical perspective of the issues.

Step Four: Identify Personal and Professional Values. When a nurse defines his or her personal and professional moral positions as they relate to ethical issues, the nurse is better prepared to understand his or her position in a particular situation. Awareness of professional codes will help identify professional values.

Step Five: Identify Values of Key Individuals. The moral values of the key people involved in the situation are as important as the nurse's values and are assessed in this step.

Step Six: Identify Value Conflicts. Value conflicts can occur within one individual or between values of the persons involved in the situation. Understanding why conflicts exist and keeping track of how conflicts have been resolved in the past assists with the final decision.

Step Seven: Determine Who Should Decide. Many people are available to assist in making the final decision. The physician, nurse, social worker, patient, and patient's family are all involved in health care ethics. At this point, it must be decided who should be responsible for the decision or action.

Step Eight: Identify Range of Actions with Expected Outcomes. A clear list of alternatives helps the nurse recognize possible consequences of a decision and identify a course of action.

Step Nine: Decide on the Course of Action and Carry It Out. The person(s) must decide on the course of action.

Step Ten: Evaluate Results of the Decision. The final step involves evaluating the decision made to determine if the outcome was the one anticipated. Evaluation also provides information that assists in future ethical decision making.[54]

Every problem does not have a solution. Unsolvable problems do exist. For example, "when a health care professional performs triage, that is, rations care at the scene of an accident, some are helped and some neglected. This is the damned-if-you do, damned-if-you-don't situation; the essence of the human tragedy"[44] (p. 11). Even the environment in which a health care professional makes decisions can be difficult, if life and death decisions are involved.

Ethical decision making involves not only critical thinking and critical analysis, but also the intrinsic aspects of decision making. When the nurse anesthetist considers legal requirements or social expectations relevant to the situation, the professional is considering extrinsic issues. "They are extrinsic to the ethical analysis and should not be confused with right and wrong. What is legal and/or what is expected are not necessarily right and wrong"[7] (p. 61).

To use already developed ethical decision-making models or to develop a personal working model, the nurse anesthetist needs knowledge of the topics involved in ethics, practice in developing skills involved in recognizing ethical dilemmas, ability to develop an ethical stance, and confidence to act from that stance. The CRNA, as a responsible health care professional, is best prepared when preparation occurs prior to the need. Preparation involves understanding the premise of critical thinking and critical analysis, regular discussion of ethical topics with peers and at professional meetings, and staying abreast of new information in the field of ethics.

PERTINENT ETHICAL ISSUES IN ANESTHESIA

There are three primary ethics-related areas of concern that CRNAs should be mindful of; all of which have the potential to affect their clinical practice. The first is related to informed consent, which is discussed in detail in Chapter 15. The other two areas of concern are advanced directives and do not resuscitate (DNR) orders. Each is discussed in detail in this section.

Advanced Directives

For the past several decades, medical technology has undergone explosive growth, ever widening the array of choices that a provider or patient may select as part of therapy. Inherent to these technologic advancements are new problems associated with the ethical principle of respecting the autonomy of patients. New advances in medical technology have caused conflicts with older traditional attitudes and practices society currently holds concerning both the living and the dead. For instance, new life-sustaining treatments have resulted in the prolongation of life for some persons who otherwise would have died. Commensurate with the development of these new techniques was the realization that their effective and ethical use should be defined by some sort of operational guidelines.

Consequently, over the past several decades, a trend has developed that encourages individuals to have some sort of advanced directive (living will or a durable power of attorney).[55] The advanced directives enhance the principle of autonomy; that is, they are documents that allow a person to exercise a preference regarding health care decisions if it later becomes impossible for them to make a decision. The person's wishes on health care matters are made at a time when he or she is capable of making decisions, and these decisions are recognized by state law. These directives also guide future treatment decisions. The advanced directive authorizes competent adults to make decisions concerning their care should they be rendered incompetent or become comatose.[56] The Patient Self-Determination Act of 1989 became law on December 1, 1991.

The living will, also called a directive to physicians, was written and published in 1974 by the Euthanasia Educational Council, which later became Concern for Dying and the Society for the Right to Die. This directive was not initially a legal document.

> The best known type of document is the living will, which in its generic form constitutes a refusal to undergo medical interventions if a patient is in a terminal, irreversible state. It is designed to prevent prolongation of the dying process. . . . Variations include: 1. Permitting or prohibiting minors from making a valid document, 2. invalidating a "will" in case of pregnancy, 3. including or excluding nutrition and hydration as a refusable option, 4. witness or notarization requirements, 5. periodic updating, 6. modern formats or exact forms which must be used, and 7. restrictions or requirements which local political considerations impose[41] (p. 206).

The living will is an instructional type of advanced directive, developed to direct the provider, under designated conditions, to exclude specific or heroic measures from use on the patient when the patient is not competent, even though such medical measures would likely prolong the patient's life. An ongoing difficult issue for living wills is the vague and often imprecise wording. It has also been suggested that living wills often fail to anticipate new or additional medical options that may have evolved after the document was executed. The living will is still not recognized by statute in all states, but State Natural Death Acts do provide legal means to use living wills with terminally ill patients. Protection is offered that gives criminal and civil immunity to the health care professions who follow the directives. There are still difficult issues associated with this directive, such as varied interpretations of the act and concern over the determination of competence.

The other component of these directives was the durable power of attorney for health care, sometimes called the durable power of attorney in health matters. This provided a more flexible instrument by which the patient's autonomy is secured.[57] This instrument is similar to the living will in that it preserves decision making for the patient on cardiopulmonary resuscitation and life support systems in case of future incompetence or coma. This rather simple document authorizes a proxy to make legally binding decisions for the patient. The proxy may act if the patient's preferences are not clear or if the desires have not been implemented. The durable power of attorney is not limited to terminal illnesses. The proxy has the same authority as the patient with reference to individual autonomy. The authority for treatment always initially originates with the patient, which is the intent and purpose of a directive. It is durable, in that it continues even when the patient who initiated it becomes incompetent. The first durable power of attorney was adopted in California in 1984.

Several news stories and at least two movies have recently highlighted the plight of patients without advanced directives. Perhaps the case of Nancy Beth Cruzan brought to light the serious ethical and legal issues involved in medical situations pertaining to autonomy. Ms. Cruzan was a woman in her twenties who was involved in a serious automobile accident. The accident left her in a vegetative state in the Missouri State Hospital, where she remained for several years. Her parents sought termination of her treatment, but her doctors refused. The courts upheld the medical community, stating that there needs to be clear and convincing evidence to discontinue feedings of an incompetent patient. Serious debates over the ethical and legal issues of this type of case are ongoing. The issue, the determination, and the allowance of death have become ethical issues and concerns.

The Missouri Supreme Court framed the debate not as one between life and death; but as one concerned with the quality of life and death. Necessary evidence was provided by the Cruzans, and the tube was removed. Nancy Beth Cruzan died 12 days later, at the age of 33.

The courts have made it clear that a competent person may refuse medical or surgical treatment even when it is life-saving. *Natanson v. Kline* exemplified this point stating: "Anglo-American law starts with the premise of thoroughgoing self-determination. It follows that each man is considered to be master of his own body, and he may, if he be of sound mind, expressly prohibit the performance of life-saving surgery or other medical treatment."[58] Difficulties occur when incompetence is determined. Dilemmas about which treatments are humane and appropriate are particularly difficult when patients are mentally incompetent.[41] Patients may not be mentally competent to give informed consent or refusal.[59] "In acute care hospitals, about one-half of the decisions about DNR orders involve incompetent patients. . . . The challenge is to grant incompetent patients the same rights to refuse treatments as competent patients, while giving them additional protection because they are vulnerable."[41] The caregiver's task is always to educate, counsel, negotiate, and check that the patient or surrogate is informed.

Some of the unresolved issues concerning advanced directives are: (1) Many states do not have statutes that explicitly authorized the durable power of attorney for health care. (2) Statutory law about advanced directive may conflict with case law about withholding care. (3) Statutes about advanced directives may conflict with administrative regulations. (4) A patient's advance directives may conflict with a physician's professional ethics or personal conscience. (5) The duty of caregivers to protect incompetent patients needs to be clarified.[41] For the nurse anesthetist the best defense is a good offense. The nurse anesthetist must know the subject matter and the law and ask questions to clarify issues or concerns before instituting care in cases involving advanced directives.

Do-Not-Resuscitate Orders

The DNR order has become well accepted and widely used in American hospitals.[60] Studies suggest that a DNR order is written for as many as 68 percent of patients dying in a hospital setting.[61] Recent studies offer some eye-opening information concerning DNR orders. The *Journal of Family Practice* cites two relevant studies.[62] In one, 86 percent of families, but only 22 percent of patients, were involved in the decision to assign DNR status to a patient.[63] The other study of hospitalized patients found that whereas 47 percent wanted to discuss resuscitation with their physician, only 16 percent actually did so.[64] There appears to be a need for better communication in health care regarding this difficult issue.

DNR is a medical order, made by a physician and recorded in the patient's chart, to withhold resuscitation in case of cardiac or respiratory arrest. Cardiopulmonary resuscitation after cardiac and/or respiratory arrest has been one of the most dramatic innovations of medicine in the 20th century.[65] CPR has both positive and negative potential. The potential good, the sustaining of life, is obvious, but the potential harms include anoxic encephalopathy, permanent ventilator dependence, or severe functional disability.[66] This negative side of the issue has brought experts in medicine, bioethics, and medical law together. Special orders, No CPR, No Code, or most commonly, DNR, have been established to ensure that CPR is not performed inappropriately.[67] Many experts contend that a DNR order is fully compatible with aggressive care and should not imply that other life-sustaining treatment be withheld or withdrawn.[68] The standard DNR order pertains to procedures performed during CPR, including precordial compression and/or cardiac massage, endotracheal intubation, mechanical ventilation, defibrillation, and administration of vasoactive drugs.[69] The order also may be limited or modified to include all CPR procedures except intubation and protracted mechanical ventilation.[70] In clinical practice, DNR orders are often associated with withholding or withdrawing life-sustaining therapies other than CPR, and thus may lead to less intensive care.[63] DNR orders are standard for patients with a life expectancy in terms of days, weeks, or months.

Health care professionals engage in ethical decision making when they aggressively resuscitate a patient, carry out a "slow code," or withhold treatment from a terminally ill patient. A slow code involves a verbal order to staff members to respond slowly when the patient has a cardiac arrest.

There are also "partial codes." Partial codes involve omitting some medical interventions and employing others. Each code has some serious implications. Likewise, a DNR order involves ethical decision making.

> Cessation of treatment is done under the converse presupposition: 1. a technical judgment that treatment does not have a reasonable chance of technical success (e.g., that restarting the heart is useless because it cannot continue beating) or 2. an ethical judgment that even if there is technical success, the patient's ability to profit from this life is nonexistent or perhaps that prolonging life would lead only to suffering (e.g., that restoring the heartbeat might be successful for a given length of time but that the patient is hopelessly ill and that restoring the heartbeat would either result in intolerable suffering or would be irrelevant to a permanently insentient patient).[42]

People used to die in their homes; today, most die in hospitals. "Dying has become institutionalized and therefore public, necessarily hedged with a multitude of restrictions. Deciding to allow a patient to die peacefully and to withhold treatment or support is far less easy"[42] (p. 131). As both disciplines of medicine and nursing consistently admonish their own to act aggressively in emergency situations, the DNR order, for some, has become problematic. Writing a DNR order is a judgment made on the technical grounds that doing something is useless. Once a DNR decision is made, comfort measures become the primary goal.[71] DNR orders need to be well thought out; they are a necessary part of medical practice.

In the late 1980s it was reported that approximately 1.6 million persons were potential candidates for CPR each year. Eighty percent of the 2 million persons who die each year in the United States die in acute or chronic care facilities, and a common feature in the dying process is the administering of CPR.[31] It has been suggested that resuscitation efforts are successful in only 5 to 20 percent of the institutionalized persons who undergo CPR; the figures are based on the survival rate of hospitalization. It is recognized that CPR should be withheld in some patients who have chronic, progressive, or end-stage disease that is irreversible.[72]

The report from the President's Commission for the Study of Ethical Problems in Medicine and Biomedical Research advocates the need for decision making by patients or their surrogates regarding life-sustaining and resuscitation measures.[55] The DNR order is issued with the consent of the patient or an appropriate surrogate. A current debate among medical ethics experts centers around whether the physician can issue a DNR order without patient consent when there is medical consensus that CPR would be futile.[73] It is reasonable to expect health care professionals to discuss CPR and the option of a DNR order whenever the patient or appropriately designated surrogate wishes, or whenever one of the following categories applies: (1) there is some reason to question the presumption of consent to CPR, (2) the patient is terminally ill, (3) the patient has a severe or irreversible illness or disabling condition, (4) the patient has suffered an irreversible loss of consciousness, or (5) the patient is reasonably likely to suffer cardiac or respiratory arrest.[68] Many propose (and the Joint Committee on the Accreditation of Health Care Organizations [JCAHO] now requires for accreditation) that hospitals and nursing homes establish formal resuscitation policies. The following provisions are important for institutional DNR policies.[31]

> 1. DNR orders should be documented in writing in the patient's medical record.
> 2. DNR orders should specify the exact nature of the treatment to be withheld.
> 3. Patients, when they are able, and families should participate in DNR decisions.
> 4. Decisions to withhold CPR must be discussed with other staff, especially nurses.
> 5. DNR status should be reviewed on a regular basis.
> 6. DNR is not equivalent to medical or psychological abandonment of patients—a distinction the staff must understand and patients be reassured of.[55]

DNR orders can be misinterpreted as implying or suggesting more than just the avoidance of CPR. Three patient care categories have been suggested to accurately delineate decisions and desires of patients[74]: (1) Full support, including CPR (in a case of cardiopulmonary arrest, full resuscitative measures are implemented); (2) full support, excluding CPR (if cardiopulmonary arrest occurs the patient is permitted to die without CPR); and (3) modified support, excluding CPR (terminally or critically ill patients for whom the institution or continued provision of the best available medical care would provide no reasonable prospect of meaningful recovery would not receive CPR in the event of cardiopulmonary arrest).

> These categories are assigned according to the following guidelines: First, a care category should be indicated on each patient's admitting orders. If no category is indicated, the patient is automatically assigned to the first category. Patient placement in either of the no-CPR categories requires discussion with the patient, or if this is not possible, with the responsible family or guardian. Competent patients must understand the risks, benefits, and alternatives of any decision reached and decide if family is to be involved in the decision. If the patient is incompetent, a consensus must be reached between the physician and the patient's responsible family or guardian.
>
> Patient placement in a no-CPR category can be done only with the approval of the attending physician or a member of the medical service staff substituting for the attending physician; this assignment must be fully outlined in the patient's chart. The attending physician's approval may be obtained by the resident via phone, in which case the resident must indicate the attending physician's name and phoned approval on the signed order. The attending physician must then countersign the order and corresponding chart note as soon as reasonably possible.
>
> Patient placement in a no-CPR category requires a care category note in the chart, written at the same time as the order. The note must include the following: the patient's diagnosis, care, response to care provided, and reason why CPR is inappropriate; a statement defining the patient's competency; a statement outlining discussions with the patient (if possible) or with responsible family or guardian; a summary of any consultations obtained; and if necessary, a statement of the phone discussion with the attending or staff physician. For patients assigned to the third category, the patient's chart notes should define the care modifications as clearly as possible; if therapy is intended only to promote the patient's comfort, this should be stated. Or, for example, if it is decided that further transfusion or blood gas determinations or other specific diagnostic or therapeutic measures are not warranted, it should be so stated. The attending or staff physician must also countersign the care-category note as soon as possible. Finally, an order to place a patient in a no-CPR category must be rewritten every 96 hours.[74]

The following stepwise approach to deciding not to resuscitate has been offered.[75]

1. If patient is competent, honor patient's wishes.
2. If patient is unable to understand condition or express wishes:
   a. Establish likelihood of reversing illness;
      (1) If reversible, no DNR order.
      (2) If prognosis unclear, no DNR order.
      (3) If illness irreversible, a DNR order may be considered.
   b. Discuss decision with other physicians with expertise in establishing prognosis; physicians in training should discuss such decisions with attending physician or chief resident.
   c. Discuss decision with family, if available.
   d. If primary physician, consultants, and family agree, a DNR order may be written; if significant disagreement exists, further discussions are indicated before recording a DNR order.
   e. If strong disagreement persists, a hospital ethics committee may be helpful in reaching a resolution.

DNR decisions and written orders are necessary for humane and ethical care. Humane and ethical care are interpretive concepts. From an ethical point of view, principles involved in a DNR order would be autonomy (self-determination); respect for persons (consideration for patients' values and goals); and nonmaleficence (do no harm: the trauma or pain of treatment clearly outweighs any potential benefits to patients).[76] As a humane gesture, the DNR might be viewed as "an intimate final freedom."[77] Questions still do persist, even with such an attitude. Several studies have shown that DNR orders are often associated with a more global decrease in the degree of care provided.[61,63,70,78,79] Even so, as many as 15 percent of patients with DNR order undergo palliative surgical procedures.[80] Typical operations are tracheotomy, gastrostomy, and insertion of central venous catheters for administration of analgesics and other medications.[50] "While most believe it is acceptable to allow a patient to die for a terminal disease, many feel it is inappropriate for a patient to die as a result of an anesthetic complication. On closer scrutiny, however, it is difficult to rationalize any distinction between what happens in the operating room and what happens in the ward or the intensive care unit (ICU)."[50]

There are at least three arguments offered for supporting suspension of DNR orders during surgery or anesthesia.

> First, any patient who requests an operative procedure agrees to a series of interventions, including administration of anesthesia, that is hoped will lead to a desirable benefit. . . . In other words, any general anesthetic involves the deliberate depression of vital signs systems followed by their resuscitation. Separating the administration of anesthesia from resuscitation is therefore difficult and somewhat artificial. A second reason for suspending DNR order during anesthesia and surgery stems from the difference between a cardiorespiratory arrest that occurs spontaneously (as with cerebral or cardiac embolus) and one that results from therapeutic intervention. . . . DNR orders are sometimes written to account for this distinction by specifying that resuscitation will be performed if the precipitating event is likely to be easily reversible. . . . CPR during anesthesia and surgery is sufficiently different from CPR outside of this setting that the usual considerations regarding DNR orders should not automatically apply to the former. Finally, (Thirdly) . . . every anesthetic agent available promotes some degree of cardiovascular instability. Administration of an anesthetic to a physiologically unstable patient often involves a delicate balance between the goals of analgesia and amnesia, and cardiovascular collapse.[50]

Even though DNR orders have become common, it is still a difficult concept. The impetus for much of the current reexamination of aggressive policies, including CPR and DNR orders, was seen in the Karen Ann Quinlan case.[81] On April 15, 1975, Karen Ann Quinlan ceased breathing for at least two 15-minute periods. She was found comatose, with evidence of decortication. She required a respirator to assist her breathing. She was legally and medically alive, but had lost all ability to function on a human, sapient level. Her parents filed a petition that her father be appointed as her legal guardian, for the express purpose of withdrawing all extraordinary means of sustaining vital processes. The petition was opposed by Karen Ann Quinlan's doctors, the hospital, the Morris County Prosecutor, the State of New Jersey, and her guardian ad litem. Eventually, extraordinary means of sustaining the vital processes were removed. Karen Ann Quinlan lived for several more years in a vegetative condition.

This case forced the courts to examine the issue of withdrawing life-sustaining treatment. The New Jersey Supreme Court recognized the right of incompetent patients. The court's interpretation of the Ninth Amendment, which pertains to the fundamental constitutional right of privacy, allows the treatment to be withdrawn from the incompetent patient because withdrawing treatment is seen to be in the patient's best interest.

Withholding and withdrawing life-sustaining support from hopelessly ill patients is a complicated and controversial topic. The ethical issues are withholding or withdrawing artificial nutrition and hydration, ordinary versus extraordinary care, artificial nutrition and hydration versus medical treatment, and killing versus allowing to die. Feeding the hungry has been cited as the most fundamental of all human relationships and "the perfect symbol of the fact that human life is inescapably social and communal."[82] Medicine now has the ability to sustain life indefinitely by means of artificial ventilation, drugs, intravenous nutrition, and hydration. Topics to consider concerning withholding and withdrawing of treatment are: (1) indications for medical intervention, (2) objectives that can be achieved by medical intervention, (3) patient autonomy, (4) quality of life, and (5) extrinsic factors. Medicine can offer benefits. Ventilation assures that blood gases are maintained and intravenous lines can provide access for fluid, nutrients, and medication. The President's Commission Report,

Deciding to Forego Life-sustaining Treatment (1983), stated that whatever considerations justify not starting should justify stopping as well.[83] There are many intervention decisions to make.

The obligation to be involved in DNR orders and withholding of treatment decisions is grounded in the professional code. The ANA's 1985 Code for Nurses states: "Each nurse has an obligation to be knowledgeable about the moral and legal rights of all clients and to protect and support those rights."[84] The issues of this topic can no longer be bypassed. Decisions that are made by the health care professional must be made with more than just reasons—they must be made with good reasons.

GLOSSARY

Absolute duty: An obligation or responsibility owed to another; an obligation to a conduct of life (i.e., codes).

Act deontology: Knowing in each situation what ought to be done (i.e., the act); of central importance.

Act utilitarianism: Judging each situation individually according to its utility.

Allocation of scarce resources: The distribution of what is available.

Applied Ethics (normative ethics): Applying theory to situations.

Belief: A doctrine or an attitude held by the individual.

Beneficence: Doing the good; preventing or restraining harm.

Bioethics: Health care ethics; ethical concepts applied to the health care profession.

Biomedical technology: The advancements of medications, devices, procedures, and machinery in medical science.

Categorical imperative: Immanuel Kant's principle that one ought never to act on a maxim that cannot be willed as universal law.

Code of ethics: Rules by which a profession governs itself.

Confidentiality: Not repeating private information or secret knowledge that has been given.

Deontology: Viewing some actions as morally obligatory regardless of the outcome.

Dilemma: A difficult problem that has no satisfactory solution.

Distributive justice: Equality of treatment in conditions of scarcity.

Duty: An act held or seen as morally obligatory.

Epistemology: Truth-seeking.

Ethical theory: Attempting to understand the idea of ethics.

Ethics: The reasons behind the "ought" and "should" of society; asking the "whys"; distinguishing right from wrong in behavior or attitude.

Extraordinary treatment: Treatment that may be done but treatment that is not required to be done. (A difficult distinction for clinical practice.)

Fidelity: Truth-telling; veracity.

Informed consent: The uniting of the principles of autonomy and self-determination with the legal concept of the inviolability of the human person; the right to know and to make decisions.

Judgment: An opinion, decision, or conclusion about a particular action.

Justice: Allocating to people their due; fairness or impartiality.

Logic: Rules for correct reasoning.

Medical ethics: The moral obligations in the practice of medicine.

Metaethics: Suggesting that there are higher standards than the law (i.e., natural law or the will of God).

Morals: The "ought" and "should" of society; the concern for what is right and wrong in attitudes, character, and behavior.

Natural law: Related to intuitionism; knowing right from wrong without external instruction; innate knowledge.

Nonmaleficence: Do no harm or evil.

Nursing ethics: Ethics applied to nursing; referred to as an ethics of caring.

Paternalism: The treating of others as childlike; an external attitude where the health care provider assumes the dominant role.

Philosophy: Attempting to offer a unified view of existence through systematic reflection.

Principles: Basic reasons; the origin or cause or reason given for attitudes or behaviors.

Quality of life: The task of attempting to state value on varying stages of existence.

Retributive justice: Reparation for harm done.

Rights: Claims on others; ethical, legal, or both.

Rule deontology: The systematic valuing of some ethical rules.
Rule utilitarianism: Claims that some ethical rules have greater utility.
Rules: Grouping together actions of a certain kind and suggesting these actions should be done.
Situational ethics: Right or wrong is determined by, or in relation to, the situation.
Teleology: Focusing on the consequences of the action; an emphasis on the outcome.
Theories: A systematic approach to an idea or various ideas.
Utilitarianism: Viewing morality from the principle of utility (the greatest possible balance of what is valued as good over what is not valued as having worth).
Virtue: Admirable qualities of mind or character.

REFERENCES

1. Davis, AJ and Aroskar, MA: Ethical Dilemmas and Nursing Practice, ed 2. Appleton-Century-Crofts, Norwalk, CT, 1983.
2. Closer, KD: Medical ethics: some uses, abuses, and limitations. N Engl J Med 293:384, 1975.
3. Rollins, BE (ed): The Experimental Animal in Biomedical Research: A Survey of Scientific and Ethical Issues for Investigators, Vol 1. Boca Raton, FL, 1990, p. 27.
4. Anderson, E: The Schweitzer Album. Harper & Row, New York, 1965, p. 43.
5. Aquinas, T: Summa Theologica: A Concise Translation. McGraw-Hill, New York, 1991, p. 79.
6. Flight, MR: Medical ethics; reach out and touch everyone. The Professional Medical Assistant, November/December, 1987, p. 21.
7. Curtin, L and Flaherty, MJ. Nursing Ethics Theories and Pragmatics. Robert J. Brady, Bowie, MD, 1982.
8. Frankena, WK: Ethics, ed 2. Prentice-Hall, Englewood Cliffs, NJ, 1973.
9. McConnell, TC: Moral Issues in Health Care: An Introduction to Medical Ethics. Wadsworth Health Sciences Division, Monterey, CA, 1982.
10. Titus, HH: Ethics for Today, ed 3. American Book Co, New York, 1957, pp. 17–19.
11. Helm, A: Ethical dilemmas and nursing. Aviat Space Environ Med 55:754, 1984.
12. Englehardt, HT: The Foundations of Bioethics. Oxford University Press, New York, 1986.
13. Brody, B: Ethics and Its Applications. Harcourt Brace Jovanovich, New York, 1983.
14. Thompson, JE and Thompson, HO: Ethics in Nursing. Macmillan, New York, 1981.
15. Hancock, RN: Twentieth Century Ethics. Columbia University Press, New York, 1974.
16. Thompson, JE and Thompson, HO: Bioethical Decision Making for Nurses. Appleton-Century-Crofts, East Norwalk, CT, 1985, p. 6.
17. Murphy, C: The changing roles of nurses in making ethical decision. Nurse Law Ethics 4(a):173, 1984.
18. Beauchamp, TL and Childress, JF: Principles of Biomedical Ethics, ed 2. Oxford University Press, New York, 1983, p. 1.
19. Wilbur, DL: The Heritage of Hippocrates. JAMA 208 (5):840, 1969.
20. Burns, CR (ed): Legacies in Ethics and Medicine. Science History Publications, New York, 1977.
21. Konold, DE: A History of American Medical Ethics, 1847–1912. University of Wisconsin, Madison, 1962.
22. Reich, WT (ed): Encyclopedia of Bioethics. Free Press, New York, 1987, pp. 1750–1751.
23. Aikens, CA: Studies in Ethics for Nurses, ed 4. WB Saunders, Philadelphia, 1937.
24. Deloughery, GL and Gebbie, KM: Political Dynamics: Impact on Nurses and Nursing. CV Mosby, St. Louis, MO, 1975.
25. Webster's Collegiate Dictionary. Merriam, Springfield, MA, 1974.
26. Bandman, EL and Bandman, B. Nursing Ethics in the Life Span. Appleton-Century-Crofts, East Norwalk, CT, 1985.
27. Beauchamp, TL and Childress, JF: Principles of Biomedical Ethics. Oxford University Press, New York, 1979, p. 5.
28. Churchill, L: Ethical issues of a profession in transition. Am J Nurs 77:874, 1977.
29. Callahan, D: Minimalist ethics. Hastings Cent Rep 11:19, 1981.
30. Murphy, C: The moral situation in nursing. In Bandman, EL and Bandman, B (eds): Bioethics and Human Rights. Little, Brown, Boston, 1978, p. 313.
31. Youngner, SJ: Do-not-resuscitate orders: No longer secret, but still a problem. Hastings Cent Rep 17(1):16, 1987.
32. Kant, I: On a supposed right to lie from altruistic motives. In Mappers, TA and Zembaty, JS (eds): Biomedical Ethics. McGraw-Hill, New York, 1981, p. 61.
33. Bok, S: Lying: Moral Choice in Public and Private Life. Vintage Books, New York, 1978.
34. Bulecheck, G and Aydelotte, M (eds): Nursing Interventions: Treatment for Nursing Diagnoses. WB Saunders, Philadelphia, 1985, p. 365.
35. Gert, B and Culver, C: The justification of paternalism. Ethics 89(2):199, 1979.
36. Daniels, N: Cost-effectiveness and patient welfare. In Basson, M (ed): Rights and Responsibilities in Modern Medicine. Alan R. Liss, New York, 1981, pp. 162–163.
37. American Bar Association Special Committee on Evaluation of Disciplinary Enforcement: Problems and Recommendations in Disciplinary Enforcement, Section 1, The Present Status of Disciplinary Enforcement. Chicago, 1970, p. 1.
38. Norton, ML: Ethics in medicine and law—standards and conflicts. Medi Trial Tech Quarterly 26(4):381, 1980.
39. Beauchamp, TL: Ethical theory and bioethics. In Beauchamp, TL and Walters, L, (eds): Contemporary Issues in Bioethics, ed 2. Wadsworth, Belmont, CA, 1982, p. 1–12.
40. Sigman, P: Ethical choice in nursing. Adv Nurs Sci 1979; 1:38, 1979.
41. Monagle, JF and Thomasma, DC: Medical Ethics. Aspen Publishers, Rockville, CA, 1988.

42. Loewy, EH: Textbook of Medical Ethics. Plenum Publishing, New York, 1989. 16–17, 130–131.
43. Frankena, WF: Beneficence in an ethics of virtue. In Shelp, EE (ed): Beneficence and Health Care. D Reidel, Dordrecht, The Netherlands, 1982.
44. Garrett, TM, Baillie, HW, and Garrett, RM: Health Care Ethics, Principles and Problems. Prentice-Hall, Englewood Cliffs, NJ, 1989.
45. Fowler, MD: The role of the clinical ethicist. Heart and Lung 15 (3):319, 1986.
46. Meldon, AI (ed): Ethical Theories, ed 2. Prentice-Hall, Englewood Cliffs, NJ, 1967.
47. Brown, KC: Effective decision making. Am Assoc Occup Nurs J 38(3):139, 1990.
48. Thompson, JE and Thompson, HO: Ethical decision making: Process and models. Neonatal Network 9(1):69, 1990.
49. American Nurses Association: Code for Nurses with Interpretive Statements. American Nurses Association, Kansas City, MO, 1976.
50. Truog, RD: Do-not-resuscitate orders during anesthesia and surgery. Anesthesiology, 74(5):606, 1991.
51. Thompson, JE and Thompson, HO: Bioethical decision-making: Who owns the problem? Appleton & Lange, East Norwalk, CT, 1985.
52. Brody, H: Ethical decisions in medicine. Michigan State University Press, East Lansing, 1976.
53. Thompson, IE: The implications of medical ethics. J Med Ethics 2:69, 1976.
54. Watson, RL: Application of an ethical decision making model. Emphasis: Nursing 2(2):94, 1987.
55. President's Commission for the Study of Ethical Problems in Medicine and Biomedical and Behavioral Research. Deciding to Forego Life-sustaining Treatment. U.S. Government Printing Office, Washington, DC, 1983, 493–545.
56. Areen, J: The legal status of consent obtained from families of adult patients to withhold or withdraw treatment. JAMA 258:229, 1987.
57. Areen, J: The legal status of consent to withhold treatment. JAMA 258:2696, 1987.
58. *Natanson v. Kline*, 186 Kan. (1960).
59. Roth, LH, Meisel, A, and Lindz, CW: Tests of competency to consent to treatment. Am J Psychiatry 134:279, 1977.
60. Tomlinson, T and Brody, H. Ethics and communications in do-not-resuscitate orders. N Eng J Med 318:43, 1988.
61. Jonsson, PV, McNamee, M, and Champion EW. The "Do not resuscitate" order: A profile of its changing use. Arch Intern Med 148:2373, 1988.
62. Ebell, MH: The do-not-resuscitate order: Outpatient experience and decision-making preferences. J Fam Pract 31(6):630, 1990.
63. Bedell, SE, et al: Do-not-resuscitate orders for critically ill patients in the hospital: How are they used and what is their impact? JAMA 256(2):233, 1986.
64. Frankl, D, Oye, RK, and Bellamy, PE: Attitudes of hospitalized patients toward life support: A survey of 200 medical inpatients. Am J Med 86:645, 1989.
65. Kouwenhoven, WB, and Jude, JR: Knickerbocker GG: closed-chest cardiac message. JAMA 173:1064, 1960.
66. Abramson, NS, et al. Neurologic recovery after cardiac arrest: Effect of duration of ischemia. Crit Care Med 13:930, 1985.
67. Franklin, C: When and how to write do-not-resuscitate orders. J Crit Illness 5:938, 1990.
68. The Hastings Center. Guidelines on the Termination of Life-sustaining Treatment and the Care of the Dying. The Hastings Center, Briarcliff Manor, NY 1987.
69. Franklin, C: Do not resuscitate policies. Acute Care 11:208, 1985.
70. Zimmerman, JE, et al: The use and implications of do not resuscitate order in intensive care units. JAMA 255:351, 1986.
71. Loewy, EH: Treatment decisions in the mentally impaired: Limiting but not abandoning treatment. N Engl J Med 317:1465, 1987.
72. Jonsen, AR, Siegler, M, and Winslade, WJ: Clinical Ethics. Macmillan, New York, 1982.
73. Tomlinson, T, and Brody, B: Futility and the ethics of resuscitation. JAMA 264:1276, 1990.
74. Davila, F, Boisaubin, EV, and Sears, DA: Patient care categories: An approach to do-not-resuscitate decisions in a public teaching hospital. Crit Care Med 14(12):1066, 1986.
75. Lee, MA and Cassell, CK: The ethical and legal framework for the decision not to resuscitate. West J Med 140:117, 1984.
76. Martin, DA and Redland, AR: Legal and ethical issues in resuscitation and withholding of treatment. Crit Care Nurs Quarterly 10(4):4, 1988.
77. Gostin, L: A right to choose death: The judicial trilogy of Brophy, Bouvia, and Conroy. Law Med Health Care 14:198, 1986.
78. Lipton, HL: Do-not-resuscitate decisions in a community hospital. Incidence, implications, and outcomes. JAMA 256:1164, 1986.
79. Stolman, CJ, et al: Evaluation of the do not resuscitate orders at a community hospital. Arch Intern Med 149:1851, 1989.
80. La Puma J, et al: Life-sustaining treatment: A prospective study of patients with DNR orders in a teaching hospital. Arch Intern Med 148:2193, 1988.
81. Robertson, JA: The Rights of the Critically Ill. Bantam Books, New York, 1983.
82. Callahan, D: On feeding the dying. Hastings Cent Rep 13(5):22, 1983.
83. U.S. Congress, Office of Technology Assessment: Life-sustaining Technologies and the Elderly. U.S. Government Printing Office, Washington, DC, 1987.
84. American Nurses Association: Code for Nurses with Interpretive Statements. American Nurses Association, Kansas City, MO, 1985, p. 1.

GENERAL RESOURCES FOR THE STUDY OF ETHICS

Journals

American Journal of Law and Medicine
Bioethics
Bioethics Quarterly
The Bulletin of the History of Medicine
Ethical Currents
Ethics
Ethics and Medics
Ethics and Values in Health Care

Ethics in Science and Medicine
Frontlines
Hastings Center Report
Hospital Ethics
Hospital Progress
Journal of Literature and Medicine
Journal of Medical Ethics
Journal of Medicine and Philosophy
Lancet
Law, Medicine and Health Care
Linacre Quarterly
Medical-Moral Newsletter
Medicine and Law
Nursing Forum
Nursing Law and Ethics
Nursing Mirror
Nursing Outlook
Nursing Times
Perspectives in Biology and Medicine

Journal Articles

A code of ethics. Am J Nurs 26:261, 1926.
Adamson, EH: The right to refuse life sustaining medical treatment and the noncompetent nonterminally ill patient: An analysis of abridgment and anarchy. Pepperdine Law Review 17:461, 1990.
American Nurses Association, Committee on Ethical Standards: A suggested code. Am J Nurs 26:599, 1926.
American Nurses Association, Committee on Ethics: Guidelines for Implementing the Code for Nurses. American Nurses Association, Kansas City, MO, 1980.
American Nurses Association: Code for Nurses with Interpretive Statements. American Nurses Association, Kansas City, MO, 1976.
Annarino, L and Zucker, A: New York Decision (Right to Die). Death Studies 13:84, 1989.
Annas, GJ: The Quinlan case: Death decision by committee. New Physician 28(2):53, 1979.
Armstrong, PW: New Jersey—still the nation's proving ground? Hastings Cent Rep 19:25, 1989.
Aroskar, MA: Anatomy of an ethical dilemma: The practice. Am J Nurs 80:661, 1980.
Aroskar, MA: Are nurses' mind sets compatible with ethical practice? Topics in Clinical Nursing 4:22, 1980.
Bandman, E: Why ethics in nursing practice. Imprint. 26:34, 1979.
Brakes, P: Bioethics and informed consent in american health care delivery. J Adv Nurs 4:23, 1979.
Bennett, J: Nurses talk about the challenge of AIDS. Am J Nurs 87:1150, 1987.
Bindler, R: Moral development in nursing education. Image 9:18, 1977.
Bishop, VA: Taking a stand on ethics. Nursing Mirror 149:22, 1979.
Bliss, BP and Johnson, AJ: Communicating ethics during medical training. Nursing Mirror 136:23, 1973.
Brearley P: Confidentiality—the need for a code of practice. Nursing Times 74:505, 1978.
Broadhurst, J: Ethics of nursing. Am J Nurs 17:792, 1917.
Cabaniss, SH: Ethics. Am J Nurs 875, 1903.
Carnegie, ME: The patient's bill of rights and the nurse. Nurs Clin North Am 9:557, 1974.
Childress, JF: Dying patients: Who's in control? Law, Medicine & Health Care. 17:27, 1989.
Cohn, SD: The living will from the nurse's perspective. Law, Medicine and Health Care 11:121, 1983.
Cole, JJ: Moral dilemma: To kill or allow to die? Death Studies 13:393, 1989.
Coletta, SS: Values clarification in nursing: Why? Am J Nurs 78:2057, 1978.
Curtin, L: Informed consent: Information or exploitation? Update on Ethics 1:1, 1977.
Drane, JR and Roth, RB: Institutional ethics committees: What, how, and why. Health Progress 66(8):30, 1985.
Dugan, DO: Masculine and feminine voices: Making ethical decisions in the care of the dying. Journal Med Hum Bioethics 8(2):129, 1987.
Edwards, B and Haddad, A: Establishing a nursing bioethics committee. J Nurs Adm 18:30, 1988.
Ellis, K: The slow code dilemma. RN 50:28, 1987.
Galton, M: Emergency Resuscitation: Ethics and Legalisms. Australian Nurses Journal 10:44, 1980.
Gilbert, C: The what and how of ethics education. Topics in Clinical Nursing 4:49, 1982.
Humphrey, D: Legislating for active voluntary euthanasia. The Humanist. 48:10, 1988.
Johnson, DE: Withholding fluids and nutrition: Identifying the populations at risk. Issues in Law & Medicine 2:189, 1986.
Lyon, EA: The right to die: An exercise of informed consent, not an extension of the constitutional right to privacy. University of Cincinnati Law Review 58:1367, 1990.
Lynn, J and Glover, J: Cruzan and caring for others. Hastings Cent Rep 20:10, 1990.
Okrand, F: Elizabeth Bouvia v Superior Court (California). Los Angeles Lawyer 9:31, 1986.
Rothwell, C: Euthanasia. Journal of Family Law 28:336–340, 1990.
Russell, R: Death without dignity: This atrocity forced me from nursing. RN 44:87, 1981.
Sandroff, R: Is it right? To turn off life support . . . to keep a body alive for its organs? To give illegal narcotics to the dying? RN 43:24, 1980.
The next Cruzan case. U.S. News & World Report, January 14, 1991, p. 8.
The President's Commission: The need to be more philosophical. Journal of Medical Philosophy 14:369, 1989.
Young, EWD: Assisting suicide: An ethical perspective. Issues in Law and Medicine 3:281, 1987.

Books on Biomedical Ethics

Bandman, EL and Bandman, B (eds): Bioethics and Human Rights. Little, Brown, Boston, 1978.
Barry, V: Moral Aspects of Health Care. Wadsworth, Belmont, CA, 1982.
Beauchamp, TL and Childress, JE: Principles of Biomedical Ethics, ed 2. Oxford University Press, New York, 1983.
Beauchamp, TL and Perlin, S: Ethical Issues in Death and Dying. Prentice-Hall, Englewood Cliffs, NJ, 1978.
Beauchamp, TL and Walters, L (eds): Contemporary Issues in Bioethics, ed 2. Wadsworth, Belmont, CA, 1982.

Mappes, TA and Zembaty, JS (eds): Biomedical Ethics, ed 2. McGraw-Hill, New York, 1986.
Brody, H. Ethical Decisions in Medicine, ed 2. Little, Brown, Boston, 1981.
Califano, J: America's Health Care Revolution: Who Lives? Who Dies? Who Pays? Random House, New York, 1986.
Vestch, RM (ed): Cases in Bioethics From the Hastings Center Report. Hastings Center, Hastings-on-Hudson, NY, 1984.
Childress, JF: Priorities in Biomedical Ethics. Westminster, Philadelphia, 1981.
Clouser, KD: Teaching Bioethics: Strategies, Problems, and Resources. The Hastings Center, Hastings-on-Hudson, NY, 1980.
Beauchamp, TL and Walter, L (eds): Contemporary Issues in Bioethics, ed 2. Wadsworth, Belmont, CA, 1982.
Daniels, N: Just Health Care. Cambridge University Press, Cambridge, England, 1985.
Duncan, AS, Dunstan, GR, and Welbourn, RB (eds): Dictionary of Medical Ethics. Crossroad, New York, 1981.
Engelhardt, H: The Foundations of Bioethics. Oxford University Press, New York, 1986.
Francoeur, RT: Biomedical Ethics: A Guide to Decision Making. John Wiley & Sons, New York, 1983.
Gorovitz, S, et al (eds): Moral Problems in Medicine. Prentice-Hall, Englewood Cliffs, NJ, 1976.
Harrison, BW: Our Right to Choose: Toward a New Ethic of Abortion. Beacon Press, Boston, 1983.
Jonsen, AR, Siegler, M, and Winslade, WJ: Clinical Ethics: A Practical Approach to Ethical Decisions in Clinical Medicine. Macmillan, New York, 1982.
Kubler-Ross, E: On Death and Dying. Macmillan, New York, 1969.
Ladd, J (ed): Ethical Issues Relating to Life and Death. Oxford University Press, New York, 1979.
McCormick, RA: How Brave a New World? Dilemmas in Bioethics. Doubleday, Garden City, NY, 1981.
Midgley, M: Heart and Mind: The Varieties of Moral Experience. St. Martin's Press, New York, 1981.
Munson, R: Intervention and Reflection: Basic Issues in Medical Ethics, ed 2. Wadsworth, Belmont, CA, 1983.
Murphy, CP: The moral situation in nursing. In Bandman, EL and Bandman, B (eds): Bioethics and Human Rights. Little, Brown, Boston, 1978, p. 313.
Purtillo, RB and Cassell, CK: Ethical Dimensions in the Health Professions. WB Saunders, Philadelphia, 1981.
Ramsey, P: Ethics at the Edges of Life: Medical and Legal Intersections. Yale University Press, New Haven, 1978.
U.S. Congress: House Committee on Energy and Commerce. Subcommittee on Health and the Environment. National Organ Transplantation Act. U.S. Government Printing Office, Washington, DC, 1990.
U.S. Task Force on Organ Transplantation: Organ Transplantation: Issues and Recommendations. Health Resources and Services Administration, U.S. Department of Health and Human Services, Rockville, MD, 1986.
Veatch, RM: Case Studies in Medical Ethics. Harvard University Press, Cambridge, MA, 1977.
Veatch, RM: A Theory of Medical Ethics. Basic Books, New York, 1981.
Walton, DN: Ethics of Withdrawal of Life-Support Systems: Case Studies on Decision Making in Intensive Care. Greenwood Press, Westport, CT, 1983.

Media Materials

Bioethics in Nursing Practice (video, five video cassettes). Robert J. Brady, Bowie, MD, 1981.
Code Gray: Ethical Decisions in Nursing (video). Fanlight Productions, Jamaica Plains, MA, 1983.
Dax's Case, Unicorn Productions, The University of Texas Medical School, Galveston, TX, 1984.
Death and Dying (Biomedical Ethics Series) (video). University of Texas Health Science Center, Dallas, 1977.
Discussions in Bioethics (video). National Film Board of Canada, Montreal, Canada, 1985.
Dignity of Death (video). ABC News, New York, 1973.
The Ethical Challenge: Four Biomedical Case Studies (slide/tape/phonograph record programs). Science Mankind, White Plains, NY, 1975.
Ethics of Organ Transplantation (Biomedical Ethics Series) (video). University of Texas Health Science Center, Dallas, 1977.
Ethics Trigger Tape (audio). Office of Interdisciplinary Education, College of Applied Health Professions, University of Kentucky, Lexington, KY, 1983.
Hard Choice Series (video). PBS, 1980. *Boy or Girl: Should the Choice Be Ours. Genetics Screening: The Ultimate Preventative Medicine. Human Experiments: The Price of Knowledge. Behavior Control. Death and Dying. Doctor, I Want . . . Justice and Medical Care.* 1980.
PBS Frontline Show, Better Off Dead? [Public Broadcasting Service (PBS) video], 1984.
Professional Ethics. Health Media Corporation, Hillcrest Medical Center, Tulsa, OK, 1978.
The Right to Die (motion picture or 3/4-inch. video recording). Carle Medical Communications, Urbana, IL, 1985.
Tomorrow's Child (video). Landmark Films, Falls Court, VA, 1982.
Whose Life Is It Anyway? (film). Granada Television, London, England, 1975.

19

Chemical Dependency

Diana S. Quinlan

OUTLINE

OBJECTIVES

On completing this chapter, the reader will be able to:

1. Discuss the history and incidence of substance abuse, as well as define key terms related to chemical dependency.
2. Describe the differences between several theoretic models of addiction and delineate factors that put an anesthesia provider at risk.
3. Discuss predominant coping mechanisms and explain the roles of co-workers and managers in the recognition of a chemically dependent colleague, including enabling behaviors.
4. Describe the documentation process required for an effective intervention, including preferred personnel and key elements.
5. Outline a drug and alcohol program as mandated by federal law for nurse anesthesia training programs.
6. Describe the complete treatment process including programming and cost.
7. Discuss reentry and relapse among anesthesia providers and what constitutes an effective aftercare plan for a recovering colleague.
8. Discuss legal and ethical issues that impact on the chemically dependent anesthetist and explain disciplinary alternatives for the chemically dependent CRNA.

One of the most prevalent, yet least understood diseases among health professionals is chemical dependency. As the demands of the field of anesthesiology increase, and newer and more potent drugs play a greater role in clinical practice, the rate of addiction will likely increase among providers.

Any other disease afflicting 1 in 10 individuals of a select society would be considered an epidemic, a disaster of great proportion. Sadly, health care professionals, who seek to restore health and prolong life, are often among the last to receive assistance. Only through support, education, and research can one begin to comprehend the scope of this disease and its impact on the professional.

Chemical dependency has existed for centuries, perhaps even since the beginning of humankind. Knowledge of the attempt of human beings to pharmacologically manipulate their perception of the world dates back to ancient history. Wine, henbane, mandragora, opium, cocaine, and countless other mood-altering substances brought comfort and escape during the Roman Empire and probably to every other major civilization through recorded history.

In early America, abuse of medicinal substances was commonplace. Dr. Crawford Long and his contemporaries of the mid-1800s frequently held ether sniffing parties in Atlanta and Philadelphia. Other physicians of the 19th and early 20th century had a similar history of abuse. Many used themselves as subjects in an attempt to discover the therapeutic potential of certain substances. Simpson and Halstead are among the more notable physicians who became addicted during their attempts to gain first-hand knowledge about the properties of anesthetic agents.[1] Sigmund Freud used cocaine extensively and even recommended it for the treatment of morphine and alcohol dependence.[2]

Medical professionals were not the only ones to innocently succumb. The Civil War played a major role in contributing to the morphine addiction of thousands of soldiers. Early patent medicines contained opium or morphine salts so that even "nice little old ladies," like those who took Lydia Pinkham's Compound for Women, were exposed to addictive substances. Coca-Cola, as it was dispensed at soda fountains at the turn of the century, contained addicting amounts of cocaine. It was eventually reformulated under federal law.

Historically, attempts have been made to address the issue of addiction among health care providers. In 1910, a report by Flexner[3] prompted state medical associations and legislatures to regulate medical practice and to pass laws that required physicians to be free of "vice, moral turpitude, and the intemperate use of alcohol and drugs." By 1920, England passed the Dangerous Drugs Control Act that sought to register addicts. That attempt revealed that nearly 25 percent of those listed were doctors, dentists, nurses, or veterinary surgeons.[4]

Despite this early knowledge of the addictive behavior of certain health care professionals, it is rare to find literature citations concerning addiction among nurses before 1975. The Program Committee of the American Association of Nurse Anesthetists (AANA) in 1962 asked their executive director, and a prominent anesthesiologist, to prepare a paper on the professional hazards of narcotics to anesthetists. Although their search of the literature was exhaustive and yielded many revelations that still hold true, one major exception of that time was the belief that addiction was caused by an underlying emotional disturbance.[5]

The author wishes to acknowledge her indebtedness to those who have served as role models during her career, as well as to those who have assisted in the preparation of this chapter.

Sincere gratitude to Dr. Joachim Gravenstein, who raised the consciousness of all anesthesia providers about chemical dependency, who nurtured nurse anesthesia even at professional risk, and who believed in the Serenity Prayer.

Deep admiration for LTC Clement Markarian, CRNA, ANC ret., who became a mentor, collaborator, and friend, without whose encouragement little would have been accomplished. Appreciation to Scott Sheppard, whose ability to teach computer skills and lend technical support made the project manageable; and to the Nemours Children's Clinic, which lent the secretarial assistance of Mrs. Angela Bradley, and funded multiple searches of the literature.

Lasting respect for all recovering nurse anesthetists, and to those who live as examples that treatment works; and to the American Association of Nurse Anesthetists (AANA) for continued support to the concept of peer assistance.

Thankfulness for the examples of family and colleagues; especially for Bill and Kristen Quinlan; Wanda Marquardt, CRNA; Maggie Olsen, CRNA; and the pediatric anesthesiology staff of Nemours Children's Clinic.

A more contemporary "disease concept" of predisposition to addiction being biogenetically transmitted has been proposed. Numerous reports have confirmed that less than 5 percent of impaired health professionals had any psychiatric problems that contributed to their disease.[6]

Sullivan and associates[7] mention multiple studies that suggest dual impairment, psychopathology and addiction, may exist in some cases. The depressant effects of alcohol, for example, may manifest in anxiety and depression. Other emotional, social, and family problems may develop as addiction progresses, masking the primary disease. For this reason, it is essential to diagnose and treat chemical dependency *before* other psychologic problems are investigated. Treatment will likely be ineffective for other disorders if the individual is still actively using drugs.

Bissell estimated in 1978 that there were more than 40,000 alcoholic nurses in the United States.[8] Beck and Buckley[9] stated in their 1983 *Newsweek* expose that nearly 4 percent of doctors and nurses were narcotic dependent.

Despite well-intentioned attempts to determine estimates, there were no reliable data relative to the incidence of alcoholism and drug addiction within the nursing profession. One reason for this lack of information was inherent in the nature of the disorder. Since self-delusion and denial are primary characteristics of addiction, most nurses were not aware of their own plight.[10] Additionally, co-workers forged what Talbott[6] coined a "conspiracy of silence." Even when a colleague was a suspected abuser, their peers perpetuated the "conspiracy" by covering up the abusing nurses' poor work performance. A fear that confrontation attempts would result in loss of licensure, and thus loss of livelihood for their colleagues, was weighed heavily by those who would have liked to help.[11]

One index of the increasing number of chemically dependent nurses has been the rise in addiction-related disciplinary actions taken by state boards of nursing. In a survey reported in 1981, 35 of 37 participating boards commented that drug addiction was significant and increasing seriously.[12] During the same period the National Council of State Boards of Nursing determined that for a 1-year period, 67 percent of 971 actions against licenses were for chemical dependency.[11] Today that figure is reportedly in the 90th percentile.

Older statistics were likely to be misleading since most hospitals, wary of bad publicity, were reluctant to report abuse. Most hospitals fired the offending nurses, leaving them untreated and free to seek employment elsewhere. Since the initiation of the National Practitioner Data Bank (NPDB), most credentialing bodies, currently mandated to report chemically dependent physicians, are similarly reporting nurses to their licensing body.

INCIDENCE OF SUBSTANCE ABUSE

Despite the lack of confirmative data specific to nurses and physicians, well-documented trends in the general population put the problem of chemical dependency into perspective. The U.S. Department of Health and Human Services in June 1980 published a report of a national survey that examined the nonmedical use of drugs among more than 7000 Americans 12 years of age and older. Between 1972 and 1979, frequency of experience with marijuana and cocaine had doubled among those older than 25 years of age. The percentage of people between the ages of 18 and 25 reporting experience with cocaine had tripled, and experience with marijuana had increased from 48 to 68 percent.[13] These results are particularly alarming since this represents the generation of the largest sector of health care workers.[14]

Gravenstein[13] conducted a survey of 15 southeastern academic anesthesia departments for the period between 1974 and 1979. The survey asked chairpersons to recall information on the incidence of, and the outcome from, drug abuse by their personnel. It also asked all anesthesia personnel and a control group of medical students to respond to certain statements assessing attitudes toward drugs. The results of the reports indicated a 1 to 2 percent abuse rate (abuse significant enough to come to the chairperson's attention). Of that group of 44 identified abusers, 7 succumbed to their disease—a high mortality rate for any disease.

A study of all U.S. anesthesia training programs by Ward and Saidman[15] found that 30 of 235 confirmed anesthesia personnel abusers died of their disease. Three were not even suspected abusers until their deaths. This retrospective survey included the 10-year period ending in 1980. Questionnaires were distributed to 289 resident and nurse anesthetist training programs with an 85.5 percent response rate. Of the 247 respondents, 168 (68 percent) indicated at least one incident of suspected abuse; of those suspected respondents, approximately 80 percent were confirmed.

Initial suspicion of abuse was raised by a staff anesthesiologist in 47 percent, and by a staff CRNA in 31 percent of cases. The three most prevalent instances that prompted suspicion were behavioral changes, inappropriate drug requests, and mood swings. Suspected abusers were more likely to be residents and student nurse anesthetists.

A 1983 analysis of the Medical Association of Georgia's Impaired Physicians Program (MAG-IPP) placed alcoholism and drug addiction at 10 to 14 percent with anesthesiologists included among the group with the highest rates of incidence by specialty. Of the first 507 physicians treated by this program, 9.6 percent were anesthesiologists who were chemically dependent.[16] A more recent review of MAG-IPP data shows that anesthesiologists are still overrepresented as a physician specialty in the program. Of the more than 1200 physicians seen, 11.9 percent were anesthesiologists, yet they only represent 4 percent of all U.S. physicians.[17]

Of the anesthesia providers initially mentioned in the MAG-IPP in 1983, 49 were anesthesiologists and 21 were nurse anesthetists. It has often been stated that the rise in the rate of narcotic addiction among nurses clearly paralleled that among medical doctors.[18] Garb[19] suggests that the equivalent of three medical school classes and 10 nursing school classes are lost to narcotic addiction each year. A review of five state Impaired Physician Programs in the early 1980s revealed 79 to 87 percent of cases were for substance abuse as compared to physical or psychologic impairments. There was a similar correlation for nurses when comparing the reasons for disciplinary action by state boards of nursing. By the 1990s that figure jumped to over 95 percent of actions being drug related.

There is no general consensus regarding the incidence of chemical dependency among health care providers. Some authors suggest an addiction rate 30 to 100 times that of the general population.[20] A former director of the Haight-Ashbury Clinic of San Francisco believes that prescription drug dependence is two to three times higher among health care professionals than among those in other occupations.[21] Yet others feel that estimates of lifetime occupational prevalence is only slightly higher than that of the general population. One significant difference is that the history of alcoholism in professionals includes other drugs, or "dual addiction," presumably a result of increased drug availability.[1] Easy access of drugs is but one of the factors that put health professionals at risk.

THEORETIC MODELS OF ADDICTION

Factors that put individuals at risk for chemical dependency may be postulated by several theoretic models that help one understand addictive behavior.[22]

Genetic/Biologic

This theory suggests a physiologic predisposition caused by multiple factors, which influence metabolism of substances. This genetic link is supported by several studies of the general population. One survey of chemically dependent nurse anesthetists found that 71 percent reported a relative, usually a father, who was also chemically dependent.[23]

Studies of twins adopted during infancy have demonstrated that children born of alcoholic parents are four times more likely to become alcoholics regardless of the environment in which they are raised. The incidence of substance abuse is similarly much greater in children of addicts. Racial differences may also account for other biogenetic causes. One such example is acetaldehyde, a breakdown product of alcohol, which is poorly metabolized by Asians and Native Americans.[24]

Disease

Chemical dependency is now widely accepted as a primary disease. Studies have linked neurotransmitter deficiencies to a variety of addicting substances and even deviant behavior. One such study conducted on rapists in one southern prison system found the same neurotransmitter substance deficient in the entire group. Many are thus concluding that, like Parkinson's disease, a biochemical deficiency in the brain may be a real culprit in chemical addiction.

Psychologic

This theory views addiction as a function of personality disorders or traits. One such example would be the correlation between the excitement-seeking tendencies and addictive behavior seen in certain health care workers.[25] Studies have drawn a parallel between these personalities and vocational choices like working in the emergency room (ER), intensive care unit (ICU), and anesthesia. Other traits common to substance abuse include extraversion, impulsiveness, and nonconformity.[26] Substance abuse is often seen concurrently with other psychologic manifestations. Mullan[27] found that 32 percent of alcoholics were also neurotic. Abuse may mask or precipitate an underlying, preexisting disorder.

Familial

The social pathology of family dynamics may have a strong impact on addictive tendencies. Family illness or dysfunction may be prevalent for generations and have long-lasting effects on primary family members. Issues like codependency, sexual addiction, incest, and child abuse have detrimental effects on the entire family unit. They may elicit latent responses decades after the incident or offending behavior is discontinued.

The disease model is now the most widely accepted rational model for chemical dependency among medical professionals. When linked with certain genetic predispositions, or familial dysfunctions,the risk of becoming addicted escalates dramatically. Studies conducted at several facilities that predominantly treat health care professionals have revealed that less than 5 percent have any underlying psychologic disorder.[6]

RISK FACTORS IN ADDICTION

Multiple risk factors for addictive behavior have been identified for the anesthesia provider. Talbott commented on certain similarities among anesthesiologists and nurse anesthetists treated in the MAG-IPP that he labeled as "anesthesiology trigger mechanisms."[16]

Primary mechanisms of addiction related to anesthesiology include ease of drug availability, prior experimentation with mood-altering drugs, job-related stress of a highly specialized vocation, respect not equivalent to responsibility, and intimate knowledge of the "powers" of drugs.

More specific stress-related risk factors include life and death decision making, long working hours, and altered sleep patterns associated with on-call responsibilities. Depression may also manifest itself in the professional due to fatigue, stress, death of a patient, and the juggling of family and social life with a demanding career.[28]

Similar risk factors exist for the nurse anesthesia student, the most predominant being stress. Students have high expectations of their own performance in both the classroom and the clinical arena. Perception of poor performance, be it accurate or not, may put them at risk because of decreased self-esteem.[29] Other factors for students may be related to increasing financial problems, decreasing time for self and family, lack of coping skills, and depression from being overwhelmed by the associated demands.

Attitudes about alcohol, which is highly acceptable in our society and almost mandatory in certain social situations, bring added pressure. Another factor continues to be the lack of education in the health professions regarding substance abuse. Such education should be offered to all health personnel and integrated into new staff orientation.[30]

BEHAVIORS ASSOCIATED WITH CHEMICAL DEPENDENCY[2,31]

Anesthesia personnel may exhibit a wide variety of behavioral symptoms associated with chemical dependency. They include isolation and withdrawal from peers, increasing or unexplained tardiness or absenteeism, unwillingness or inability to communicate feelings, increasing mood lability with frequent, unexplained anger, overreaction to criticism, and frequent illness or physical complaints.

The profile of a chemically dependent anesthetist may include a myriad of symptoms or behaviors. Suspicion of chemical dependency should not be presumed by a single sign or symptom, but rather by increasing changes in behavior. Because the career is so sacred to the health care professional, evidence of the disease on the job usually indicates a late stage.

Other behaviors include dishonesty, often over trivial or unimportant matters; increasing difficulty with peers, supervisors, and authority; frequent home crises, family illnesses, and situational problems; gradual and subtle deterioration of routine work performance; and inappropriate dress and hygiene. In addition, the following may manifest as predictive behaviors.

1. Disappears and disappoints patients and peers during work
2. Evidence of alcohol or drug use, odor of alcohol on breath, heavy perfume or mouthwash
3. Exhibits tremors or "Monday morning shakes"
4. Waits until alone to open narcotics cabinet
5. Wears long sleeves all the time
6. Consistently signs out more narcotics than do peers
7. Is forgetful and unpredictable
8. Requires frequent bathroom breaks
9. Makes preoperative rounds or visits at unusual hours
10. Comes to work during scheduled time off and loiters around departmental drug supply
11. Is intoxicated at social functions
12. Chooses inappropriate type or amount of drug
13. Uses infrequently used drugs or narcoleptic drugs on simple cases

Denial and Addiction

There are many misconceptions about the disease of chemical dependency, by both the addict and co-workers. In a profession at risk for substance abuse, it is alarming that colleagues know so little about an occupational hazard that will likely affect them at some time in their career, either directly or indirectly. A study conducted for the Alabama Association of Nurse Anesthetists in 1985 revealed both a negative bias on the part of nurse anesthetists who had worked with impaired anesthetists as well as poor performance on a knowledge test about the disease. The anesthetists who were most knowledgeable were recent graduates and those within the 30 to 39 age group. Over 60 percent of those responding to the mailed survey had some exposure to a chemically dependent individual, and over 70 percent listed "co-worker" as their relationship to that individual. When respondents were asked if they would be able to recognize chemical dependency in themselves, almost 80 percent answered in the affirmative; yet less than 8 percent had any confidence in their ability to recognize dependency in a colleague. These responses support the frequently cited characteristic of the disease, *denial,* and furthermore emphasize the fact that CRNAs may not know how to handle the problem of chemical dependency alone.[14]

Denial is the most difficult obstacle to overcome for chemically addicted health care workers and their colleagues. The worker often performs adequately while impaired, and some accounts attest that there are those who actually excel at their tasks while under the influence of drugs. Even when job performance deteriorates most managers and colleagues are quick to accept excuses like stress, fatigue, and use of cold remedies. Employers sustain denial even at termination by offering rationales that have nothing to do with addictive behavior. One such account tells of an employer who, on finding a nurse on the bathroom floor with a narcotic syringe in her thigh, dismissed her on the grounds that she was late reporting from lunch.[7]

Despite the fact that alcoholism is designated a primary disease by the American Medical Association (AMA), the health care industry and the public continue to view alcohol and drug use as a personal choice, manageable by willpower.[7] Nurses are expected to maintain a composure in the face of disaster. When able to do this despite other questionable behaviors, the problem of abuse is often ignored.

Medical professionals are trained to perceive medication and its applications as beneficial. Therefore many colleagues may fail to question a workers drug use, and instead, assume they are knowledgeable about its effects and addictive potentials. Even more, professionals are trained to look for the physical symptoms of dependency. By the time these features are evident co-workers have generally supported the impaired colleague's dependency through denial and enabling.

An often forgotten contributor to the denial of addiction is the family. One of the reasons health care professionals are so highly esteemed by our society is the personal sacrifices made by many of them. Coupled with enormous responsibilities, long hours, and a deep commitment to patient care, one wonders why anyone would pursue such a vocation. The family unit understands this sense of commitment from the inside. They are therefore apt to accept changes in personal behavior as job-related without questioning.

ROLES OF COLLEAGUES

Addiction manifests itself in many ways in an individual's life. For the health care professional, the workplace is usually the last area affected because the career is so highly cherished and protected. Co-workers and managers are in an influential position to identify impairment and encourage a colleague to seek help.

Nurse anesthetists are caregivers and naturally want to help people. However, even the best of intentions may lead to the wrong kind of help. Chemically dependent colleagues who fail to provide their share of the work increase stress for their co-workers and managers and may ultimately affect patient safety.

In attempts to rescue, co-workers often pick up the slack created by the increasing inability of the chemically dependent professional to cope. This only covers up the problem and begins a vicious cycle of emotions (Fig. 19–1). Assumption of these responsibilities often leads to frustration and resentment. The co-worker may feel more like a victim, trapped in the role of rescuer. He or she may become overburdened, feel taken advantage of, and become angry. Anger soon turns to guilt as the co-worker remembers the plight of the colleague and assumes

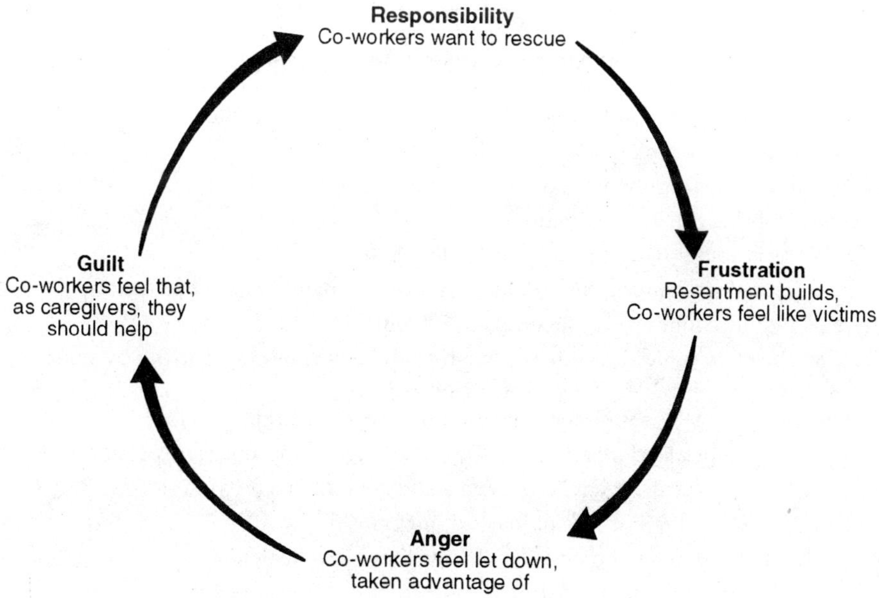

Figure 19–1. Co-workers' cycle of emotions.

responsibilities once again. The cycle continues, rescuing escalates, the problem is covered up, and the chemically dependent health care professional is inadvertently encouraged to continue the behavior.[32]

Enabling an Abuser

Co-workers and managers often enable impaired colleagues to continue bad behavior and poor performance. By making excuses, ignoring problems, covering up mistakes, and accepting incomplete work, co-workers and managers become enablers. The message sent to the chemically dependent health care professional is that his or her behavior is acceptable and a change in performance is not needed.

To be a part of the solution co-workers need to stop enabling and talk clearly about the behaviors seen at work. They need to acknowledge that a problem may exist for the colleague and put the colleague on notice that the co-worker will no longer be responsible for the addicted health professional's share of the workload. In a study of chemically dependent nurse anesthetists, Norris[23] found that 75 percent believed their colleagues knew they were actively abusing while administering anesthesia *and did nothing*. Box 19–1 lists common behaviors of health care providers who enable chemically dependent colleagues.

The Role of the Supervisor

Managers and instructors generally are even further removed from observations of poor performance. They may not be aware of a problem until it is brought to their attention by a colleague. Supervisors may also enable by ignoring poor performance and assigning co-workers to complete the tasks of the impaired; they may also overlook staff complaints of patient pain or inappropriate drug dosage.

To be an effective manager, one must be alert to the signs of chemical dependency: increasing absenteeism, patient complaints, missing drugs, poor record keeping, and changes in behavior. A supervisor must know the policies of the workplace, including personnel policies and legal responsibilities. Becoming familiar with all available resources in and out of the workplace are key and, it is hoped, are undertaken before a problem arises. Employee assistance programs, state nursing associations, diversion programs, and even the medical staff office or risk management department of the facility are excellent resources that may offer information and guidance.

BOX 19–1
COMMON ENABLING BEHAVIORS

1. Accepting chemically dependent person's responsibilities and duties
2. Repressing one's own feelings, reacting defensively
3. Feeling superior, self-righteous about chemically dependent colleague
4. Avoiding, withdrawing from situation
5. Believing one is able to fix chemically dependent behavior
6. Moralizing, judging, blaming chemically dependent person for own bad feelings
7. Denying condition, minimizing severity of problem
8. Protecting the chemically dependent person from consequences of using by lying, covering up, protecting chemically dependent colleague's image
9. Believing the chemically dependent person can control use and behavior
10. Accepting the chemically dependent person's rationalizations, excuses, promises
11. Reasoning with, enduring behavior of chemically dependent co-worker
12. Confronting with generalities, opinions, judgments
13. Expressing vague, general demands for change that provoke denial
14. Failing to follow through on ultimatums

Documenting the Facts of Abuse

Documenting performance and behavior of a suspected employee is essential to objective evaluation of the situation, as well as being crucial to an effective resolution or intervention. When a manager or colleague has strong suspicion, they may want to initially keep a personal journal recording date, time, place, and behavior to document a pattern. When these suspicions appear valid it would be appropriate to begin a thorough record review to lend support and credence to a confrontation and/or ultimate action. Box 19–2 provides an example of data included in this personal employee journal.

Confronting the Abuser

As managers prepare for the eventual confrontation or disciplinary action, they should anticipate that the worker will likely deny any allegations and will be highly caustic and defensive in the process. This is a typical reaction of the substance abusing health care worker who will also be armed with elaborate excuses. It is essential that a caring, supportive tone be communicated while substantiating all of the allegations with appropriate documentation. The goal of the confrontation is to help the individual acknowledge the problem and make plans for treatment.

There may be two different approaches to the resolution of the problem associated with an abusing employee. The first offers progressive discipline beginning with a verbal and then a written warning. It proceeds to a formal meeting and eventually disciplinary action if the performance expectations are not met. This method is standard in mediating most employee-employer problems. This may be appropriate for the student anesthetist not yet assigned to a clinical rotation, or for a CRNA educator or administrator who has no patient contact. However, managers should intervene in a more expeditious manner when dealing with individuals who have direct patient care responsibilities. Indeed, a delay of action may place managers or co-workers at risk for disciplinary action if mandatory reporting is a condition of nursing licensure of the state.

INTERVENTION

An alternate approach to resolving the problem is preferred. This method helps the

BOX 19–2
EXAMPLE OF PERSONAL EMPLOYEE JOURNAL DATA COLLECTION AND DOCUMENTATION OF SUSPICIOUS BEHAVIOR

Record Review

1. Narcotic records noting discrepancies and wastage with stock supply
2. Anesthesia records are legible and complete with appropriate use of drugs
3. Postoperative notes demonstrate pain relief medication given is congruent with clinical picture of patient
4. Employee records demonstrate clear and accurate prior work history, absence of germane disciplinary actions, incident reports, attendance records
5. Record of driving under the influence/driving while intoxicated (DUI/DWI)

Behavior

1. Unusual behavior at work
2. Inappropriate behavior with staff and patients
3. Documented mood changes/poor performance
4. Demonstrated lack of judgment
5. Increasing somatic complaints, declining appearance
6. Significant change in usual work schedule, visits hospital on days off, refuses breaks for lunch
7. Physical symptoms including tremors, diaphoresis, pupillary changes

individual receive appropriate treatment rather than just solve a dilemma for the workplace. It necessitates a full-scale professional intervention. For chemically dependent anesthetists who are clinically active, and therefore have greater availability to their drug of choice, nothing short of well-planned intervention should be attempted. When practicing anesthetists recognize that they have been detected, he or she will feel trapped. Fearing the loss of the most important thing in their lives, their careers, many flee the job; still others attempt suicide. Either way the employer is then too late to be in a position to help the individual. It is imperative that an intervention be well planned and rehearsed, since it is rare to ever be afforded a second opportunity.

When a facility is preparing for an intervention, consultation should be sought from those with expertise in all phases of intervention. The consultant must be knowledgeable about the ethical and legal issues of the locality, hospital facility dynamics, and the roles of all the health professionals who will be essential to the identification and intervention process.[33] Major hospitals and universities often have access to employee assistance programs (EAP). Other facilities may have established networks with regional peer assistance programs or other specialized facilities.

The consultant coordinates the intervention activities by gathering data (establishing probable cause), selecting the team members, determining the leverage to be used, verifying employee benefits and insurance coverage, acting as facilitator during the intervention meeting, closing the process by getting the impaired professional evaluated and/or started in treatment, and notifying appropriate regulatory agencies.

Prior documentation by managers and coworkers becomes the foundation of information needed to establish probable cause. Other supporting data may be asked for and reviewed at this time to provide evidence during the actual confrontation. The chemically dependent nurse is typically not willing to accept the data without dispute or submit easily to evaluation. The two key elements likely to bring about admission of abuse are the impact of the actual team members' testimony and the leverage used to bring about compliance.

The impact team members have is vital to successful intervention. Therefore, team member selection is of great importance. The list should include colleagues who have directly witnessed the suspicious behavior, the immediate supervisor, family members or significant others, EAP counselor or human resources director, others that may be essential to providing support in the treatment period (business partner, financial advisor, clergy, employer), and a recovering addict, preferably another health care professional.

Team members need to be coached on how to stay focused on the dominant theme of caring and wanting the individual to be well again. They need to remain nonjudgmental and offer examples only of behavior they have witnessed that they believe causes the chemically dependent individual to be negatively affected. The coordinator's role is to also disqualify potential team members if they appear to be excessively emotional or vulnerable to the chemically dependent individual.

For most health care professionals, the job or career is highly coveted. Because nurse anesthetists earn more money than most nurses, few would want to return to general nursing. Retaining their position, or at the very least, their license to practice, generally provides significant enticement to comply with the intervention. Using options that would protect the license while the chemically dependent nurse is in treatment would add a great incentive during the intervention. This option varies in each state but is growing in popularity as the success of diversion programs is reported across the nation. Another condition that gives the consultant a great deal of leverage is the promise to retain a position, or reinstate the individual, if he or she submits to medical evaluation and/or treatment.

The actual meeting that brings the team and the chemically dependent nurse together for the intervention has been compared to an inquisition. Those in recovery relate that it is a horrifying, intimidating, vulnerable event that brought about the first day of their new life. The impaired nurse should not be alerted to the intervention but rather told that he or she will meet with his or her supervisor for a conference. The team will have already met an hour before to review what the coordinator has asked each of them to share during the meeting. The "script" also contains the data collected and reminders to remain nonjudgmental and nonthreatening during the process.[33]

The meeting place should be in a comfortable, private, unintimidating area. The consultant states the purpose of the meeting, that those present want to share their concerns about the anesthetist's practice. The participants are introduced to the chemically dependent nurse and each presents his or her data and observations in a supportive, caring tone, above all else, *conveying a message of hope*. Despite being forewarned, the participants will be surprised at the anger, rage, denial, hostility, rationalization, and manipulation that may emanate from the nurse.

Intervention should focus on evaluation (and possibly treatment) of a colleague suspected of abuse. Very few interventions, planned thoroughly with a professional consultant, ever reveal a negative history of substance abuse. The extensive documentation and record review generally reveal enough evidence to provide a high degree of confidence in the decision to intervene.

Advance planning should include an inpatient facility ready to admit the individual immediately on conclusion of the intervention. The impaired nurse should be physically escorted by friends or family directly to the facility to be placed under the care of someone from the treatment center. The chemically dependent nurse who requests time to first run errands, make arrangements, or visit family members may be seeking an opportunity to flee or worse, to end his or her life.

Once the team has succeeded in getting the nurse to admit to the abuse and to submit to evaluation, the goal of intervention has been reached. Since most interventions last from 1 to 2 hours and are emotionally draining, everyone will require time for decompression at its conclusion. The coordinator helps the team explore its feelings and perceptions. Emotions may include anger, guilt, hopelessness, anxiety, fear, and denial. Short-term follow-up may even be required to adequately deal with all the emotional turmoil.

The last step in resolving the situation is the formal notification of appropriate authorities. Ideally the nurse who has opted for treatment will have immunity from prosecution and no negative action on their license while in recovery. This nonpunitive approach is the essence of the diversion programs. Unfortunately this varies with each state. The nurse who has refused this alternative and those licensed by a state without a diversion program face formal hearings through the state licensing body, and possibly criminal charges if narcotics were involved. Nurses have been escorted from the workplace in handcuffs and jailed for drug violations. This need not happen.

With the recent national shortage of nurses, the profession is beginning to value the individual worker and the cost-effectiveness of recognizing chemical dependency early enough to treat and retain the professional nurse. It is only with the last decade that nursing is "finally becoming an army that does not shoot its wounded" (author unknown).

Currently, in over 40 states, a laborer belonging to a union has a better chance of being offered treatment and job security than the professional nurse. Each state in this country has a functioning committee for the impaired physician either through the state medical association or the regulatory agency. Yet fewer than 10 states have any formal programs that afford the same rights to professional nurses.

The federal government is taking an active role in addressing the issue of substance abuse. One legislative act established a national clearinghouse for the reporting of adverse actions against licenses or credentials. This NPDB, which formally opened in 1991, targets licensed health care professionals. The second activity focused on the student and resident population and called for the creation of programs within formal training facilities.

REGULATION AND DISCIPLINE

In 1991, the U.S. government mandated that any training program which in any way benefits from federal funds must have a *Drug and Alcohol Program*. Requirements of these federal provisions are outlined in Box 19–3. Anesthesia co-workers and managers

BOX 19–3
REQUIRED COMPONENTS OF A DRUG AND ALCOHOL PROGRAM

1 Outline the school drug policy and philosophy

2 State the purpose of the drug and alcohol program
- a. Provide information
- b. Provide standards of conduct
    1. Cite state law (nurse practice act)
    2. Cite institutional standards
    3. Cite AANA standards of conduct and practice
- c. Offer mechanisms of peer support
- d. Suggest treatment modalities
    1. Employee assistance programs
    2. Diversion programs for nurses
    3. Treatment facilities for health professionals

3 Provide educational opportunities on addiction through
- a. School curriculum
- b. In-service to faculty, employees
- c. Availability of other workshops

4 Investigate legal and institutional sanctions for screening
- a. Screen students prior to admission with consent
- b. Draft program policy that permits testing of students or faculty on request and for just cause. (A signed form that grants prior consent and release of test results should be witnessed and cite dates that would be inclusive of the expected length of training.)
- c. State institutional policy on accountability

5 State methods for intervention referral to treatment
- a. Private consulting center
- b. AANA Hotline to Peer Assistance Advisors
- c. State diversion or impaired nurse program
- d. Private physician referral

6 State method for evaluation of the program

7 Include a statement requiring self-reporting by the student or faculty in accordance with the Drug-Free Workplace Act.
- a. Report of a conviction must be made by the student or faculty to their department head within 5 days of the conviction
- b. The department head must notify the funding agency within 10 days of this notice

should be instrumental in the recognition of substance abuse in the workplace and deeply concerned about the treatment and retention of their colleagues in the profession.

Disciplinary actions taken by state boards of nursing for abuse of drugs or alcohol range from 67 percent to as high as 90 percent.[34] These boards have varying philosophies regarding their role as it relates to the impaired nurse. Despite the ANA Resolution of 1982, which advocates offering treatment *antecedent* to disciplinary action, many boards continued to take a caustic approach to addiction. A study conducted by the boards of nursing in 1986 confirmed that the majority believed their primary obligation was to the public and therefore took a very punitive posture toward the addicted nurse. Few state boards expressed any interest in developing programs for impaired nurses or believed they had little latitude for alternatives to discipline.[35] To date less than 10 states have any formal legislation or programs that permit treatment without an adverse judgment upon the license.

In 1985, the National Nurses Society on Addiction (NNSA) offered a legislative model that would allow the establishment of a diversion program.[36] This process fulfills the intent of the ANA Resolution adopted in 1982 in that it provides an avenue for treatment before any disciplinary action. Nurses diverted into these rehabilitation programs agree to enter treatment and may return to the work force without the loss of licensure, provided they continue to comply with prescribed conditions. The phase immediately posttreatment, referred to as *aftercare,* is a continuation of the recovery process. Compliance to the conditions of a formal, written aftercare agreement enables the chemically dependent nurse to return to the workforce. States that have enacted diversion legislation report much success in retaining, treating, and returning nurses to productive careers.

In 1990, the ANA published a monograph on "Suggested State Legislation: Nursing Disciplinary Diversion Act" that included a rehabilitation model with an immunity provision that is helpful in negotiating agreements for reentry into practice.[37]

One of the more relevant examples of disciplinary actions occurred in the state of Maryland. Because they were without an established committee to advocate for the impaired nurse, the Board of Examiners of Nurses issued a charge letter that offered the nurse an opportunity to negotiate a settlement prior to a full evidentiary hearing. (Licenses were suspended or revoked but with a stay of action that placed the individual on probation.) As long as the nurse complied with the terms of probation (treatment and aftercare) the stay protected the license. Nurses actually returned to work with the stay in place under close monitoring. It was the board's view that this nonpunitive approach served both the public and the professional.[38]

TREATMENT FOR ADDICTION

Chemical dependency is a treatable disease. Those who suffer from it, and their families, should be entitled to the same care as those who suffer from any other disease. Treatment should be found in the mainstream of the American health care system with a full range of services. Unfortunately, the health care provider is just beginning to be afforded the same treatment as any other patient.

Treatment of an addictive disease is different from any other disease for multiple reasons.[1] The major symptom is denial; guilt and shame inhibit the individual from asking for help. In addition, the disease cannot be eradicated with traditional medical therapies; few laboratory tests can predict the progress of treatment. Success in treatment requires the complete commitment of the patient.

TREATMENT PROGRAMS

The predominant format for facilities in the treatment of chemical dependence is abstinence-oriented, with the introduction of a 12-step program. Box 19–4 outlines the elements of modern inpatient programs. The approach outline in that table is holistic in nature as it attempts to address the physical, emotional, and spiritual needs, and wounds, of the addict. Anesthesia providers seem best served in programs that are geared specifically to health professionals. These innovative treatment programs use other recovering health care professionals in the process. "Mirror image therapy," a concept pioneered by Dr. Talbott of MAG-IPP, helps the newest arrivals to treatment see the progress made by other addicts with the same professional background. Goals become tangible when seen through the eyes of a professional colleague who has had a similar experience.

The cost of this type of treatment is currently \$20,000 to \$30,000. It usually includes one 28-day inpatient course and 2 years of follow-up (aftercare). Most major health plans are accepted by treatment facilities. Once health insurance pays this expense, it is considered a one-time coverage. Treatment for relapse, lost wages, and random screening tests are generally not compensated by any health insurance plan.[39]

Because treatment is so costly, yet vital to survival, it is imperative that managers and employers permit a leave of absence during this time. In most cases, this ensures continued health insurance coverage. Employers who react by terminating the chemically dependent nurse create a situation in which the nurse may perceive his or her only options as fleeing to another job or suicide.

Disability coverage is often difficult to obtain, or maintain, after treatment. Apparently malpractice insurance has not been

BOX 19–4
COMMON ELEMENTS OF A DRUG TREATMENT PROGRAM

1 Detoxification from alcohol and drugs
2 Monitored abstinence from mood-altering agents
3 Treatment of current medical ailments
4 Positive health habits in diet, exercise, sleep
5 Participation in supervised group and community therapy
6 Diagnostic evaluation and self-revelation
7 Evaluation and intervention within the family
8 Mediation with the employer and authorities
9 Introduction of Alcoholics Anonymous or Narcotics Anonymous (AA or NA)
10 Short-term limited objective counseling
11 Instruction in short-term recovery skills
12 Discharge planning and continued aftercare

Source: Talbott Recovery System, Atlanta, GA, 1987. Used with permission.

affected by the diagnosis of addiction, since there has been no public record of patient injury directly resulting from the drug use of an anesthesia provider.[39]

REENTRY TO CLINICAL PRACTICE

The American Society of Anesthesiologists (ASA) has addressed the issue of whether successful reentry is possible in the field of anesthesiology. Citing a 60 to 80 percent recovery rate for physicians, and having no specific data for anesthesiologists, many wonder if returning to the work environment is in the addict's or the patient's best interest. A survey of residency program directors by Menk revealed a success rate of only 34 percent for anesthesiology residents who were narcotic addicts compared to 70 percent for those with nonnarcotic addictions.[39]

Gray, a certified addictionologist and an anesthesiologist at the University of Texas at San Antonio, attributes the fact that all of the anesthesiologists he has treated have successfully returned to work to strong institutional policies and rigid aftercare contracts. The follow-up care includes the usual regimen of abstinence from mood-altering substances, regular Alcoholics Anonymous (AA)/Narcotics Anonymous (NA) meetings, and random drug screens. It also includes naltrexone therapy for opioid abusers and a sample collection protocol that is strictly adhered to. Additionally, recovering anesthesiologists must pay for their own drug screens, a fee that currently costs about $150 for fentanyl assays.[39] The ASA is also partially funding the development of an inexpensive screening test for fentanyl that should be available sometime in 1993.[39]

In 1985, Adler and colleagues described a narcotics control program in use in anesthesia training. This model supposes that narcotics and other drugs of potential abuse pose an occupational risk to physicians and nurses. They advocated a system that limits access and encourages strict accounting.[40] The ASA is currently conducting a prospective study based at the University of Virginia to track all anesthesia residents who enter treatment for substance abuse. The Peer Assistance Committee of the AANA conducted a retrospective survey of nurse anesthesia programs in 1992 replicating the Ward survey for the decade of the eighties.

Relapse

The relapse rate anecdotally appears to be higher for opioid abuse, with a fatality rate of about 10 to 30 percent for anesthesiology residents, according to Miller of the University of California at San Francisco. He believes that residents who abuse opioids should be counseled into working in another area of specialization.[39] Hornbein of the University of Washington developed a policy where residents and staff anesthesiologists are granted one chance to reenter practice after treatment but are not allowed to return if they relapse. The Medical Society of New Jersey will "not advocate anesthesia residents in recovery to return to their programs, and will give practicing anesthesiologists only one chance at reentry into the specialty."[39]

Aftercare

Returning to the workforce after appropriate treatment is challenging for both the recovering anesthetist and the employer. To make reentry smooth for both parties, a contract is recommended that clearly states the expectations of both. The contract is necessary for the employer and the agency overseeing the recovery process, for example, treatment facility, state diversion program, and impaired nurses committee. Figure 19–2 provides a composite of an *aftercare contract* that demonstrates the range of expectations.[7,41]

In addition to the contract, there also should be mechanisms for ongoing evaluation of work performance. These assessments should be more frequent at first, then weekly, then tapered to monthly. The recovering anesthetist should also contribute to the process by providing written objectives for his or her own progress.

All reporting and assessments should remain confidential; however, colleagues should know that the anesthetist is in recovery. This is beneficial for several reasons. It actually assists the anesthetist to remain compliant when supporting staff are knowledgeable about the disease. It also decreases enabling behaviors of well-meaning col-

Date______________

I, ______________________ recognizing that I suffer from a life-long disease of addiction, desire to return to work during my recovery process, and agree to:

1. Abstain from all mood-altering substances.
2. Grant observed urine/blood sample collections and screening tests on demand.
3. Inform my personal physician, Dr. ______________________ of the conditions of this agreement and request that any potentially addicting medication prescribed for me be with the knowledge of my employer.
4. Obtain initial, then annual, physical examinations with the results released to my employer.
5. Participate in an approved peer assistance program for a period of not less than 2 years following treatment.
6. Attend and become active in self-help group meetings (AA, NA, or impaired health professional support group) at least twice a week and to obtain a sponsor from said groups.
7. *Not* handle or administer any narcotics or potentially addicting substances for a period of 6 months, and then to only administer these drugs under supervision by a designated monitor for a minimum of 3 months.
8. Inform my spouse, sponsor, and/or significant other, ____________________, of the conditions of this agreement.
9. Inform of any relapse, and re-enter treatment.
10. Give permission for the regular reporting of my progress to the state licensing body and facility credentialing body; and further understand that any impairment in my practice *will be reported* to those bodies.

I agree to comply with the terms of this contract for a period of 1 year, at which date, ______________________ the contract will be reviewed.

(The contract is dated and signed by the impaired anesthetist and witnesses.)

Figure 19–2. Aftercare contract. (Data from Sullivan et al[7] and Robbins.[41])

leagues, and explains the unusual need for rigid supervision of narcotic administration.

The reentry to practice can also be facilitated by educating the staff about alcoholism and drug addiction. Initial reentry should be as free of stress and temptation as possible. Therefore, it is highly desirable that the anesthetist be assigned only to duty on the day shift and without night call. Rotating shifts or overtime are best avoided early in recovery as well. Because this may add a burden on other department members, it would be therapeutic to have a session that allowed colleagues an opportunity to express their feelings and concerns.

Narcotic Accountability

Many departments find the need to evaluate the efficacy of their narcotic accountability. The use of a satellite pharmacy within the operating room has met with great success. Another method requires that all unused portions of narcotics be returned for "wasting" in a central drop-box location. The term "drop-box" refers to the fact that deposits cannot be withdrawn from this locked repository except by someone officially designated. This designee, usually a departmental narcotics control officer, should consistently be the same person rather than someone assigned on a changing basis.

It is the officer's responsibility to account for all scheduled substances that were signed out by his or her department. He or she should check for record completeness, trends in usage, and the amount used versus the amount wasted. This supply is then randomly assayed for content. These random assays may raise suspicion of other department members and should be followed up by observations of their behavior and audits of their anesthesia records.

Having a recovering member within the department should encourage employers to make certain that they have written policies governing fitness for duty, health benefit coverage for drug dependency, and effective evaluation mechanisms for overall performance. These adjustments in policies and procedures make a department stronger and better prepared to respond to the occupational hazard of chemical dependency.

LEGAL ASPECTS RELATING TO ADDICTION

The legal issue considered by many to be foremost is the nurse's rights versus patient or public responsibility. Confidentiality of information and records concerning substance abuse is addressed by the Department of Health and Human Services under Part 2 of Section 42 of the Code of Federal Regulations (CFR).[42,43]

When the facility employing the recovering health care provider (patient) is a recipient of federal funds, information obtained during that patient's management may only be disclosed with written consent of the patient. The regulation permits "communication of information within a program" during management of the patients care and between a program and a "qualified service organization," which would include impairment committees or state diversion programs. The intervention process could also be interpreted as patient management and therefore disclosure of this information, except to a treatment program, could be illegal.

Disclosing Information

It is wise to secure a written consent from the recovering addict before disclosing anything related to the substance abuse. A letter of recommendation, for example, should be composed only after up-to-date permission has been obtained. This consent must include "the name of the person making the disclosure, the recipient of the information, the name of the patient, the need for disclosure, the extent of information to be disclosed, and a statement that permission may be revoked at a later date."[42]

It must also include a declaration indicating that its confidentiality is protected by the above federal regulation and that further disclosure without the written approval of the addict is prohibited.

Institutional Liability

Regulations found in Title 45 of the CFR Part 84 concerns the rights of handicapped individuals. Under those regulations, "handicap" applies to "any person who has a physical or mental impairment which substantially limits one or more major life activities" including work or employment. The term "mental impairment" is defined as "any mental or psychological disorder" and includes both alcoholism and drug addiction.

The regulations state that any individual who "can perform the essential functions of the job in question" is considered by law to be "*qualified handicapped.*" Furthermore, the regulations state: "No other qualified handicapped individual shall solely by reason of his handicap be excluded from the participation in, be denied the benefits of, or be subjected to discrimination under any program receiving federal assistance." This is broadly interpreted to include hospitals reimbursed under Part A of Medicare.[42,44]

This law raises the question as to whether a recovering addict may be a "qualified handicapped." That judgment must be made individually based on the facts surrounding the abuse, the job to be performed, and the risks involved for the employer.[43] The history of substance abuse makes the issues difficult. A case could be made for the recovering provider not being trustworthy. Recovering anesthesiologists who have been addicted to opiates are more likely to relapse than are those who have been addicted to alcohol or nonopiates, including cocaine.[42] If the potential employer "can demonstrate that the accommodation would impose an undue hardship on the operation of its program" then they are in compliance by refusing to hire.[44] Nevertheless, 45 CFR Part 84 prohibits discrimination based solely on a history of substance abuse. Legal recourse is available if employment is refused, although none have been used in any legal challenge to date.

Wrongful Determination

Ward addressed the issue of liability for wrongful determination during an ASA panel discussion of the impaired anesthesia provider. Unless a secondary diagnosis, such as a personality disorder, masks the disease or clouds the judgment of the accuser, it is highly unlikely that a defamation case would be supported. If the colleague's and the patient's safety are the paramount reasons for pursuing action, and the intervention has been conducted in a confidential manner, the accused, in Dr. Ward's judgement, would probably not risk publicizing the case by bringing suit. "In either event, liability is much more likely to be due to NOT taking action when a colleague and his patients are in jeopardy because of the disease."[39]

PREVENTION

Talbott, a pioneer in the treatment of addiction among health professionals, feels chemical dependency should be "managed like cancer, with careful attention to host and environmental factors, screening programs, investigation of alternative methods of induction and maintenance of remission, prompt detection and treatment of recurrence, and long-term follow up."[1]

As newer, more highly addicting synthetic drugs become part of the armamentarium of the anesthetist and the demands on the profession increase, it becomes vital that studies be conducted that continue to identify risk factors, causality, and treatment. Education about chemical dependency in the professions should begin in nursing school, continue in nurse anesthesia program curricula, and be mandated as a part of continuing education for the CRNA. Many states now require mandatory biannual courses on hepatitis and acquired immunodeficiency syndrome (AIDS) because they believe the health care worker bears a significant risk. The anesthesia provider, who has a 10 percent higher risk of becoming chemically addicted than their nursing colleagues, should be encouraged to participate with the same educational vigor.

RESOURCE ORGANIZATIONS AND EDUCATIONAL AIDS

Box 19–5 lists a number of resource organizations for chemical dependency problems. Table 19–1 presents some educational aids available from various organizations. The AANA Position Statement on Chemical Dependency is presented in Box 19–6.

BOX 19–5
RESOURCE ORGANIZATIONS

Al-Anon Family Groups
P.O. Box 862 Midtown Station
New York, NY 10018-0862
(212) 302-7240

Alcoholics Anonymous (AA)
475 Riverside Drive
New York, NY 10115
(212) 870-3400

American Association of Nurse Anesthetists (AANA)
Peer Assistance Advisor
222 S. Prospect Ave.
Park Ridge, IL 60068
(708) 692-7050

American Nurses' Association (ANA)
Publications Fulfillment Center
600 Maryland Ave. SW, Suite 100 W
Washington, DC 20024-2571
(202) 554-4444

American Society of Addiction Medicine (ASAM)
5225 Wisconsin Avenue NW, Suite 409
Washington, DC 20015
(202) 244-8948

American Society of Anesthesiologists (ASA)
520 N. Northwest Highway
Park Ridge, IL 60068-2573
(708) 825-5586

Anesthetists in Recovery (AIR)
Randy Ratliff, CRNA
2205 22nd Avenue, South
Minneapolis, MN 55404-3131
(612) 724-8238 (home)
(612) 347-3157 (work)

Association for Medical Education and Research in Substance Abuse, Center for Alcohol and Addiction Studies
Box G-BH, Brown University
Providence, RI 02912
(401) 863-3173

Drug and Alcohol Nursing Association, Inc. (DANA)
113 West Franklin St.
Baltimore, MD 21201
(410) 752-3318

National Council on Alcoholism
12 West 21st Street
New York, NY 10010
(212) 206-6770

National Institute on Drug Abuse
Room 10 A-39
5600 Fishers Lane
Rockville, MD 20857
(301) 443-1124

National Nurses Society on Addictions (NNSA)
Impaired Nurse Committee
5700 Old Orchard Road
Skokie, IL 60077-1024
(708) 966-5010

GLOSSARY

Aftercare: The period of time following formal outpatient or inpatient treatment during which performance, conduct, and compliance with an established plan of recovery from abuse or addiction are closely monitored.

Cage test: A questionnaire that asks four basic questions regarding alcohol consumption. A score of two or more positive responses requires further evaluation.

Have you ever felt that you had to cut down on your drinking?
Have people annoyed you by criticizing your drinking?
Have you ever felt bad or guilty about your drinking?
Have you ever had a drink first thing in the morning to steady your nerves or get rid of a hangover?

DSM-III: *The Diagnostic and Statistical Manual of Mental Disorders*, ed. 3 (Washington, DC, 1980; revised 1987 as DSM-III-R), of the American Psychiatric Association. This manual defines diagnostic criteria for psychoactive substance abuse and psychoactive substance dependence.

TABLE 19–1

EDUCATIONAL AIDS

Organization	*Available Media*
American Society of Anesthesiologists (ASA) 520 N. Northwest Highway Park Ridge, IL 60068-2573 (708) 825–5586	Patient Safety Videotape No. 12—The Impaired Practitioner
Burroughs Wellcome Company (local representatives)	"The Impaired Practitioner" (Videotape No. 12)
Florida Nurses Association P.O. Box 536985 Orlando, FL 32853-6985 Phone (407) 896–3261 Fax (407) 896–9042	"Managing Chemical Dependency and Impairment in the Work Place: A Guide for Nurse Administrators" (manual) "A Guide for Assisting Colleagues Who Demonstrate Impairment in the Workplace" (manual) March 1991
Grandview Hospital and Medical Center (producer), Johnson, E, (director). Dayton, OH, 1986	"Chemical Dependency and Nurses: The Deadly Secret" (video)
Janssen Pharmaceutica Product Director, Anesthesia 1125 Trenton-Harborston Road P.O. Box 200 Titusvill, NJ 08560-0200 (800) 253–3682	"Unmasking Addiction: Chemical Dependency in Anesthesiology" (video)
Johnson Institute (producer) Minneapolis, MN (612) 374–2905	"I'll Quit Tommorrow" "The Intervention" "The Enablers" (video)
Krames Communications 1100 Grundy Lane San Bruno, CA 94066-3030 (415) 742–0400	"Chemical Dependency: Reaching Out to the Impaired Caregiver" (brochure)
National Clearinghouse for Alcohol Information (NCALI) P.O. Box 2345 Rockville, MD 20852 (301) 468–2600	*Alcohol and Drug Abuse Teaching Methodology Guide for Medical Faculty* *Obtaining a Medical Education in Alcohol and Drug Dependence: A Student's Guide*
NIAAA 6500 Fishers Lane Rockville, MD 20857	*A Resource Manual for Alcohol and Other Drug Abuse Education in Family Medicine Medical School and Residency Programs*
National Nurses Society on Addictions (NNSA) 5700 Old Orchard Road Skokie, IL 60077-1024 Phone (708) 966–5010 Fax (708) 966–9418	*Addictions and Psychological Dysfunctions in Nursing: The Profession's Response to the Problem* [NNSA, American Nurses Association (ANA), Drugs and Alcohol Nursing Association (DANA) jointly in 1984] monograph
Public Relations Department Ridgeview Institute (producer), Verdery, VL and O'Sullivan, P (directors)	"Intervention: Rescue from Destruction" (video) "Addiction, R.N." (video)

Diagnostic Criteria for Psychoactive Substance Dependence (DSM-III-R, 1987)

A. At least three of the following:

(1) Substance often taken in larger amounts and over a longer period of time than the person intended [using more than intended]

(2) Persistent desire of one or more unsuccessful efforts to cut down or control substance use [unsuccessful efforts to control use]

(3) A great deal of time spent in activities necessary to get the substance (e.g., theft), taking the substance, or recovering for its effects [excessive time involvement]

(4) Frequent intoxication or withdrawal symptoms when expected to fulfill major obligations at work, school, or home (e.g., does not go to work because hung over, goes to school or work "high," intoxicated while taking care of his or her children), or when substance use is physically hazardous (e.g., drives when intoxicated) [use interferes with responsibilities or safety]

(5) Important social, occupational, or recreational activities given up or re-

BOX 19–6
AMERICAN ASSOCIATION OF NURSE ANESTHETISTS POSITION STATEMENT ON CHEMICAL DEPENDENCY

The American Association of Nurse Anesthetists (AANA) expresses its commitment to the promotion of the profession of nurse anesthesia, to the support of all members of the AANA, and to the practice of competent anesthesia care for all consumers. Chemical dependency poses potential threats to these goals, therefore, the AANA recognizes that education, research and resources are the responsibility of the profession in seeking to resolve the issue of chemical dependency.

"Chemically dependent" is defined as the use or abuse of a substance which the person is unable or unwilling to stop the use of, therefore interfering with safe anesthesia practice and personal relationships with family, profession, health, and self. The AANA supports the concept of helping nurse anesthetists identified as "chemically dependent" to become "chemically independent."

The AANA affirms that nurse anesthetists are legally and ethically accountable to the consumer and the profession for the quality of anesthesia care rendered.

The AANA recognizes that a safe, supportive, and confidential atmosphere is essential to protect the rights of those seeking assistance with chemical dependency.

The AANA has a responsibility to identify and recommend the means of educating anesthesia practitioners to the inherent problems of the chemically dependent, to investigate the availability and effectiveness of treatment modalities, to provide information on the mechanisms of peer support, and to make recommendations for the provision of care by providing names of available, qualified rehabilitation centers.

Adopted by the AANA Board of Directors, November 11, 1984. Source: American Association of Nurse Anesthetists, Park Ridge, IL. Used with permission.

duced because of substance use [lifestyle change due to use]

(6) Continued use despite knowledge of having a persistent or recurrent social, psychologic, or physical problem that is caused or exacerbated by the use of the substance (e.g., keeps using heroin despite family arguments about it, cocaine-induced depression, or having an ulcer made worse by drinking) [uses knowing it causes other problems]
(7) Marked tolerance: need for markedly increasing amounts of the substance (i.e., at least a 50 percent increase) in order to achieve intoxication or desired effect, or markedly diminishing effect with continued use of the same amount
(8) Characteristic withdrawal symptoms [withdrawal symptoms]
(9) Substance often taken to relieve or avoid withdrawal symptoms [medicating withdrawal]

B. Some symptoms of the disturbance have persisted for at least 1 month, or have occurred repeatedly over a longer period of time.

NOTE: A change in diagnostic criteria has been proposed for the upcoming International Classification of Diseases (ICD-10). The new language asks for clear evidence and specific situations to document abuse. Dependence criteria relate to more contemporary terms like compulsion, loss of control, and progressive neglect.

Diagnostic Criteria for Psychoactive Substance Abuse (DSM-III-R)

A. A maladaptive pattern of psychoactive substance use indicated by at least one of the following:
   (1) Continued use despite knowledge of having a persistent or recurrent social, occupational, psychologic, or physical problem that is caused or exacerbated by the use of the psychoactive substance [uses knowing it causes other problems]
   (2) Recurrent use in situations in which use is physically hazardous (e.g., driving while intoxicated) [use interferes with safety]

B. Some symptoms of the disturbance have

persisted for at least 1 month, or have occurred repeatedly over a longer period of time.

Physical dependence: Occurs when a user cannot stop taking the drug without experiencing withdrawal. These symptoms, including tremors, vomiting, delirium, cramps, convulsions, or even death vary according to the specific drug, the amount used, and length of time abused.[2]

Psychologic dependence: May be characterized as an intense craving, compulsion to use, and preoccupation with the taking of drugs. It is more difficult to treat than physical dependence since treatment must be focused on underlying behavior.

Recovery: A lifelong process of abstaining from the drugs or triggers that brought about substance-abusing behavior. For the health professional this begins the moment he or she admits being chemically dependent and continues with compliance to a program designed to maintain a drug-free life.

Substance abuse: May be defined as the consumption of "mood-altering agents in dosages sufficient to result in physical, situational, or emotional harm."[1] "When such behavior continues over time, a biological, physical and behavioral process of addiction will occur in about three out of five individuals, and chemical dependence will develop."[1]

Tolerance: Indicated by the user requiring larger amounts of a substance to achieve a given level of effect.

REFERENCES

1. Talbott, GD and Wright, C: Chemical Dependency in Health Care Professionals. Occupational Medicine: State of the Art Reviews 2:581, 1987.
2. Health Communications: Do You Know the Facts About Drugs? Health Communications, Deerfield Beach, FL, 1983.
3. Flexner, A: Medical Education in the United States and Canada: A Report to the Carnegie Foundation for the Advancement of Teaching. Carnegie Foundation, New York, 1910.
4. Stimson, GV, Oppenheimer, BA, and Stimson, CA: Drug abuse in the medical profession. Br J Addict 79:395, 1984.
5. Lundy, JS and McQuillen, FA: Narcotics and the Anesthetist: Professional Hazards. AANA Journal 30:147, 1962.
6. Talbott, GD: Mirror image therapy. Address at the Annual Meeting of the American Association of Nurse Anesthetists, New Orleans, LA, August 1983.
7. Sullivan, EJ, Bissell, L, and Williams, E: Chemical Dependency in Nursing: The Deadly Diversion. Addison-Wesley, Menlo Park, CA, 1988.
8. Isler, C: The alcoholic nurse: What we try to deny. RN 41:48, 1978.
9. Beck, M and Buckley, J: Nurses with bad habits. Newsweek, August 22, 1983, p. 54.
10. Bissell, L and Jones, R. The alcoholic nurse. Nursing Outlook 29:96, 1981.
11. Green, PL: The impaired nurse: Chemical dependency. Focus on Critical Care 11:42, 1984.
12. Mereness, D: Protect your patients from nurse addicts. Nursing Life 1:71, 1981.
13. Gravenstein, JS, Kory, WP, and Marks, RG: Drug abuse by anesthesia personnel. Anesth Analg 1983;962:467–472.
14. Quinlan, DS: A study of the opinions of Alabama Certified Registered Nurse Anesthetists regarding selected factors related to chemical dependency. University of Alabama at Birmingham, Unpublished thesis, 1985.
15. Ward, CF and Saidman, LJ: Controlled substance abuse: A survey of training programs 1970–1980. Anesthesiology 55:A345, 1981.
16. Farley, WJ and Talbott, GD: Anesthesiology and addiction (editorial). Anesth Analg 62:465, 1983.
17. Gallegos, KV, et al: Addiction in anesthesiologists: Drug access and patterns of substance abuse. Qual Rev Bull, April: 116, 1988.
18. Bissell, L and Haberman, PW: Alcoholism in the Professions. Oxford University Press, New York, 1984.
19. Garb, S: Narcotic addiction in nurses and doctors. Nursing Outlook 13:30, 1965.
20. Jefferson, LV and Ensor, BE: Help for the helper: Confronting a chemically impaired colleague. Am J Nurs 4:574, 1982.
21. Naegle, M: Drug and alcohol abuse in nursing, an occupational hazard? Nursing Life 8:42, 1988.
22. Swain, EA and Stasiak, DB: Chemical dependency and the student nurse anesthetist: A strategy for caring. CRNA: The Clinical Forum for Nurse Anesthetists 1:50, 1990.
23. Norris, J, Pierson, F, and Waugaman, W: Critical factors associated with substance abuse and chemical dependency in nurse anesthetists. Journal of Alcohol and Drug Education, Winter: 6, 1988.
24. Arnold, WP: Disease or not disease, that is the question. ASA Newsletter 53:7, 1989.
25. McDonough, JP: Personality, Addiction, and Anesthesia. AANA Journal 58:193, 1990.
26. Forgays, DG: Personality Characteristics and Self-Abusive Behavior. NIDA Monograph Series, Rockville MD, 1986.
27. Mullan, M, et al: The relationship between alcohol and neurosis. Br J Psychiatry, 48:435–441, 1986.
28. The impaired physician in anesthesiology: An overview. ASA Newsletter 53:4, 1989.
29. Kless, JR: Use of a student support group to reduce student stress in a nurse anesthesia program. AANA Journal 57:75, 1989.
30. Clark, MD: Preventing drug dependency, Part 1, Recognizing risk factors. J Nurs Admin 18:12, 1988.

31. Hyde, GL: Management of the impaired person in the OR. Plastic Surgical Nursing 10:77, 1990.
32. Krames Communications: Chemical Dependency: Reaching Out to the Impaired Caregiver. Krames Communications, San Bruno, CA, 1989.
33. Crosby, LR and Offer, PL: Intervention with chemically dependent nurses: A paradigm for professional retention. Qual Rev Bull 111, 1988.
34. Fowler, MD: Doctoring or nursing under the influence. Heart and Lung 15:205, 1986.
35. Markarian, CJ and Quinlan, DS: A Study of Disciplinary Attitudes of State Boards of Nursing. Unpublished research, 1986.
36. National Nurses Society on Addictions: Statement on Model Diversion Legislation for Chemically Impaired Nurses. NNSA, Evanston, IL, 1985.
37. Nursing Disciplinary Diversion Act. ANA, Kansas City, MO, 1990.
38. Dorsey, DM and Scheer, R: Licensing boards and impaired professionals. M Med J 36:238, 1987.
39. Polk, SL: Substance abuse in anesthesia: Patient safety among issues. Anesthesia Patient Safety Foundation Newsletter 6:1, 1991.
40. Adler, GR, et al: Narcotics control in anesthesia training. JAMA 253(21):3133, 1985.
41. Robbins, CE: A monitored treatment program for impaired health care professionals. J Nurs Admin 17:17, 1987.
42. Arnold, WP: Legal aspects of chemical dependence. ASA Newsletter 55:2, 1991.
43. Department of Health and Human Services: 42 CFR Part 2: Confidentiality of Alcohol and Drug Abuse Patient Records. Federal Register, June 9, 1987, p. 21796.
44. Department of Health, Education and Welfare: 45 CFR Part 84: Nondiscrimination on the Basis of Handicap. Federal Register, May 4, 1977, p. 22676.

20

Departmental Management

Lynne M. Van Wormer

OUTLINE

OBJECTIVES

On completing this chapter, the reader will be able to:

1. Understand the emerging role of the CRNA as a manager.
2. Describe the preparation of the CRNA manager with regard to education, general experience, and accepted employment practices.
3. Discuss management theory.
4. Understand management responsibilities and the range of activities related to such responsibilities.
5. Explore future opportunities for the CRNA in the field of management.

UNDERSTANDING THE EMERGING ROLE OF THE CRNA AS A MANAGER

Anesthesia services are provided within the context of health care institutions or facilities that combine technology with human and financial resources. Within these organizations, nurse anesthetists are increasingly assuming management positions where decisions rendered may have a substantial effect on the overall operation of the organization. When nurse anesthetists assume such leadership positions they must be conversant with the multifaceted aspects of management and the skills required to implement organizational goals. This chapter provides a brief overview of the responsibilities of managing an anesthesia department or a specific section of a larger health care organization relating to the delivery of anesthesia services.

As has been described in previous chapters, professional roles within the discipline of nurse anesthesia are quite diverse. Health care has become vastly more complex as the knowledge and skills of practitioners increase. This situation is coincident to a time when federal, state, and local governments demand increasing compliance with growing numbers of statutes and regulations. Consequently, Certified Registered Nurse Anesthetists (CRNAs) are assuming proportionately larger responsibilities for functions related to departmental management. For example, a few arenas in which the CRNA manager may be involved could potentially include insurance billing, continuous quality improvement, risk management, labor union negotiation, personnel development, and resource acquisition and management. Hospital and other health care facilities are now requiring that CRNAs assume greater participation and responsibility to provide services and expertise in all areas.

The CRNA, as an officially recognized manager, is becoming more common in health care facilities throughout the country. In some instances, these responsibilities within the organizational structure of an anesthesia department carry the title of chief nurse anesthetist, director of anesthesia services, or departmental administrator. In other cases, the CRNA has assumed some or all of the functions of a departmental manager without benefit of formal education or title.

In addition to fulfilling requirements of agencies external to the health facility, CRNAs, as departmental managers, are involved in policy and procedure development, budget preparation, hiring, training, evaluating, long-range planning, advocacy, and quality improvement activities. CRNA managers are chairpersons or participants on numerous facility committees. In some anesthesia departments, the CRNA manager may also be the individual responsible for securing anesthesia equipment and supplies.

As the reader can appreciate, just as the profession of nurse anesthesia is diverse, so too is the responsibility of the anesthesia departmental manager. In 1988, the American Association of Nurse Anesthetists (AANA) board of directors recognized the need to "provide direction in establishing and organizing nurse anesthesia services within a management structure and to assure quality anesthesia service through the provision of professional leadership and management functions by and for Certified Registered Nurse Anesthetists." To that end they issued position statement No. 1.4 (contained in the Professional Practice Manual), which defines a CRNA as the "most appropriate health professional qualified to fulfill the direct management role involving CRNA's functioning within a clinical organizational chart."

This chapter initially discusses the preparation of the CRNA manager and definitions of popular management and organizational theories. Statutes and regulations governing employment practices are also addressed. This is followed by a profile of typical management responsibilities. The chapter concludes with a discussion of management opportunities for CRNAs in the future.

PREPARATION OF THE CRNA MANAGER

General Experience

CRNAs and student nurse anesthetists have often gained cursory leadership experience prior to embarking on a career in nurse anesthesia, typically in critical care nursing roles. Curriculum requirements addressing leadership skills, role modeling, and decision making are all inherent to most generic nursing programs, especially those at the baccalaureate level. The professional registered nurse frequently functions as a team leader, charge nurse, head nurse, supervisor, or director of nursing services. All of the above-mentioned positions require some degree of management skills. At this stage of their careers, nurses routinely perform these duties with little or no additional preparation other than their nursing education courses.

Some nurses may attend organization or facility-sponsored management development seminars. Unfortunately, these facility-specific workshops are frequently limited in their breadth and scope. Other nurses may have had formal credit courses in association with undergraduate or graduate degrees, which is becoming much more commonplace in the population of nurse anesthesia students.

CRNAs working as solo anesthetists or in small group practices may find themselves assuming extensive management responsibilities simply because no one else is doing it. In such situations, three areas of responsibility can usually be identified: scheduling of personnel, ordering of anesthesia equipment and supplies, and maintaining and assessing quality improvement activities. It is not uncommon in a small department for these responsibilities to be divided within the group. "Management by committee" is often the result of such an arrangement. Formal structure is frequently lacking.

The larger and more complex an anesthesia department becomes, the more likely it will need an individual who assumes primary responsibility for management of all or a large portion of its administrative functions. With increasing frequency the individual who assumes such responsibility is a CRNA.

Education

The Council on Accreditation of Nurse Anesthesia Education Programs, in its *Standard and Guidelines for Accreditation of Nurse Anesthesia Educational Programs,* at one time specifically delineated "Departmental Management" as part of its academic requirements.[1] However, in 1990, when the "standards" were revised, broader categories of requirements were listed. Most program directors included the teaching of some aspects of departmental management under the division of "Professional Aspects of Nurse Anesthesia." The total number of contact hours for this broad category is 45 hours. In view of time constraints, and the necessity of discussing other pertinent professional topics, only a superficial treatment of the subject is addressed in most educational programs.

During the late 1980s and early 1990s, as increasing numbers of CRNAs found themselves in management positions, many felt the need for education in this area. They turned to the AANA for guidance and leadership. In response to membership request, the AANA board of directors in 1989 formed a management task force specifically to develop a curriculum and workshop to educate managers with respect to business skills needed to manage an anesthesia department. Focus sessions at both the 1990 and 1991 AANA annual meetings addressed educational needs of managers. These focus groups also served as a catalyst for networking on the part of the managers present at those sessions.

In addition to the focus sessions, management workshops were held at the 1990, 1991, and 1992 AANA annual meetings. In 1991, there were actually two separate offerings at the annual meeting. In addition to the agenda described below, a second session addressing management assessment was held.

It was a direct result of the actions taken in the focus groups at the meetings mentioned above that led to a joint venture by the AANA and a major university school of business. This pilot program was the first of an annual offering of this nature. Additionally, the same university is expected to offer managerial education yearly at the AANA annual meeting.

In 1990, the Council on Public Interest in Anesthesia in cooperation with the AANA and A Plus (AANA subsidiary dealing with liability insurance) worked with the St. Paul Companies to conduct a human factor survey of all AANA members. The survey revealed that CRNA-physician relationships were the single most important source of workplace stress and employment dissatisfaction among CRNAs.

The results of the survey became the emphasis for the management workshop held at the 1991 and 1992 AANA annual meetings. This session addressed identifying factors that impact on anesthetist-physician relationship, with emphasis on dysfunctional relationships. The purpose of this particular workshop was to expose the CRNA manager to different perspectives and approaches used in bringing about resolution to common management problems that require interaction within the facility.[2]

As increasing numbers of CRNAs assume management roles, additional needs for educational offerings will exist. Since government agencies will likely continue to enact new regulations and restraints for health care facilities and practitioners, CRNA managers need guidance in how to comply with new requirements. The AANA must continue to address the needs of this growing number of specialists.

Other options for education in management exist within degree programs of business administration. Many CRNAs have pursued this avenue successfully. However, when all nurse anesthesia educational programs are offered at the graduate level by the end of this decade, an MBA may become a less viable option due to financial and time constraints. Professional seminars, workshops, and other similar educational offerings will serve as the primary methods used to prepare CRNAs as departmental managers.

STATUTES AND ACCEPTED EMPLOYMENT PRACTICES

Many CRNAs and student nurse anesthetists may not be familiar with the laws that affect all aspects of their practice. Irrespective of the size of a department of anesthesia, or the employment relationships that exist, the scope and range of laws affecting the rights and responsibilities of both management and staff are extensive.

Employment-related laws as they pertain to anesthesia practices address such areas as[3]

- Regulation of entry into practice
- Employment practices regarding nondiscriminatory hiring, pay, and other areas.
- Circumstances surrounding firing of employees
- Formation of unions
- Provision of financial assistance in association with job loss or disability
- Job safety standards
- Private pension plans regulations
- Social security administration

In addition to the above areas, since the practice of anesthesia is an integral part of the health care system, all of the statutes and regulations pertaining to health care practices and reimbursements have an impact on the day-to-day management of an anesthesia department. This includes mandates from such entities as the Health Care Financing Agency, the Occupational Safety and Health Administration, the Centers for Disease Control, state licensing boards, and state health departments, to name a few. One must also appreciate that facility-specific bylaws, practice agreements, medical staff decisions, and corporate policies also have an impact on how a department is to be managed.

Although it is not within the scope of this chapter to give an in-depth analysis of the nuances of all the areas enumerated above, the author describes some particular statutes and employment practices to enable the reader to visualize the scope of responsibilities assumed by a departmental manager.

Occupational licensing laws as they pertain to the practice of anesthesia are straightforward. In all states, a requirement for practice as a CRNA dictates that the individual must first be licensed as a nurse. Additional requirements regarding licensure or state certification as an anesthetist vary from state to state. In addition, many facilities require certification/recertification by the AANA Council on Certification/Recertification as a condition of employment. It is frequently the departmental manager who is responsible for making sure that all employee credentials are current. If a CRNA manager's responsibilities include verification of physician staff credentials, then the CRNA must be conversant with physician licensure and certification requirements.

Since drug addiction is an area that involves considerable patient safety issues, a manager of an anesthesia department must be aware of any practice restrictions that may have been placed on the license of any recovering anesthesia practitioner the department employs. It is the responsibility of the manager to enforce any conditions of employment for this category of practitioner.

Many employment relationships can be terminated at any time for any reason. This is known as an "employment at will." However, employment contracts or work agreements can also exist. One of the terms of such agreements usually includes the agreed upon length of time the employment will last. Hunt[3] has outlined federal laws that place restrictions on an employer's right to terminate employees. One such law is the National Labor Relations Act (NLRA). The NLRA places prohibitions on employers from discharging employees due to their activities with regard to unions. Title VII of the 1964 Civil Rights Act deals with discriminations based on race, color, religion, sex, or national origin.

Other federal laws forbidding discharge of employees under certain conditions include the Age Discrimination in Employment Act, Americans with Disabilities Act, Occupational Safety and Health Act, and Judiciary and Judicial Procedure Act. Many states have laws restricting employee termination. A CRNA manager must be sure not to violate any of these statutes when terminating an employee. Above all, facility procedure should be carried out to the letter when dealing with employee termination, and all communications between the parties should be in writing. It should be noted that the extent to which a health care facility must comply with any or all of the provisions of statutes described above usually depends on whether or not it is a publicly or privately supported institution *and* whether or not it receives federal and/or state financial support. The exact terms of compliance, and under what conditions, is a primary role the CRNA manager must assume.

Privacy in the workplace is a right afforded both employers and employees. This right is also limited in some circumstances by government requirements. With respect to the employer, (i.e., departmental manager) potential legal liability may require investigation of an employee's background. Health facilities are required to access the National Practitioners Data Bank with respect to physicians and other health care practitioners with regard to their malpractice liability history. Nurses, CRNAs included, are being phased into this system.

If CRNA managers are the individuals responsible for employee hiring, they may contact an applicant's previous employers or references for information concerning the applicant's work and character history. Although this may be viewed by some as an invasion of privacy, the practice is routine and permitted by law. It is also essential for documentation of the credentialing process. In addition to any responsibility for confidentiality, there also exists a potential issue of legal liability for employing individuals with documented deviant practice patterns. Conversely, when an employer provides information about a former employee, the information must be true and not derogatory.

With increasing frequency, states are investigating the propriety of limiting the number of consecutive hours a resident in training may be on duty. New York state currently has in place such a restriction. CRNA managers may wish to consider the implications such restrictions may have regarding scheduling hours of work for employees.

The Federal Occupational Safety and Health Act (OSHA) requires employees to provide working conditions that are free from recognizable hazards to the workers' safety and health. Recent OSHA requirements address the area of blood-borne pathogens. Although the overall administration of OSHA's requirements is the responsibility of the facility, certain portions of these mandates would be delegated to departmental managers. Identifying job-specific tasks that carry increased risk for employees, delineating necessary protective equipment, educating employees as to safe practice within their work area, and assuring compliance within a particular department are all departmental manager's responsibilities.

Other OSHA standards CRNA managers need to be familiar with include fire protection and equipment maintenance. Hunt[3] lists some of the areas in which states can assume the enforcement of job safety with OSHA's approval. They include workers' rights, standards, inspectors, and appeals.

A working knowledge of disability benefits may or may not be the responsibility of a CRNA departmental manager. In many facilities the implementation of these benefits is overseen by the human resources department. CRNAs who assume this responsibility need to know that two principal programs provide this service. They are Social Security and Workers' Compensation; Hunt[3] provides a comprehensive discussion of this topic.

Equal employment opportunity (EEO) laws are well known and will not be discussed in depth at this time. Suffice it to say that as a manager a CRNA must be cognizant of the federal and state mandates as they apply to employment discrimination with respect to race, color, religion, sex, or national origin and handicapped workers.

With regard to the Fair Labor Standards Act, which addresses such issues as minimum wage and overtime rates above a 40-hour work week, CRNAs are generally considered exempt professionals. These standards may be governed at both the federal and the state level.

Hunt[3] again provides a fairly extensive overview of labor unions. The activities and rights of a union are regulated by federal law. Under the auspices of the Labor Department's Management Services Administration, the requirements of the federal Labor Management Reporting and Disclosure Act are administered. The rights of union members in the workplace are protected by the National Labor Relations Board (NLRB). A violation of these rights by an employer is called an "unfair labor practice(s)."

The CRNA manager, in a facility with union representation, must be cognizant of the fact that any disciplinary or termination procedures in place may be restrained by the collective bargaining contract. During such a procedure, the manager may be dealing with individuals other than the employees, that is, the union representative(s).

If a facility is not unionized but attempts are being made to do so, the CRNA manager should be aware of the fact that this action calls into play sophisticated areas of labor law. For that reason, it would be wise to consult the facility counsel or an attorney conversant in labor law before taking any action. Table 20–1 provides a chronologic listing of federal labor laws. The title and section numbers of the U.S. code containing these laws are also noted.

In addition to all the previously mentioned statutes and regulations, which generally govern employer-employee relationships and employment practices, there are additional regulations CRNA managers must adhere to. The Joint Commission on Accreditation Health Organizations (JCAHO), although a voluntary accrediting agency, has quasigovernmental authority insofar as Medicare and other federally administered reimbursement programs are

TABLE 20–1

FEDERAL LABOR LAWS

1983	Civil Service Act, 5 U.S.C. 2101
1926	Railway Labor Act, 45 U.S.C. 151
1935	Davis-Bacon Act, 40 U.S.C. 276A
1935	National Labor Relations Act, 29 U.S.C. 151 (amended by the Labor Management Relations Act in 1947)
1936	Social Security Act, 42 U.S.C. 301
1938	Fair Labor Standards Act, 29 U.S.C. 201 (amended by the Equal Pay Act in 1963)
1959	Labor Management Reporting and Disclosure Act, 29 U.S.C. 401
1962	Work Hours and Safety Act, 40 U.S.C. 327
1964	Title VII, 1964 Civil Rights Act, 42 U.S.C. 2000e
1965	McNamara-O'Hara Service Contract Act, 41 U.S.C. 351
1967	Age Discrimination in Employment Act, 29 U.S.C. 621
1970	Occupational Safety and Health Act, 29 U.S.C. 651
1972	Vietnam Era Veterans Readjustment Assistance Act, 38 U.S.C. 2011
1973	Vocational Rehabilitation Act (handicapped employment amendment), 29 U.S.C. 793
1974	Employee Retirement Income Security Act, 29 U.S.C. 1001
1982	Job Training Partnership Act, 29 U.S.C. 1501

Reprinted with permission: Appendix D "Federal Labor Laws," from The Law of the Workplace Rights of Employers and Employees, by James W. Hunt. Copyright 1984 by the Bureau of National Affairs, Inc., Washington, DC, 20037.

available only to JCAHO-approved institutions. The manager of an anesthesia department must be familiar with and implement the standards pertaining to anesthesia services that are found in the JCAHO accreditation manual.

State health codes (or business and professions codes) frequently promulgate hospital regulations containing sections applicable to departments of anesthesia both in an inpatient and outpatient setting. These regulations vary from state to state and cover such topics as professional employee credentialing requirements, physical plant specifications, and required supplies and services as they relate to patient safety. The CRNA manager must be aware of the regulations governing the particular department he or she manages.

Environmental statutes as they pertain to anesthesia practices is another area of concern for departmental managers. The National Institute for Occupational Safety and Health (NIOSH) addresses guidelines for health care workers with respect to waste anesthetic gases. Disposal of used anesthesia products such as syringes, circuits, and so on is another area of regulation. Although responsibility for actual disposal of anesthetic waste materials may not be in the purview of the anesthesia department manager, practitioner compliance with initial handling practices and bagging of waste materials is a responsibility of the departmental management. Documents relating to both the issues of blood-borne diseases and waste gas management are available from the AANA.

The statutes and regulations governing anesthesia practice and employer-employee relations are far-reaching. A CRNA manager must have a working knowledge of the intricacies of these laws. Access to proper and current resource materials is mandatory to ensure the lawful operation of an anesthesia department.

Leadership Capabilities

Effective management is dependent on quality leadership skills. A section of Chapter 3 of this text discusses leadership skills as they relate to the CRNA in professional practice. This author will not reiterate that information. To apply these skills in the area of management is a goal of some CRNAs and student nurse anesthetists.

Since health care delivery systems have continued to evolve into increasingly complex businesses, departmental managers are dealing with increasingly complex situations. Decreasing resources, both human and economic, at a time when the health care consumer is requiring more complex procedures and more sophisticated anesthetics may mean that a departmental manager must provide more with less. It is essential that CRNAs who aspire to become departmental managers assess the behavioral characteristics that they themselves possess. Management positions in today's anesthesia departments require all the tangibles considered to be the hallmark of a good leader as well as those elusive "je ne sais quoi" qualities that are also the signature of leadership.

INTRODUCTION TO THEORY

Management Theory

Most experts in discussions of management define it in terms of a process. The literature also defines the characteristics of an effective manager in terms of that individual's leadership traits. Longest[5] defines management as "a process with both interpersonal and technical aspects, through which the objectives of the health services organization are specified and accomplished by utilizing human and physical resources and technology."

Most management theorists in the early to mid-1900s had a "closed system" view of management practice. According to Peters and Waterman,[6] early theorists did not address external factors such as the marketplace, competition, or the environment. About 1960, theorists recognized the impact of external events on internal dynamics. This was the case in corporate America. It was at that time that health care facilities began to be restructured and administered similarly to businesses. However, it would be another 20 years before health services organizations looked outward and moved into the "open system" era of management.

This chapter does not review the evolu-

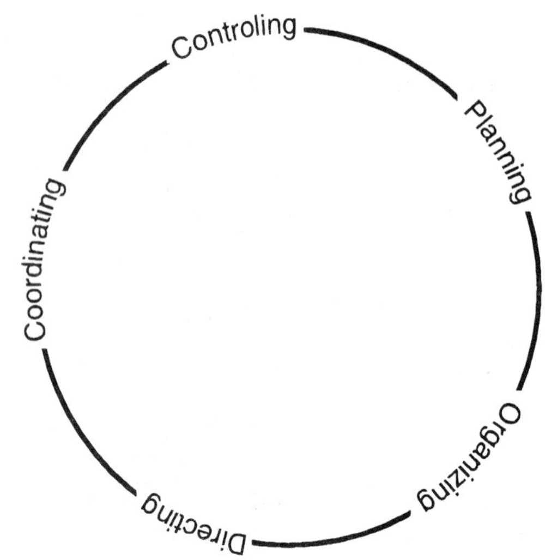

Figure 20–1. The management functions as a continuum. (From Longest, BB, Jr: Management Practices for the Health Professional, ed 4. Appleton & Lange, East Norwalk, CT, 1990, p. 37, with permission.)

tion of management theory, as volumes have been written concerning this subject. This chapter addresses managerial process, skills, and roles as they apply to the CRNA departmental manager.

Figure 20–1 depicts the management functions as a continuum. Note that separation of management functions does not occur either on the continuum or in actual practice. Separation of functions for purposes of discussion leads to the following views: planning deals with formulating objectives; organizing involves allocating resources, human and other, to attain the objectives; coordinating results in achieving harmony out of diversity; and controlling measures achievement. Functions are the means of describing the management process.

The skills needed to be an effective manager are those previously used to describe the characteristics of a leader. The role of the CRNA departmental manager is discussed later in this chapter.

Organizational Theory

The literature explaining organizational theory is as diverse as that addressing both leadership and management theory paradigms. Once again it is best left to those experts to extensively analyze the topic. This discussion briefly examines organizational theory as it applies to health care organizations, more specifically departments of anesthesia.

Concepts important to managers within health services organizations (HSO) are those of effectiveness and efficiency. To date there is no one design model of HSOs that guarantees the attainment of the stated goals. While in their discussion of organizational concepts, Rakich and colleagues[7] divide their approach into two broad categories, classic and modern, and readily indicate that "concepts about organizations are part of an evolutionary process and constant adaptation to organizational dynamics in health services delivery is necessary."

Most HSOs are defined as matrix organizations. They combine favorable aspects of project organizations and functional organizations. An additional concept that applies to HSOs is the fact that they are considered systems. A *system* is defined as a set of interrelated and interdependent parts forming a complex whole.[7] HSOs are further defined as open systems since they interact with their environment. It is the successful interaction with outside entities such as patients, suppliers, and government agencies that is important for the viability of the organization. Advancements in technology lead to increasing complexity of organizations and difficulties in management. This is true for health care systems, in general, and anesthesia departments, in particular. A final concept regarding organizations that CRNA departmental managers must be cognizant of relates to the existence of an informal organization within the department. Informal organizations are those relationships that develop within the facility that are not delineated on the organizational chart. They are usually social as well as work-oriented and may be tapped as a resource to achieve management objectives.

MANAGEMENT RESPONSIBILITIES

Understanding the profile of a leader and manager is the first step in delineating the role of a CRNA departmental manager. A working knowledge of the complexity of today's health care delivery system helps one visualize the range of responsibilities afforded a departmental manager in the context of the present health care delivery system.

This section examines many of the management responsibilities of a CRNA departmental manager. As has been alluded to before, the reader must keep in mind the fact that organizational charts of departments of anesthesia will vary with their size. CRNA managers may find themselves accountable for all or some of the duties delineated herein.

Policy and Procedure Development

Little has been written in management literature regarding the development of policies and procedures, and even less in relationship to the anesthesia department. Policy and procedure statements address such areas as preoperative evaluations, anesthesia records, infection control practices, job descriptions, and operating room attire. Drafts of proposed policies and procedures must be approved by the facility's attorney and board of governors.

Whenever possible, policies should be developed that are broad in scope and act as a guide for the anesthesia practitioner. A generic item should be referenced to facility policies and then address the unique aspects concerning the anesthesia department. For example, the section of the policy manual covering infection control would first refer to the hospital infection control policy. Following that reference, statements would address the decontamination of anesthesia equipment and other aspects of infection control that pertain specifically to the practice of anesthesia.

Budget Preparation

Given the sophistication of today's health care delivery system, financial management within such a facility is a complex process. Berman and associates[8] state that the operating plan of the entire institution must first be developed. This involves defining operating activities and projects expected to implement the corporate strategy. The next step involves interpreting these activities in financial terms. That is the process of budget preparation. Usually executive management sets a limit on the total expense budget. This limit is determined by an estimate of revenues versus decisions concerning maintenance of operating margins and reserve levels. Division managers are given a framework of financial parameters. These managers, in turn, set the level of constraints within which departmental managers must prepare the departmental budget. Frequently, these budgets are itemized very specifically. Each individual area of expenditure and expected revenue is listed. For example, the budget for an anesthesia department would include such items as full-time employee (FTE) positions, expected per diem individuals needed (if applicable), educational expenses, cost of malpractice insurance, equipment, and so forth. Equipment may be handled in the capital budget instead of the departmental budget. The decision concerning this area of expense would depend on such factors as local policies, tradition, and the specified cost of the equipment involved. With respect to revenues, such particulars as income from pain service, reimbursement for obstetric anesthesia services, and monies received for services performed outside of the operating room would all be itemized. Figure 20–2 depicts an overview of budget preparation within a health service organization. Not shown in the schematic is the ongoing process of evaluating the various steps.[9]

Preparing a budget may or may not be the responsibility of the CRNA departmental manager. However, even if the anesthesia department has a fiscal officer, that individual often seeks input from the CRNA manager regarding such budget items as number of staff positions and replacement equipment.

If an institution is large, the CRNA manager may be required to make suggestions concerning other departmental budgets. An example of this would be if the facility had a school of nurse anesthesiology. Some of the operating costs of that program may be supported by departmental funds. In that case, the dollar amount would appear on the anesthesia department's budget as an expense item while it would read out on the educational program's budget as revenue received from the department.

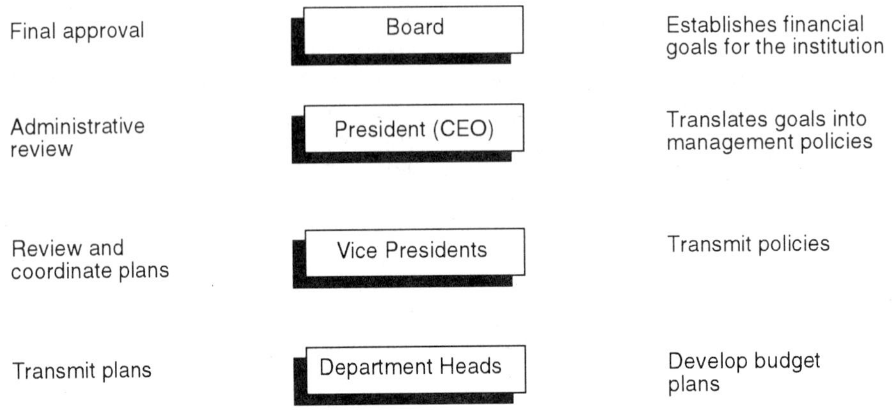

Figure 20–2. Budget preparation. (From Fottler, MD, Hernandez, SR, and Joiner, CL: Strategic Management of Human Resources in Health Services Organizations. John Wiley & Sons, New York, 1988, p. 22, with permission.)

The reader should note that many facilities have instructions regarding the institution-specific technique of budget preparation in the procedure manual. In addition, many institutions provide an administrative or budget packet for use in developing a departmental budget.

An integral part of the budget process is an ongoing review of departmental operations with respect to target projections. Included in this process is the need for justification of expenditures. As health care dollars decrease, this step becomes more important and accountability becomes more critical. At regular intervals throughout the fiscal year, departmental activities must be assessed with respect to their impact on budget projections. This exercise serves to ensure the ongoing evaluation of how a department is operating within its target projections.

Personnel Management

A considerable amount of time and energy are expended by departmental managers in dealing with personnel issues. Included are such responsibilities as hiring, training, motivating, evaluation, retention, and dismissing. CRNA managers may find that they are responsible for only professional staff such as physician and nurse anesthetist employees. However, in some anesthesia departments, the CRNA manager may have a managerial oversight of support staff such as secretaries and anesthesia technicians. Many or all of the previously mentioned activities are done in cooperation with the human resources department of the facility. The human resources (personnel) department establishes organizationwide policies. It is incumbent on the CRNA departmental manager to be familiar with these policies because personnel policies form the basis for interaction between the CRNA manager and staff. In addition, personnel policies interpret legislative and judicial mandates regulating employment.

The first personnel management area of concern to CRNA managers can be classified as staffing activities. Included in this function are activities such as human resources planning, recruitment, selection, and orientation. Human resources planning should be done on a regular basis since organizational and departmental needs change. The opening of an additional operating room or the addition of a liver transplant service may require more staff. On the other hand, if a service is eliminated, the FTE numbers may be less.

Once a decision has been reached to hire additional staff, the CRNA manager may be responsible for the actual recruitment activities, or he or she may be asked for ideas and recommendations to be carried out by the human resources department. An integral part of recruitment and selection is formulation of job descriptions. Included in a job description should be such basic information as education, experience, and necessary skills. For many CRNA staff, job descriptions are tied to clinical privileging, that is, the extent to which a CRNA is able to practice to the fullest extent of his or her training will depend on the specificity of the job description. A useful document for CRNA managers to use in developing some of the above documents is *The Professional Practice Manual for the Certified Registered Nurse Anesthetist* available from the AANA. Included in the manual are scope of practice information and guidelines for granting clinical privileges to CRNAs. Although it is the individual CRNA who petitions the medical staff of a facility for clinical privileges, it is frequently the CRNA manager who acts as a facilitator in this process. Since hiring depends on privileging, it is in the anesthesia department's best interest to provide the documentation needed by the individual seeking employment.

Selection of staff personnel is usually within the purview of the departmental manager. Tools to assist the manager in this task include application forms, letters of reference, and an interview with the applicant. CRNA managers must remember that state and federal laws clearly restrict the kinds of information that may be obtained during an interview. Final selection of an employee is ideally made by the departmental manager with counsel from the human resources department. This approach ensures that both departmental and facility needs are met.

When a new staff member has been selected he or she must be oriented. Some orientation should be carried out by the human resources department. This includes facility orientation and enrollment in facility insurance programs including health, disability, and death benefits; explanation of benefits; and program and personnel services. Orientation to the specific operational activities of the anesthesia department should be done by the CRNA manager. Included in this orientation should be a review of the department policy and procedure manual, scheduling, assignments, equipment, and responsibilities of the employee. Documentation that this process has occurred should be maintained by the manager.

The second personnel management area of concern to CRNA managers is that of retaining employees. This includes such activities as performance appraisal (evaluations), training, discipline, employee assistance and counseling, safety and health, and compensation and benefits administration. Performance appraisal, or evaluation, is carried out on a scheduled basis by all departmental managers. The establishment and maintenance of an organizationwide employee performance appraisal system is the responsibility of the human resources department. Since the roles and responsibilities of the members of the anesthesia department are unique to that area, the CRNA manager will have to modify any document to reflect the activities of the members of the anesthesia department. In addition to the fact that this document is used to determine merit raises, retention, promotions, and dismissals, CRNA managers are reminded that documentation of this activity is required by JCAHO.

Of the various techniques available for employee performance appraisals, the most frequently used is the rating scale method. The advantage of this tool is that it can be individualized to the employee by simply modifying the weights afforded particular sections of the scale. Most managers use a formal performance appraisal for each staff member at least annually. It is useful, however, to give staff informal feedback more frequently than once a year as timely feedback can improve performance and document areas of potential or emerging problems.

Education and training is another area of responsibility of management. CRNA managers have the added responsibility of verifying the acquisition and recording of continuing education credits needed by nurse anesthetists staff to maintain certification and recertification. CRNA managers may wish to offer continuing education units (CEU) credit programs within their own facilities, or they may wish to offer time for CRNAs to attend educational meetings outside the hospital. A CRNA manager assumes the responsibility of assuring that the staff is familiar with the operation of new equipment and products and providing inservice education relative to changes and revisions in facility policies.

When rules are violated, the CRNA manager has the authority and the responsibility to correct the infraction and administer discipline. Protocol for the disciplinary pro-

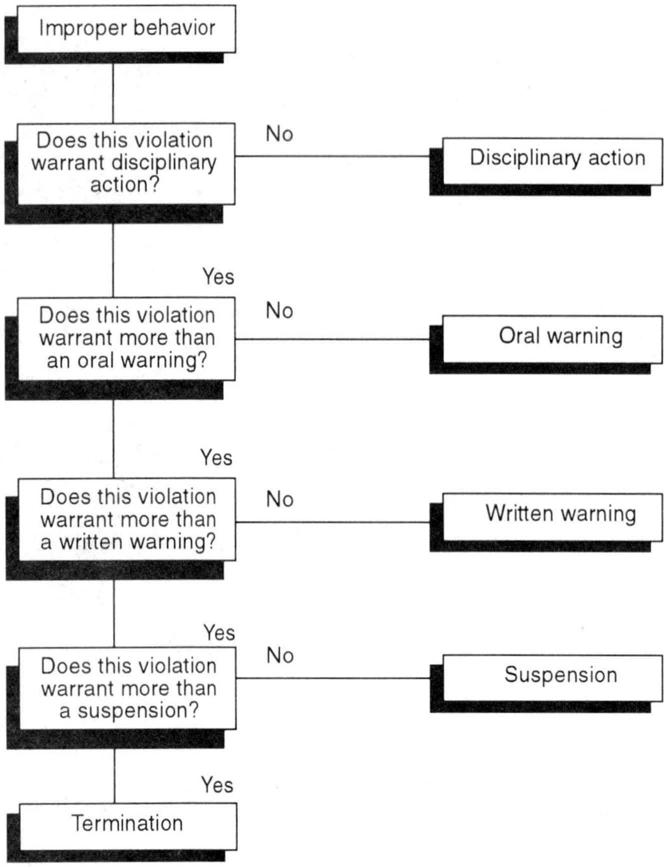

Figure 20–3. The progressive discipline approach. (From Mondy, RW and Noe, RM, III: Personnel: The Management of Human Resources, ed. 3. Allyn & Bacon, Boston, 1987, p. 630, with permission.)

cess should be established and in writing before it is needed. The human resources department and institution counsel should be appraised of a situation requiring disciplinary action. Meticulous documentation of all phases of the disciplinary process must be kept. The type of discipline administered is dependent on the severity of breach and can range from unrecorded oral warning to dismissal. Figure 20–3 illustrates the continuum of disciplinary options.

Another area of personnel activity for the CRNA manager is dealing with employees who are chemically dependent. If confronted with this situation, the CRNA manager must handle the issue without jeopardizing patient safety but also with an aim to assist the impaired practitioner. Chapter 19 addresses the issues of chemical dependency as they apply to anesthesia practice. The reader is referred to that chapter for a more extensive discussion.

Ensuring on-the-job health and safety is an additional area of responsibility for CRNA departmental managers. As stated earlier in this chapter, OSHA is the federal agency that regulates this area of management practice. To reiterate, CRNA managers are responsible for education and training of employees with regard to potential health and safety hazards of their jobs. Additionally, they are responsible for ensuring that employees have and use the protective and safety equipment necessary to decrease hazards inherent in their jobs.

An important area of responsibility of CRNA managers is the administration of compensation and benefits. Although establishment of and administering a compensation system is usually a human resources department activity, the CRNA manager has input into the system. The CRNA manager keeps abreast of market value, recruiting difficulties, and retention problems. Analysis of these areas may lead to adjustment in compensation packages. Factors influencing pay and benefit philosophies include compensation, demographics, organizational resources, and type of facility.

The decision of employee termination, although rare at the professional level, does occur. When faced with this task, CRNA managers need to remember the provisions of restriction found in some federal laws. The facility's policies regarding discipline and termination must be strictly adhered to, and the human resources department and institution's legal counsel should also be consulted during this process.

Problem Solving and Decision Making

Albert Einstein noted, "The significant problems we face cannot be solved at the same level of thinking we were at when we created them." Einstein was a forward-thinking individual, a visionary. So too must a CRNA departmental manager be when it comes to the areas of decision making, problem solving, and long-range planning. Decision making is an integral part of all of the managerial functions discussed earlier in this chapter. Several steps are used to define the process of decision making. They include

- Recognizing the need to make a decision
- Defining the problem
- Evaluating available information
- Examining alternatives
- Choosing the alternative
- Executing the decision
- Evaluating the outcome

Decisions are usually made concerning perceived problems. Problem solving is often either task-related or interpersonal in nature. Task-related problems may be questions such as, which model anesthesia machine is best for the department's needs? Or, does a newly marketed new muscle relaxant offer a better quality alternative at a cost-effective price? Interpersonal relation problems call into play a different set of leadership skills. Diplomacy, tact, listening ability, and facilitation are all assets to be used when working on interpersonal relation problems. This is an exceptionally important area of endeavor for the CRNA manager, as experience shows that most day-to-day problems dealt with as a manager involve a significant measure of personality or value conflicts.

Decision-making tools abound in management practice. A few will be mentioned here. The *decision grid* is a display of possible alternatives with elements that will affect it. This is especially useful for those CRNA managers who are visually oriented. Decision trees are useful in evaluating decisions joined together over time with various possible outcomes. The CRNA manager must recognize that decisions are not made in a vacuum. Advice from others, experience, the external environment, intuition, and a host of other variables affect and aid the decision-making process.

Long-Range Planning

Following the rapid growth of the economy after World War II, corporate America began to realize that 1-year planning projections no longer sufficed to ensure continued organizational productivity. The current climate of rapid change within the health care delivery system of this country makes long-range planning a critical feature in health care management. The shortage of anesthesia providers further exacerbates these problems and demands that CRNA managers plan carefully and systematically for future department needs.

CRNA managers must be aware of organizational goals, forecasts, and long-range plans in order to project departmental needs, direction, and orientation. The concept of strategic planning has evolved from the shortcomings of traditional patterns of long-range planning. Fottler and associates[9] describe strategic planning for the health service industry in terms of four steps: analysis of anticipated results taking into account environmental factors, competitive analyses, portfolio analysis, and diversification analysis. Strategic planning allows managers to evaluate the administrative reality of goals. As resources, both human and material, become more scarce, CRNA managers must be involved in futuristic planning both for departmental and societal needs.

Fostering Interdisciplinary Relationships

Within the health care delivery system, all professionals function via a relationship of interdependency. No one health care provider or group of practitioners manages the care of a patient in isolation. Longest[5] discusses the fact that health services organizations usually demonstrate very high levels of interdependence among their component parts. He further states that in such a situation coordination is a critical managerial task. CRNAs often share patient care responsibilities in concert with other disciplines including surgeons, radiologists, obstetricians, pediatricians, psychiatrists, operating room nurses and technicians, dentists, podiatrists, intensivists, and internists. Additionally, CRNA managers interact with other departmental managers.

As early as the 1930s, the founding members of the National Association of Nurse Anesthetists (NANA, predecessor to the AANA) recognized the need for fostering interdisciplinary relationships. Bankert's[10] history relating Gertrude Fife's recollection of the milieu surrounding the nurse anesthetists' first convention stated that one objective was: "to facilitate efficient cooperation between nurse anesthetists and the medical profession, hospitals and other agencies interested in anesthesiology." Time has not lessened the need to meet that objective.

CRNA managers need to cultivate positive interactions with other disciplines and must view every encounter with other professionals as an educational opportunity. CRNA managers must inform colleagues in other disciplines as to the particulars of CRNA education and scope of practice. As such, CRNA managers must assume an advocacy role for the profession of nurse anesthesia. Membership on a facility's various committees affords the CRNA manager a unique opportunity to foster interdisciplinary relationships. By presenting a positive professional image and participating intelligently in problem solving and planning activities, CRNA managers can lay the groundwork for productive liaisons with colleagues in other disciplines.

THE FUTURE OF MANAGEMENT OPPORTUNITIES FOR THE CRNA

Health care delivery in this country continues to change at an unprecedented rate. Change presents opportunity for growth. This applies to the practice of anesthesia and anesthesia management as well as to other areas of health care. A number of opportunities for the CRNA manager currently exist and will continue to expand.

Continuing Attention to Public Accountability

The profession of nurse anesthesia has been a leader in demonstrating public accountability since its inception. According to Bankert,[10] "to promulgate an educational program to enlighten the general public as to the importance of the proper administration of anesthetics, and to take all proper steps to accomplish, as nearly as possible, complete protection to the public" was a stated goal of the founders of the AANA. Chapter 4 of this text outlines the role of the AANA including ways in which the profession has held itself accountable to the public. CRNA managers' actions and daily decisions are an ongoing demonstration of that accountability. Maintaining high standards of performance for their employees, active involvement in infection control and quality assurance endeavors within the institution, staff development programs, and participation in community education seminars are all part of continuing to be accountable to the public.

The hiring of qualified, credentialed anesthesia staff is a primary responsibility of a manager. However, the CRNA manager may have the responsibility of removing staff from the clinical area who are physically or emotionally unable to perform duties safely, should that unfortunate occasion arise. At a time when work loads may be heavy and staff options limited, decisions may not always be easy, yet responsibility to the patient must remain the first priority.

Managing Challenges with Limited Resources

It has been stated and alluded to previously that health care in this country is in a state of flux. That may be an understatement. At no other time in the history of this nation have we been faced with such complex health care problems. The numbers of uninsured patients are staggering, resources are shrinking, and numbers of surgical procedures are increasing. CRNA managers are being asked to critically evaluate every purchasing decision. The challenge for the future is finding ways to maintain effectiveness (i.e., quality) while improving efficiency (i.e., cost-effectiveness).

CRNA managers have the opportunity to propose creative staffing patterns, initiate research as to cost of one anesthetic technique versus another, and study the effect of cost cutting measures on patient outcome. CRNA managers can be leaders in restructuring surgical scheduling to promote more efficiency in the utilization of material and human resources. When faced with challenges, CRNAs have always risen to the occasion, providing valuable insights into the restructuring of anesthesia care.

Attention to Continuous Quality Improvement

The discipline of risk management and quality assurance has undergone considerable evolution in recent years. The reader is referred to Chapters 16 and 17 of this text for an account of nurse anesthesia involvement in this area of practice. As the evolution continues toward an emphasis on quality improvement, CRNA managers need to take an active role in this exercise.

Information obtained from an excellent quality improvement program can impact on many other areas of practice. Data can give credence to a technique or method of anesthetizing a certain patient population. Data can demonstrate the fact that a certain age group or American Society of Anesthesiologists (ASA) classification makes up a large portion of the anesthesia department's patient population. It can substantiate the need for replacing equipment. A wise CRNA manager can use the department's quality improvement program as a tool in the day-to-day decision making and in long-range planning activities of the anesthesia department.

A WORD TO THE WISE

No chapter on management would be complete without a brief exploration of the more pragmatic issues that surround the topic, from the perspective of those who have traveled that road before. Call it helpful hints, pure opinion, or, it is hoped, sage advise, there are many pitfalls to avoid, some of which are discussed below.

1 *Seek further formalized education.* As the CRNA manager soon realizes, the tasks of management are not easy, even though there are those who appear to make it seem so. A manager should receive formal training in personnel management, organizational theory, budget construction and analysis, and conflict resolution, to name but a few areas. This coursework can be obtained informally through inservices of a health care institution or professional organization or through a formalized course of college or university study.

   In addition, the CRNA soon realizes that too many managers/chairpersons/chiefs, and so on serve in those positions not by virtue of their education or ability to manage or lead but because nobody else wants the position or the manager perceives it as an ego-fulfilling opportunity. This axiom goes for physician anesthesiologists as well as CRNAs. Just because someone holds a position of authority in no way guarantees that he or she is prepared or capable of performing competently in a leadership capacity.

2 *Accepting responsibility and authority.* When the CRNA is approached about assuming a managerial role, it should be accepted only after careful consideration of whether he or she will be afforded sufficient authority to implement the responsibilities that have been given. In other words, the manager who attempts to implement change without the authority or external ad-

ministrative support to do so will likely meet with failure. A brief example follows. You are the chief CRNA of a large hospital, and you are responsible for ordering all departmental supplies and equipment. This responsibility should not be accepted unless you have signature authority to purchase equipment, budget authority to determine the cost/benefit ratio of the equipment purchased, and decision-making authority to recommend purchase or negotiation of contract details in procuring equipment.

3 *Make expectations clear.* Within the course of the management role there are many times when misunderstandings of one sort or another occur. This usually results when the parties involved in a certain situation do not make their expectations of one another's performance clear and explicit or when the expectations are unreasonable, impossible, or inadvisable. For instance, if a departmental chief asks you for a massive change in scheduling of CRNA personnel to be completed within 48 hours, it is highly unlikely you will be successful. By accepting unquestionably an unreasonable expectation, you are like to fail in this scenerio due to unrealistic time constraints.

The same adage applies to the supervision of students in the operating room. The most often cited course of conflict between an instructor (authority figure) and student is the lack of discussion prior to the case regarding how it will be handled and what will be done should specific and likely problems arise. These types of conflicts are largely avoidable if proper planning and discussion precede the actual conduct of a case.

4 *Assuming the role of change agent.* One of the most difficult jobs for a manager is to implement change. Employees generally do not like change and often expend great energy to abort it. Nevertheless, change is the one single characteristic that makes organizations dynamic, responsive, and accountable. Change must be understood and managed well. It must be preceeded by careful planning, organization, and discussions with all parties affected, and it must be implemented systematically and fairly so that the project or change will likely succeed.

5 *Establishing personal credibility.* As has been mentioned in this chapter, a successful manager must garner the respect of colleagues. This respect is often achieved because the manager has gained the reputation of having the ability to listen, to be fair, to be accountable, to say "no" when appropriate, to resist efforts of micromanagement (the tendency to delegate responsibility without authority). The manager must also be able to perform capably what he or she asks of others who report to him or her.

A manager must be firm in his or her resolve, resist undue pressure from superordinates or subordinates, and deal effectively with nonmanagement personnel. This is of great importance as managers are often perceived as the "enemy," those who "don't work in the trenches," those who sit in big offices and lose touch with the "real world." Even though these stereotypes are often untrue, too many CRNAs in managerial roles find themselves apologizing to colleagues for their management role, the very one that takes them beyond the realm of staff personnel and provides great opportunities for personal and professional growth. A good manager understands this perspective and seeks to maintain the delicate balance between interpersonal relationships and organizational goals required of a competent leader.

SUMMARY

As health care in general, and specifically anesthesia delivery, has become more complex and as anesthesia departments have evolved into sophisticated organizations, the precedence of CRNA as managers has been established. Those who choose departmental management as their specialty must commit to the same level of professional excellence and involvement found throughout the specialty of nurse anesthesia.

REFERENCES

1. Council on Accreditation of Nurse Anesthesia Educational Programs: Standards and Guidelines for Accreditation of Nurse Anesthesia Educational Programs, Park Ridge, IL, 1990, p. 12.
2. Schedule AANA 1992 Annual Meeting, Denver, CO, Session L—Management Workshop, August 11, 1992.
3. Hunt, JW: The Law of the Workplace—Rights of Employers and Employees. The Bureau of National Affairs, Inc., Washington, DC, 1984.
4. Kouzer, JM and Posner, BZ: The Leadership Challenge: How to Get Extraordinary Things Done in Organizations. Jossey-Bass, San Francisco, 1987.
5. Longest, BB, Jr: Management Practices for the Health Professional, ed 4. Appleton and Lange, East Norwalk, CT, 1990.
6. Peters, TJ and Waterman, RH: In Search of Excellence, Lessons from America's Best-Run Companies. Warner Books, New York, 1982, p. 91.
7. Rakich, JS, Longest, BB, Jr, and Darr, K: Managing Health Services Organizations. WB Saunders, Philadelphia, 1985.
8. Berman, HJ, Weeks, LW, and Kukla, SF: The Financial Management of Hospitals, ed 6. Health Administration Press, Ann Arbor, MI, 1986.
9. Fottler, MD, Hernandez, SR, and Joiner, R: Strategic Management of Human Resources in Health Services Organizations. John Wiley & Sons, New York, 1988.
10. Bankert, M: Watchful Care: A History of America's Nurse Anesthetists. Continuum Publishing Co, New York, 1989.

APPENDIX

AANA Code of Ethics

With Interpretive Statements for the Certified Registered Nurse Anesthetist

American Association of Nurse Anesthetists
222 South Prospect Avenue
Park Ridge, IL 60068-4001
(708) 692-7050

PREAMBLE

The purpose of a Code of Ethics is to acknowledge a professions's acceptance of the responsibility and trust conferred upon it by society and to recognize the obligations inherent in this code. The Code of Ethics encompasses nurse anesthetists who are certified or recertified by the Councils on Certification/Recertification of Nurse Anesthetists and AANA professionals. Certified Registered Nurse Anesthetists (CRNAs) must strive, both on an individual and collective basis, to pursue the highest possible ethical standards.

The principles set forth define the profession's responsibilities and expectations which each member of the American Association of Nurse Anesthetists has a personal obligation to uphold and adhere to, as well as to ensure collegial conformance.

I. Patient Care

A Certified Registered Nurse Anesthetist has the responsibility to preserve human dignity, respect patient rights to self-determination, and support the well-being of the patient under his/her care.

Interpretive Statement:

The CRNA must render quality anesthesia care regardless of the patient's race, color, religion, age, sex, nationality, disability, or his or her social or economic status.

II. Competence

A Certified Registered Nurse Anesthetist demonstrates a high level of competence. Competence is a composite of the individual's professional values, knowledge, judgment, and technological and interpersonal skills.

Interpretive Statement:

CRNAs must assume the responsibility to strive for excellence and maintain that level of knowledge, judgment, technological skill, and professional values prerequisite to delivering high quality health services. CRNAs engage in lifelong professional educational activities and participate in peer review and other continuous quality improvement mechanisms as a basis for assessing quality of care/practice in order to ensure the public's protection. While there are no mechanisms which can fully guarantee competent practice in every instance, each CRNA joins the profession in constantly reviewing and practicing with nationally recognized standards for the public benefit.

III. Professionalism

A Certified Registered Nurse Anesthetist is responsible and accountable for individual professional judgments and actions. The CRNA should actively support the educational process of nurse anesthetists, other health care professionals, and the public. The CRNA shall be an advocate for the patient's rights and safety.

Interpretive Statement:

A. Responsibility—A CRNA is responsible for the anesthesia care provided.

B. Professional Judgment—A CRNA is accountable for judgments made and actions taken in the practice of nurse anesthesia. Neither physician's orders nor institutional policies relieve the CRNA of accountability for actions taken and judgments made relative to the care and well being of the patient.

C. Informed Consent—As a licensed professional, the CRNA shall verify that a valid informed consent has been obtained from the patient or legal guardian as prescribed by federal or state statute or institutional policy.

D. Safety—A CRNA shall provide quality anesthesia care and protect the patient from harm.

IV. Societal Obligation

A Certified Registered Nurse Anesthetist has an obligation to society.

Interpretive Statement:

The CRNA must be a responsible citizen to society and the community. A CRNA is obligated to be aware of environmental and global health issues.

V. Confidentiality

A Certified Registered Nurse Anesthetist protects the patient's right to privacy.

Interpretive Statement:

A CRNA must maintain confidentiality of patient information unless required by law to breach the confidence.

VI. Personal Integrity

A Certified Registered Nurse Anesthetist maintains personal integrity, and strives to establish appropriate mechanisms to protect his/her freedom of conscience as it pertains to patients and each member of the health care team.

Interpretive Statement:

A CRNA is obligated to be knowledgeable of all moral and legal rights including those of the patient, self, and other professionals. In situations where the CRNA's personal convictions prohibit participation in a particular procedure, the CRNA may withdraw from the case provided that such withdrawal does not harm the patient or constitute breach of duty. CRNAs should avoid employment situations where frequent conflicts of personal conviction occur.

Each CRNA must assume responsibility for protecting patients and health care professionals against colleagues who may exhibit incompetency, engage in substance abuse, and/or commit illegal acts. A CRNA is obligated to assume responsibility for his/her actions toward the association and the membership.

VII. Endorsement

A Certified Registered Nurse Anesthetist may endorse products and services provided that he/she assumes personal accountability for their safety and/or quality. A CRNA shall not act as an agent of the AANA unless duly authorized by the Board of Directors.

Interpretive Statement:

CRNAs may actively represent themselves in a variety of settings to include professional, personal, public, educational, media, and social. A CRNA must exercise sound judgment in matters which potentially involve conflict of interest in relation to the AANA.

VIII. Research Ethics

A Certified Registered Nurse Anesthetist protects patients or animals involved in research projects and conducts the projects according to accepted ethical research and reporting standards established by public law and institutional procedures.

Interpretive Statement:

A. The CRNA participates in research activities to expand practice and to enhance continuous quality improvement efforts.

B. The CRNA must adhere to bioethical standards in the practice setting.

IX. Practice Settings

A Certified Registered Nurse Anesthetist has the right to participate in a variety of practice settings, including private practice, institutional employment, and other variations of business organization.

Interpretive Statement:

A. Right to Practice—The CRNA has the legal right to practice in a variety of employment settings and business relationships.

B. Reimbursement Responsibility—When the CRNA is a private practitioner, he or she has an ethical responsibility to the consumer to ensure responsible reimbursement policies. Fees for professional anesthesia services should be consistent with reasonable and customary charges and should reflect actual participation in and/or consultation on the procedure.

X. Employment Relations

A Certified Registered Nurse Anesthetist supports the profession in its efforts to maintain conditions of employment, practice privileges and contractual relationships.

Interpretive Statement:

A. Responsibility for Conditions of Practice—The CRNA must practice in accordance with the standards established by the profession. These standards include the preanesthesia assessment, intraoperative management, and postanesthesia care.

B. Contractual Agreements—The agreements shall be consistent with the professional standards of practice, laws, and/or regulations pertaining to nurse anesthesia practice.

C. Ethical Business Practices—The CRNA should maintain ethical business practices in dealing with potential clients and colleagues. Dealings should be characterized by concepts of mutual regard, equity, honesty, and constructive interpersonal communication.

Approved by the AANA Board of Directors 8/92 12/92-5000

Index

An f following a page number indicates a figure, a t indicates a table, and a b indicates a box.